Imaging of CNS Infections and Neuroimmunology

Bo Gao • Hongjun Li • Meng Law
Editors

Imaging of CNS Infections and Neuroimmunology

Springer

Editors
Bo Gao
Department of Radiology
Affiliated Hospital of Guizhou Medical University
Guiyang
Guizhou
China

Hongjun Li
Department of Radiology
Beijing You'an Hospital
Capital Medical University
Beijing
China

Meng Law
Radiology and Nuclear Medicine
Alfred Health
Melbourne
VIC
Australia

Department of Electrical and Computer Systems Engineering
Monash University
Clayton
VIC
Australia

Department of Neuroscience
Monash School of Medicine
Nursing and Health Sciences
Clayton
VIC
Australia

ISBN 978-981-13-6903-2 ISBN 978-981-13-6904-9 (eBook)
https://doi.org/10.1007/978-981-13-6904-9

This Springer imprint is published by the registered company Springer Nature Singapore Pte Ltd.
The registered company address is: 152 Beach Road, #21-01/04 Gateway East, Singapore 189721, Singapore

Foreword 1

In recent years, the scope of clinical neurology seen in developed or developing countries has evolved substantially. As the world has become smaller through travel and immigration with the spread of digital media, neurologists or radiologists must have to be familiar with the immersed diseases that have been previously geographically limited. The coming decades are deemed to provide an ever-evolving landscape influenced by central nervous system (CNS) infection and neuroimmunology.

With the rapid development of modern medical imaging technology, radiology has played a more pivotal role in the diagnosis and treatment of classical or emerging infections and immunological diseases. This book primarily summarizes the imaging features in CNS infection and neuroimmunology, serving as a clinical guide and possessing a practical significance for the understanding, theranostics, and prevention of these diseases. Furthermore, with the advances of neuroimaging and microbial diagnostic techniques, the range of potential infectious etiologies of dementia and stroke is widening. Familiarity with the clinical and laboratory features of these diseases may help identify treatable entities and avoid potentially unnecessary endeavors.

This book is published in a timely fashion, as the modern imaging modalities, such as CT, MRI, and PET/CT, are now becoming widely available in China, not only in the hospitals in large cities but also in second- and third-tier cities. A large number of imaging specialists and staffs equipped with the current knowledge of radiology will be needed to meet the ever-increasing demand for medical services in China. Along with the development of telemedicine and teleradiology, even the patients in the remote areas can benefit from this rapid advancement. This book can certainly be served as a reference book for practicing neurologists and radiologists, as well as a textbook for residents and fellows in these fields.

The editors of this book, Bo Gao MD, Hongjun Li MD, and Meng Law MD, have provided thorough and illustrative reviews of these emerging and controversial topics. I am pretty glad to introduce this book to those who are addicted to the clinical practice and research of CNS infection and neuroimmunology.

Min Chen
Department of Radiology
Beijing Hospital
Beijing, China

Foreword 2

I am quite honored to have been asked by Dr. Gao to write an introduction to this intrepid endeavor. A text is long overdue that focuses solely on the imaging of CNS infections and immunology, as the spectrum of infections and classifications of autoimmune disorders have changed over the decades; thus, so must imaging and subsequent therapy evolve as well. In this regard, this excellent work covers the current understanding of pathophysiology, imaging patterns, differential diagnosis, and some therapies for CNS infections and autoimmune disorders. As many physicians in the West will attest, the knowledge of the many infectious diseases is taken for granted, as we are often stumped by an atypical presentation or imaging pattern of a once-typical infection! Hence, a textbook that incorporates updated understanding of the basic pathophysiology and imaging appearance is necessary, particularly with the myriad imaging of new techniques that have been deployed in the past decade.

Recently, evolved imaging techniques include gadolinium-based contrast and MR and CT perfusion (MRP/CTP) imaging of blood-brain barrier dysfunction from endothelial injury, diffusion imaging (DWI) to evaluate the cytotoxic effect or structure within lesions, positron emission tomography (PET) for neuroinflammatory markers, functional MR imaging (fMRI), MR spectroscopy (MRS) to detect various metabolites, susceptibility-weighted imaging (SWI) to detect hemorrhagic deposits, and utilizing imaging for imaging-guided biopsy, to name a few. This text covers the use of these recent techniques in detail as regards the imaging patterns of various infections and autoimmune disorders and provides diagnostic patterns and differentials to aid in ultimately reaching a diagnosis.

Also, the imaging appearances of emerging infections causing encephalitides or meningitis are covered herein, which include bacterial, viral, fungal, aseptic, and granulomatous disorders. Prion-related disorders are also covered, which are critical given their increasing recognition, and the classification with more recently identified various subtypes is discussed with accompanying imaging. It is also particularly helpful that this book covers classical disorders that are less often seen nowadays in some parts of the world and reviews traditional as well as newer imaging appearances.

Hence, I believe that this unique book will remain an asset and a staple in the field for years to come. I congratulate the authors on their accomplishment of this work, and I look forward to future editions. I have to believe that such future editions will be required, since we seemingly encounter new infections and autoimmune diseases every year!

Alexander M. McKinney
Department of Radiology
University of Minnesota Medical School
Minneapolis, MN, USA

Preface

Infectious and immunological diseases of the central nervous system (CNS) are often complex. It is obligatory to require knowledge of pathology, anatomy, and physiology, as well as virology, parasitology, and immunology, to make a final diagnosis with confidence. Infections of the CNS frequently involve immunocompromised patients. Neuroimmunological diseases such as multiple sclerosis account for about 10% of all neurological diseases. Advanced MR techniques such as diffusion-weighted imaging, perfusion imaging, susceptibility-weighted imaging, as well as MR spectroscopy provide adjunct evidence on differentiating between infectious, immunological diseases of CNS and other entities, such as neoplastic, metabolic, or ischemic diseases. On the other hand, the cross study of imaging with autopsy and pathology will provide valuable and scientific evidence on the understanding and research of neuroinfections and neuroimmunology. How to resolve a couple of diagnostic problems in comprehensive textbook is still a huge challenge to the clinicians and neuroradiologists. This specific textbook serves as a practical approach toward imaging diagnosis in neuroinfections and neuroimmunology.

This book primarily illustrates the neuroimaging characteristics and theory of CNS infections and neuroimmunology, serving as a practical pocketbook and clinical guidance for the understanding, prevention, and diagnosis of these entities. The book was divided into 3 consecutive parts and 19 chapters according to their different subjects. The first part briefly introduces advanced imaging modalities including multi-detector CT, high-field MRI, PET, and brain biopsy techniques, as well as diagnostic algorithm based on imaging patterns. The second part addresses in details variable CNS infections such as viral, bacterial, mycoplasmal, parasitic, and opportunistic, as well as some specific topics: cerebrovascular complications of infection, infections of spinal cord, and childhood infections. The third part covers multiple sclerosis and other demyelinating diseases, granulomatous diseases, autoimmune encephalitis, inflammatory diseases of the meninges, and inflammatory and autoimmune disorders of the spinal cord.

The personalized structure of the particular chapters would help the contributor find the way to solve the complexity of the diseases and help the reader understand the coherence of clinical, epidemiological, pathological, and radiological features of infectious and immunological diseases. The authors of each chapter have provided thorough and illustrative reviews of these emerging and controversial topics, and we are indebted to them for their hard work and expertise. The materials included in the book were collected from lots of native hospitals and were well organized with excellent organization. We sincerely appreciate all the experts who contribute to this book, although there are some overlap among the different chapters and topics, which are undoubtedly benefits to better understand some specific entities from different standpoints. Our hope is that this will serve as a reference textbook that will benefit a spectrum of readers, from medical students, radiology residents, and neuroradiology fellows to the junior and senior neuroradiologists, as well as readers in neurology, neurosurgery, and associated disciplines.

I would like to appreciate my academic mentors, Prof. Xue-jian Wang, Prof. Bin Zhao, and Prof. Gao-jun Teng, who had woken my interest on radiology and had led me to pursue this career. As friends and companions, Prof. Chi S. Zee and Prof. Meng Law inspired me not only during composing this book but also during my visiting fellowship study in Keck Medical Center, University of Southern California. Further, I also thank the project coordinators, Mr. James Hu, Mr. Vignesh Iyyadurai Suresh and Ms. Shanjini Rajasekaran from Springer PG, who patiently assisted me during collecting and editing the manuscript and advised me patiently regarding the structure and details of this book. Last but not least, I sincerely thank my parents, my wife, and my daughter, for giving me ample space and time to be myself for creating and editing this book.

The contributors and I would be grateful to the enthusiastic readers who are giving constructive criticism of this book. We would like to be kept informed if anything would need polishing in the next edition in the future.

Guiyang, China Bo Gao

Contents

Contributors

Delilah Burrowes Division of Neuroradiology, Ann & Robert H. Lurie Children's Hospital of Chicago, Chicago, IL, USA

Xiaoxi Chen Department of Radiology, Affiliated Hospital of Zunyi Medical University, Zunyi, China

Hui Dai Department of Radiology, First Affiliated Hospital of Soochow University, Suzhou, China

Orlando Diaz Neurovascular Center, Houston Methodist Hospital, Weill Cornell Medical College, Houston, TX, USA

Ke Ding Department of Radiology, Third Affiliated Hospital of Guangxi Medical University, Nanning, China

Zhongxiang Ding Department of Radiology, Affiliated Hangzhou First People's Hospital, Zhejiang University School of Medicine, Hangzhou, China

Bo Gao Department of Radiology, Affiliated Hospital of Guizhou Medical University, Guiyang, China

Kirt Gill Division of Neuroradiology, Keck School of Medicine, University of Southern California, Los Angeles, CA, USA

Meng Law Radiology and Nuclear Medicine, Alfred Health, Melbourne, VIC, Australia

Department of Electrical and Computer Systems Engineering, Monash University, Clayton, VIC, Australia

Department of Neuroscience, Monash School of Medicine, Nursing and Health Sciences, Clayton, VIC, Australia

Alexander Lerner Division of Neuroradiology, Keck School of Medicine, University of Southern California, Los Angeles, CA, USA

Hongjun Li Department of Radiology, Beijing You'an Hospital, Capital Medical University, Beijing, China

Li Li Department of Radiology, Beijing You'an Hospital, Capital Medical University, Beijing, China

Yongmei Li Department of Radiology, First Hospital of Chongqing Medical University, Chongqing, China

Chia-Shang Liu Division of Neuroradiology, Keck School of Medicine, University of Southern California, Los Angeles, CA, USA

Heng Liu Department of Radiology, Affiliated Hospital of Zunyi Medical University, Zunyi, China

Jie Lu Department of Radiology and Nuclear Medicine, Xuanwu Hospital, Capital Medical University, Beijing, China

Yubo Lyu Shanghai Jiahui International Hospital, Jiahui Health, Shanghai, China

Shandong Medical Imaging Research Institute, Shandong University, Jinan, China

Fanny Morón Department of Radiology, Baylor College of Medicine, Houston, TX, USA

Vivek Pandey Advocate Illinois Masonic Medical Center, Chicago, IL, USA

Yinfeng Qian Department of Radiology, The First Affiliated Hospital of Anhui Medical University, Hefei, China

Chenglong Ren Department of Radiology, Affiliated Hospital of Shaanxi University of Chinese Medicine, Xianyang, China

Yan Ren Department of Radiology, Huashan Hospital, Fudan University, Shanghai, China

Guiquan Shen Department of Radiology, Affiliated Hospital of Guizhou Medical University, Guiyang, China

Mark S. Shiroishi Division of Neuroradiology, Keck School of Medicine, University of Southern California, Los Angeles, CA, USA

Yan Song Department of Radiology, Beijing Hospital, Beijing, China

Jiali Wang Department of Radiology, Affiliated Hospital of Xuzhou Medical University, Xuzhou, China

Mei Wang Department of Radiology, Affiliated Hangzhou First People's Hospital, Zhejiang University School of Medicine, Hangzhou, China

Yanan Wang Department of Radiology, Affiliated Hospital of Zunyi Medical University, Zunyi, China

Mu-xi Wu Department of Radiology, Affiliated Hospital of Guizhou Medical University, Guiyang, China

Shuang Xia Department of Radiology, Tianjin First Center Hospital, Tianjin, China

Zhiming Xiang Department of Radiology, Guangzhou Panyu Center Hospital, Guangzhou, China

Jian Xu Department of Neurology, Detroit Medical Center, Medical School of Wayne State University, Detroit, MI, USA

Vivek Yedavilli Advocate Illinois Masonic Medical Center, Chicago, IL, USA

Chi S. Zee Department of Radiology, Keck School of Medicine, University of Southern California, Los Angeles, CA, USA

Zhen Zeng Department of Radiology, Affiliated Hospital of Zunyi Medical University, Zunyi, China

Tijiang Zhang Department of Radiology, Affiliated Hospital of Zunyi Medical University, Zunyi, China

Fuqing Zhou Department of Radiology, The First Affiliated Hospital, Nanchang University, Nanchang, China

Part I

Imaging Modalities and Decision-making

Multidetector Computed Tomography

1

Yan Song

1.1 Introduction

CT is the most influential technology that uses X-ray since it was introduced in 1972 by G. Hounsfield. The invention owned him The Nobel Prize in Physiology and Medicine in 1979. Then in the next 40 years, the evolution of CT technique accompanied closely with the development of medicine. From the 1970s to the 1980s, the development of CT technique concentrated on the extension of scanning position, from head extending to the body. From the 1980s to the 1990s, the scanning speed was the main character which resulted in sub-second scanning. From the 1990s to the 2000s, helical scan drew our eyes mostly, which could be considered as the milestone of CT technique progression. From then on, CT technique progressed rapidly from single-section helical CT to multi-section helical CT, even to the volume CT nowadays, with the core technology of slip ring and wide detector. At the same time, super-high-speed computers and sophisticated imaging techniques are crucial and necessary to process the images collected in this manner. Compared to traditional single-section helical CT, multidetector CT improves temporal resolution and spatial resolution in the Z-axis, increases the concentration of intravascular contrast material, decreases image noise, as well as allows efficient X-ray tube use and anatomic coverage. These merits of multidetector CT substantially increase the diagnostic accuracy in clinical examination and enable faster and accurate evaluation of patients in a wider spectrum of clinical indications. In the twenty-first century, CT technique is not restricted to the morphological examination and protrudes to the quantitative analysis, which results in the CT spectral scan and opens a new world for CT performance.

As to the CT examination modalities applied in central neural system, it provides the plain CT scan, enhanced CT scan, CT angiography, CT perfusion, and dual-energy CT scan.

1.2 Pre- and Post-Contrast CT

Plain CT scan and enhanced CT scan are the basic CT examination modalities for CNS diseases. Plain CT scan is simple, quick, and very convenient to detect the lesion. But the relatively low soft tissue resolution of plain CT scan, besides the beam hardening artifact, is the main barrier in its application in CNS infectious disease, which makes it difficult to detect some of lesions located in posterior cranial fossa, small lesions with iso-density, and the abnormalities of meninges [1]. In such conditions, contrast-enhanced CT scanning is necessary. With the administration of contrast medium, the attenuation difference between lesion and adjacent cerebral parenchyma may be enhanced (Fig. 1.1); thus it is possible to show the small lesions and meningeal abnormality. The enhancement behavior also can help to analyze the blood supply of the lesion so as to make it possible to decide the pathology staging of the infectious disease [2]. Different from the other kinds of CNS disease, some of the CNS infectious disease, especially tuberculosis, require the special consideration of delay time. Usually, the delay time of cerebral enhanced CT scan is 25 s. Many investigators found that cerebral tuberculosis lesions won't show satisfied enhancement with such a traditional delay time, which may be due to lack of blood supply or low circulation speed of the contrast agent in the lesion. Based on this hypothesis, it was recommended to prolong the delay time to 5 min [3]. By this way, we can now delineate the boundary, size, enhancement behavior of the lesion, and meningitis much better than usual.

1.3 CT Angiography

CT angiography (CTA) is a well-established medical imaging technique for the detection, evaluation, and therapy planning of intracranial vascular diseases, replacing almost completely conventional angiography. In the past decades,

Y. Song (✉)
Department of Radiology, Beijing Hospital, Beijing, China

B. Gao et al. (eds.), *Imaging of CNS Infections and Neuroimmunology*, https://doi.org/10.1007/978-981-13-6904-9_1

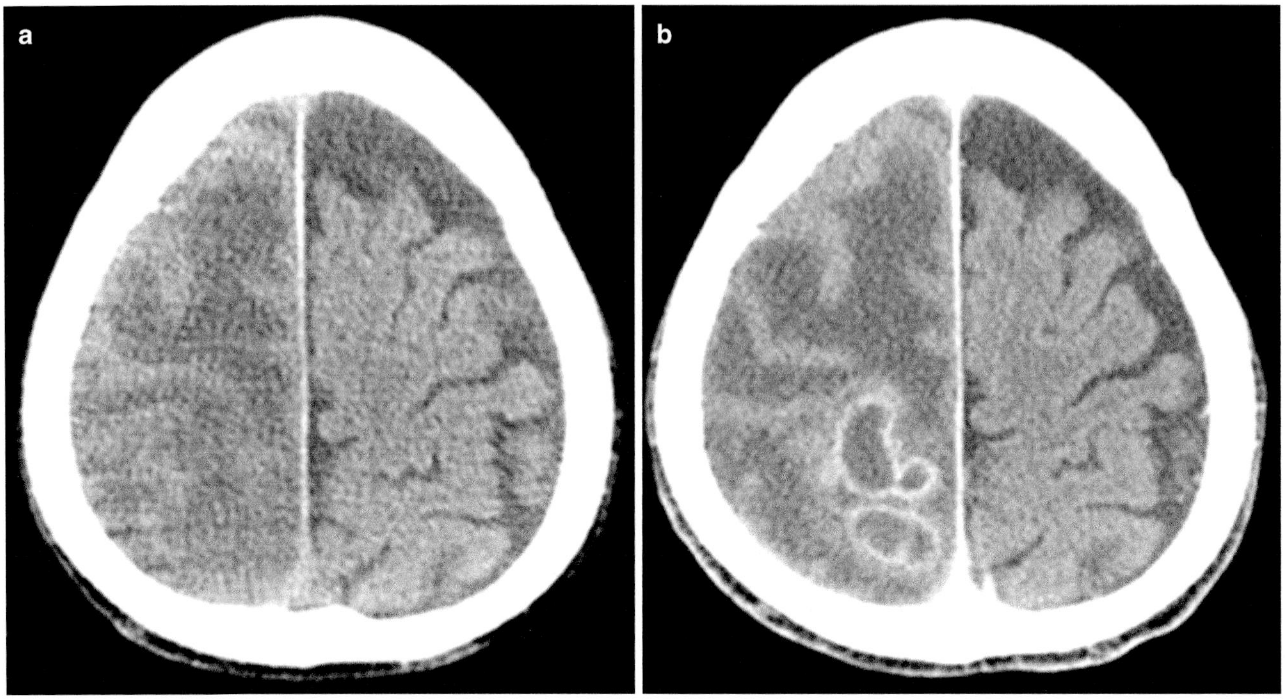

Fig. 1.1 A 59-year-old male with brain abscess. (**a**) Plain CT shows patchy low attenuation in the right cerebral hemisphere. (**b**) The lesions only could be seen on post-contrast CT when the contrast media induced the density difference between lesion and adjacent tissue

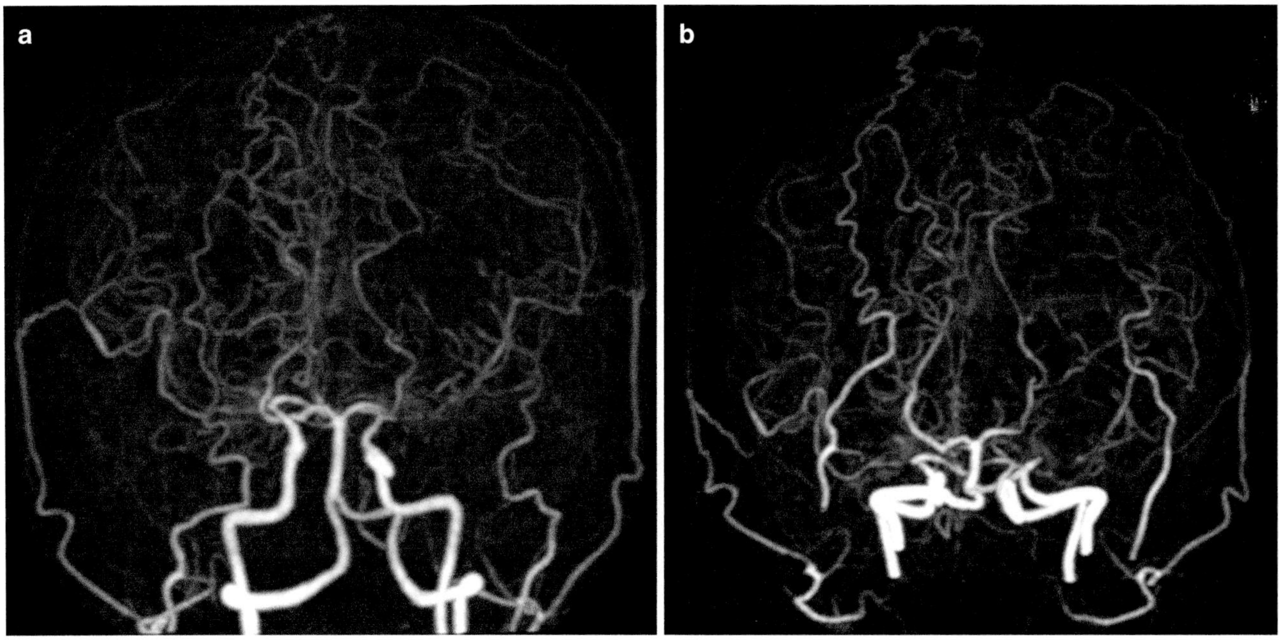

Fig. 1.2 A 54-year-old male with Moyamoya disease. (**a**, **b**) CTA shows the occlusion of bilateral MCA and abnormal vascular collateral networks that developed adjacent to the stenotic vessels

CTA has evolved tremendously and has played a dominant role in disease diagnosis, management decision, and outcome evaluation. The revolution of novel CT scanner geometries, data reconstruction strategies, and sophisticated post-processing workflow is paving the way for the further evolution of CT angiography [4, 5]. Nowadays, CTA is mostly used to assess the atherosclerotic disease and ischemic disease, intracranial aneurysm, and vasculitis (Fig. 1.2).

1.4 Computed Tomography Perfusion Imaging (CTPI)

Perfusion CT serially samples the first-pass parenchymal wash-in and wash-out of an iodinated contrast agent bolus to generate a dynamic assessment of capillary level blood flow. A series of time-concentration curves are generated for each voxel of the CT images after selection of arterial input and venous output vessels. Some of the principle data sets displayed for each voxel include cerebral blood volume (CBV), mean transit time (MTT), cerebral blood flow (CBF), time to peak (TTP), and capillary permeability (PS).

CBV represents the total volume of the blood within a given volume of parenchyma, typically referenced as mL blood per 100 g tissue (mL/100 g). MTT is derived primarily from the arterial input function and represents the average time required for blood cell passage through the parenchymal capillary network, measured in seconds. CBF is a derived rate unit reflecting the volume of blood perfusing a given volume of parenchyma per unit time. The central volume theory holds that CBF = CBV/MTT. Time to peak (TTP) describes the time required for maximum density of contrast within a particular region of brain tissue, measured in seconds. PS can be expressed as $PS = -BF \cdot \ln(1 - E)$. PS is the unidirectional diffusional flux of contrast medium from intravascular space into interstitial space through the "openings" of the permeable capillary endothelium (mL/min/100 g).

1.4.1 Determining Ischemic Penumbra and Infarct Core

PCT not only allows early detection of cerebral ischemia but also gives valuable information on ischemic penumbra which is very important in early diagnosis and treatment, allowing individualized thrombolytic therapy decisions in an extended time window based on tissue viability at presentation [6]. Perfusion CT maps characterize tissue viability by reflecting changes in parenchymal autoregulatory mechanisms following arterial occlusion. Reactive vasodilation and collateral flow recruitment attempt to normalize parenchymal blood flow (CBF) which can result in an overall increase in ischemic territory CBV (Fig. 1.3). Increased CBV is a hallmark of ischemic penumbra and is observed if collateral circulation is robust enough to maintain compensatory neurobiochemical mechanisms. When such mechanisms are overwhelmed by prolonged or severe ischemia, the CBV and CBF will decline below viability thresholds and precipitate irreversible tissue damage, resulting in the infarct core.

	MTT	rCBF	rCBV
TIA	↑	normal	↑
Penumbra	↑↑	↓	↑
Infarct	↑↑↑	↓↓	↓

Fig. 1.3 The changes of MTT, rCBF, and rCBV in different conditions

1.4.2 Diagnosis and Differential Diagnosis of Brain Tumors

Perfusion CT is dedicated to assess the blood supply and hemodynamics of brain tumors by quantifying blood flow, blood volume, and permeability surface (PS). High-grade gliomas would show higher BF, BV, and PS than those of low-grade gliomas on PCT imaging. PCT can also differentiate grade III from grade IV gliomas in specific of PS demonstrating better predictability and accuracy than BV in this regard. PCT also plays an important role in differentiating brain tumor from other intracranial masses. Tumefactive demyelinating lesions (TDLs) and primary brain lymphoma usually show significantly lower BF, BV, and PS than HGGs on PCT. However, there was no significant difference of BV and PS between HGGs and metastases. BV values in the peritumoral edema of tumors were significantly higher in HGGs than those of metastases [7, 8]. Assessing posttreatment reaction and prognosis is another important issue. Pseudo-progression and radiation-induced necrosis (RIN) are two post-radiotherapy scenarios that mimic true progression on MRI. On PCT imaging, true progression has significant higher rBF, rBV, and PS than those of TIN. PCT have been used to predict overall survival (OS) after surgery/biopsy, radiotherapy, and chemotherapy.

1.4.3 CTPI in Intracranial Infectious Lesions

Infected lesions like tuberculoma and abscess showed significant difference in perfusion parameters from high-grade tumor, lymphoma, and metastasis. CTP also can differentiate various ring-enhancing lesions like metastasis, abscess, and tuberculoma [9, 10]. The rCBV of the center of abscess showed significantly hypoperfusion compared to those of high-grade tumor, metastasis, tuberculoma on antitubercular treatment (TOT), and tuberculoma without treatment (TWT). The rCBV of enhancing portion of abscess was found to be lower compared to glioma, which was attributed to decreased neovascularity and high amount of mature collagen in abscess.

Other infectious lesions like cerebral toxoplasmosis and cryptococcomas show hypoperfusion compared to tumors like lymphoma. Capsule of TWT showed significantly hypoperfusion compared to TOT, abscesses, and metastases. TOT showed hyper-perfusion values, similar to high-grade intracranial tumors. Thus, it is difficult to differentiate TOT (less than 2 months) from high-grade glioma, solely depending on perfusion parameters. But the rCBF and rCBV in TOT (>6 months) significantly reduced compared to those of TOT (<2 months), perhaps related to the healing process of fibrosis, reactive gliosis, and calcification.

1.5 Dual-Energy CT

So far, the development of dual-energy CT can be divided into two periods, dual-energy subtraction and spectral CT imaging. Dual-energy subtraction technology can be implemented through receiving the signals generated from two tubes with different levels of tube voltages by two different detectors, whereas spectral CT imaging applied one tube and one detector with two tube voltage rapid-switching technique. Besides different principles between these two approaches, both techniques acquired high- and low-energy level projections, based on which the material decomposition images can be derived either in projection space or in image space. Further, virtual monochromatic images are derived and simulate the information of real monochromatic X-ray image. The virtual monochromatic images have less beam hardening artifacts and benefits for early detection of lesion, quantification, and quantitative analysis.

As we all know, computed tomography can screen for numerous neurological emergencies and clearly display the supratentorial region. However, due to the beam hardening artifacts and nonlinear partial volume artifacts, it is difficult for CT to display posterior cranial fossa and skull base structures, such as the visualization of brain stem and cerebellum. Since CT is applied on neuro system, the severe posterior cranial fossa artifact had been always highly focused in the field. The new devices with thinner slice, higher voltage tube, and advanced reconstruction algorithm can improve the images here for some extent, but still cannot eradicate the artifacts. The physical features of mixed energy X-ray beam lead to the inevitable reduction of image quality. Due to the mixed X-ray features, the beam hardening artifacts, such as Hounsfield dark area, always exist on CT image. A real monochromatic X-ray CT image can avoid beam hardening artifacts and averaging effect; however the real monochromatic X-ray CT cannot be applied in clinic practice at present. The virtual monochromatic image (70 keV and 65 keV) obtained by dual-energy CT can effectively reduce the image noise of the head and brain and reduce the artifacts in posterior cranial fossa [11].

For the reason of average effect, cranial conventional polychromatic CTA may be not the prime approach to evaluate the intracranial vessels. Virtual monochromatic images can provide sufficient image contrast [12]. Further, the optimal keV level could be derived to visualize the intracranial vessels and surrounding brain parenchyma due to the analysis of optimal contrast to noise ratio. According to the preliminary clinical study, there are two optimal keV levels of intracranial vessel CTA surrounding 55 keV and 65 keV, respectively. Compared with conventional polychromatic CTA, vessels reconstructed with the optimal keV may provide better image contrast and demonstrate more vascular branches (Fig. 1.4).

Another utilization of dual-energy CT in CNS is reducing the artifacts of metallic implants (Fig. 1.5). In evaluation of intracranial aneurism after spring coil implantation using conventional polychromatic CT, the metallic artifacts caused

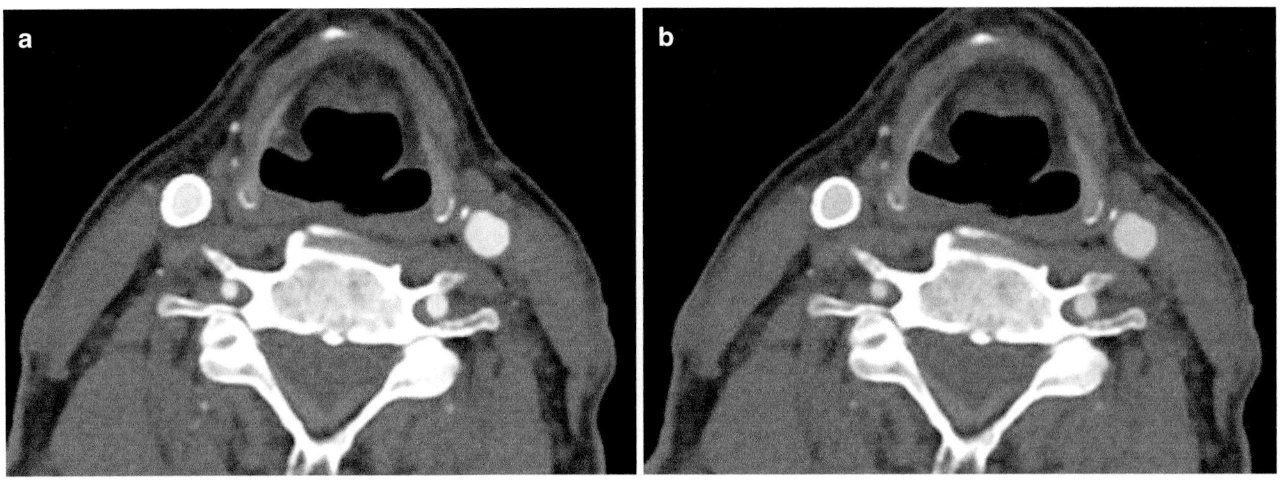

Fig. 1.4 (**a**–**d**) The reconstructed images of different keV, which were 70, 80, 90, and 100 kev, respectively. A proper keV can be chosen according to the purpose. For example, the image of 70 keV is the best to analyze the left carotid artery, while the image of 80 keV is the best to analyze the stent and intrastent lumen

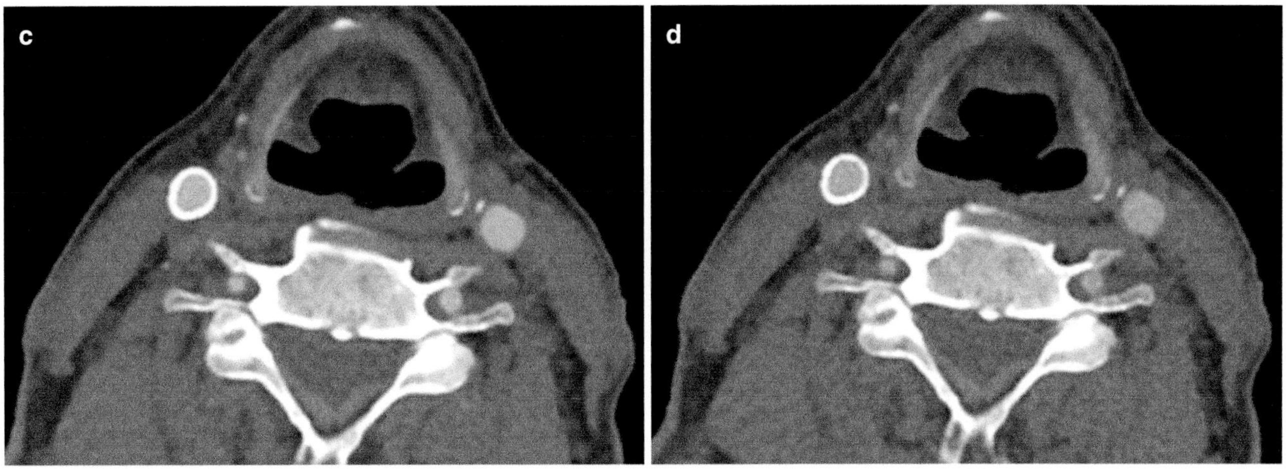

Fig. 1.4 (continued)

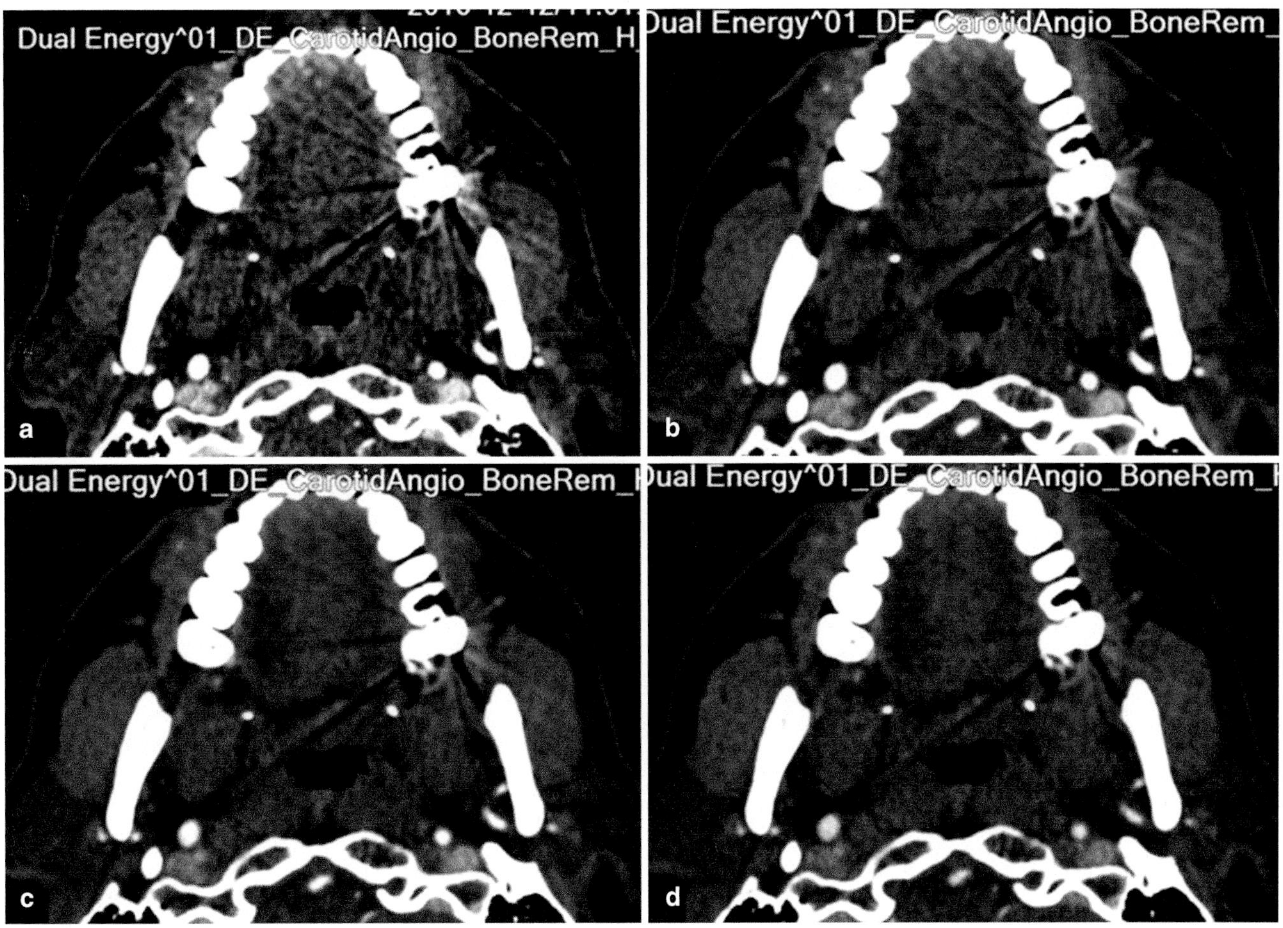

Fig. 1.5 (**a**–**d**) Images of different keV, which were 60, 70, 80, and 90 keV, respectively. The metallic implant-related artifact reduced gradually with the increase of keV

by spring coil shield adjacent structures and limit the observation of small aneurism. The dual-energy CT can improve the image quality via virtual monochromatic images and metallic artifact reduction techniques, facilitating the evaluation of aneurism after spring coil implantation [13, 14].

References

1. Sam K, Birbeck GL, Oostveen RJ, et al. Alternative oblique head CT scanning technique reduces bone artifact and improves interpretability of brainstem anatomy. Neurol Int. 2010;2(1):e14.
2. Gunness VR, Hana A, Berthold C, et al. Posterior fossa mass in immunosuppressed patient. Bull Soc Sci Med Grand Duche Luxemb. 2014;3:25–30.
3. Hou D, Qu H, Zhang X, et al. Multi-slice computed tomography 5-minute delayed scan is superior to immediate scan after contrast media application in characterization of intracranial tuberculosis. Med Sci Monit. 2014;20:1556–62.
4. Yahyavi-Firouz-Abadi N, Wynn BL, Rybicki FJ, et al. Steroid-responsive large vessel vasculitis: application of whole-brain 320-detector row dynamic volume CT angiography and perfusion. AJNR Am J Neuroradiol. 2009;30(30):1409–11.
5. Siebert E, Bohner G, Dewey M, et al. 320-slice CT neuroimaging: initial clinical experience and image quality evaluation. Br J Radiol. 2009;82(979):561–70.
6. Donahue J, Wintermark M. Perfusion CT and acute stroke imaging: foundations, applications, and literature review. J Neuroradiol. 2015;42(1):21–9.
7. Yeung TPC, Bauman G, Yartsev S, et al. Dynamic perfusion CT in brain tumors. Eur J Radiol. 2015;84(12):2386–92.
8. Kamble RB, Jayakumar PN, Shivashankar R. Role of dynamic CT perfusion study in evaluating various intracranial space-occupying lesions. Indian J Radiol Imaging. 2015;25(2):162–6.
9. Kamble RB, Jp N, Shivashankar R. CT perfusion dynamics of intracranial tuberculomas. J Clin Diagn Res. 2015;9(5):TC01–5.
10. Hiwatashi A, Togao O, Yamashita K, et al. Evaluation of glioblastomas and lymphomas with whole-brain CT perfusion: comparison between a delay-invariant singular-value decomposition algorithm and a Patlak plot. J Neuroradiol. 2016;43(4):266–72.
11. Lin XZ, Miao F, Li JY, et al. High-definition CT gemstone spectral imaging of the brain: initial results of selecting optimal monochromatic image for beam-hardening artifacts and image noise reduction. J Comput Assist Tomogr. 2011;35(2):294–7.
12. Postma AA, Hofman PA, Stadler AA, et al. Dual-energy CT of the brain and intracranial vessels. AJR Am J Roentgenol. 2012;199(5 Suppl):26–33.
13. Dolati P, Eichberg D, Wong JH, et al. The utility of dual-energy computed tomographic angiography for the evaluation of brain aneurysms after surgical clipping: a prospective study. World Neurosurg. 2015;84(5):1362–71.
14. Machida H, Tanaka I, Fukui R, et al. Dual-energy spectral ct: various clinical vascular applications. Radiographics. 2016;36(4):1215–32.

MR Imaging and Advanced MRI Techniques

2

Shuang Xia

2.1 Introduction

Sometimes it is difficult for imaging studies to make the diagnosis conclusively as of a specific pathogen, however, some of which may have characteristic features and narrow the differential diagnosis spectrum. For CNS infection, four kinds of imaging patterns can be defined, including parenchymal involvement, meningeal involvement, ventricular involvement, and abscess formation (Fig. 2.1).

Non-purulent parenchymal involvement presents abnormal hyperintensity in the parenchyma on T2WI or FLAIR without or slightly patchy contrast enhancement. Meningeal involvement is identified as abnormal hyperintensity along the sulcus on FLAIR and contrast enhancement. These two patterns are commonly seen in CNS virus and fungus infection. Basal cistern enhancement is most commonly seen in tuberculosis. Abscess formation is defined as a ringlike enhancement pattern. Ventricular involvement was diagnosed when abnormal hyperintensity on FLAIR or linear enhancement found in the subependymal regions. Empyema can also be seen in some bacterial CNS infection which shows hyperintensity fluid collection within the ventricles or subdural area on DWI and capsular enhancement. The abscess wall with its thinnest medial margin faces toward the ventricular system. Ventriculitis and choroid plexitis are commonly secondary to an abscess rupturing into the ventricular system, sometimes to hydrocephalus [1, 2, 3].

2.2 Advanced MRI Techniques

Lots of MRI sequences can be scanned including T1-weighted imaging (T1WI) and T2-weighted imaging (T2WI), T2 fluid-attenuated inversion recovery (FLAIR), susceptibility weighted imaging (SWI), diffusion-weighted imaging (DWI), MR angiography/MR venography (MRA/MRV), MR spectroscopy (MRS), arterial spin labeling (ASL), magnetic resonance perfusion (MRP) imaging, and T1-weighted post-gadolinium imaging utilizing fat saturation if needed. Routinely T1WI is used to show anatomy and T2WI to better display the etiology or pathology. The advanced MRI sequences have been used in the evaluation of new findings of infection of CNS [1–10].

FLAIR is quite sensitive to evaluate the changes after infection, especially the changes of leptomeninges. It is performed using a turbo-spin-echo-based inversion recovery which is better to show the lesions. A new modified sequence, T1-FLAIR, generates T1-weighted images by using inversion time (TI) of about 800 ms. T1-FLAIR images improves tissue contrast between gray and white matter, more suppression of signals from vessels.

DWI investigates the water diffusion characteristics within a region. It is critically important in distinguishing intracranial tumors and other mimickers from abscess, as the center of abscess shows hyperintensity with restricted diffusion. The wall of abscess all shows isointensity on T2WI and ring contrast enhancement. In suspicion of meningoencephalitis, DWI is also recommended to show abnormal limited diffusion in the early stage of purulent infection. Two pat-

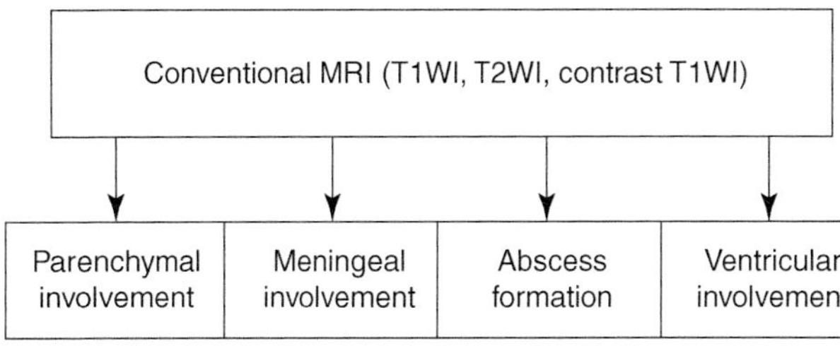

Fig. 2.1 In the brain infection, four kinds of imaging appearances can be defined on MRI

S. Xia (✉)
Department of Radiology, Tianjin First Center Hospital, Tianjin, China

B. Gao et al. (eds.), *Imaging of CNS Infections and Neuroimmunology*, https://doi.org/10.1007/978-981-13-6904-9_2

terns of hyperintensity were shown on DWI: (a) within the subarachnoid space and ventricles and (b) within the brain parenchyma. The hyperintensity of subarachnoid space is corresponding to linear contrast enhancement on post-gadolinium T1WI. Hyperintensity of brain parenchyma on DWI can indicate infection or post-infection infarction which can be confirmed by combination of routine sequences. But keep in mind that fungus infection will not show limited diffusion, especially cryptococcal infection in HIV patients [1, 2, 9, 10].

ASL is one of MR perfusion methods and has several merits, such as no use of contrast media, noninvasiveness, and convenience. ASL can be used to evaluate the whole brain perfusion in 2–5 min; CBF can be easily obtained. Some authors reported that either increased or decreased CBF can be seen in patients with CNS infection, which depends on the occurrence of immune reconstitution inflammatory syndrome. Noguchi et al. reported that 77% of patients with meningitis had hyperperfusion detected on FLAIR or post-contrast MRI. Combination ASL and FLAIR can do differentiation meningitis from subarachnoid hemorrhage and meningeal carcinomatosis which do not show hyperperfusion [4]. In clinical practice, ASL might be helpful in differentiating abscess formation from cystic glioblastoma and hyperintense lesion on DWI with a low perfusion of wall supporting the diagnosis of abscess. Muccio et al. reported low relative cerebral blood volume (rCBV) in brain abscess formation measurements with dynamic contrast enhanced MRI (DSC-MRI) [5]. This pathological finding may also apply to some abscess lesions with hypoperfusion on ASL.

MRS can provide metabolic information of brain lesions by detecting the changes of specific chemical metabolites. It is feasible to detect a microorganism pending on the expected products of reflected in the metabolic peak. MRS is suggested to be added in the examination when it is difficult to differentiate tumors such as recurrent lymphoma from abscess in an immunocompromised patient. Abscess could not contain N-acetyl aspartate but may include amino acids. When evaluating the metabolites of brain abscess, short echo (TE = 35 ms) is suggested to be employed in protocols. The amino acid peak at 0.9 parts per million (ppm) [inverted peak at time of echo (TE) = 136 ms] may indicate valine, leucine, and isoleucine. The detection of succinate (2.4 ppm) and acetate (1.92 ppm) is indicating the presence of anaerobic organisms. Elevations of lactate and myoinositol had been reported in the early stage of subacute sclerosing panencephalitis [6]. Lipid peaks at 0.9, 1.3, 2.0, and 2.8 ppm are commonly seen in tuberculosis, and the presence of lipids without other amino acids, lactate, and succinate strongly supports tuberculosis.

References

1. Hunter JV, Goerner L. Infections. Handb Clin Neurol. 2016;136:1173–98.
2. Reiche W, Schuchardt V, Hagen T, et al. Differential diagnosis of intracranial ring enhancing cystic mass lesions--role of diffusion-weighted imaging (DWI) and diffusion-tensor imaging (DTI). Clin Neurol Neurosurg. 2010;112(3):218–25.
3. Tan K, Wijaya L, Chiew HJ, et al. Diffusion-weighted MRI abnormalities in an outbreak of *Streptococcus agalactiae* Serotype III, multilocus sequence type 283 meningitis. J Magn Reson Imaging. 2017;45(2):507–14.
4. Noguchi T, Yakushiji Y, Nishihara M, et al. Arterial spin-labeling in central nervous system infection. Magn Reson Med Sci. 2016;15(4):386–94.
5. Muccio CF, Esposito G, Bartolini A, et al. Cerebral abscesses and necrotic cerebral tumours: differential diagnosis by perfusion-weighted magnetic resonance imaging. Radiol Med. 2008;113(5):747–57.
6. Tekşam M, Cakir B, Ağildere AM. Proton MR spectroscopy in the diagnosis of early-stage subacute sclerosing panencephalitis. Diagn Interv Radiol. 2006;12(2):61–3.
7. Ances BM, Sisti D, Vaida F, et al. Resting cerebral blood flow: a potential biomarker of the effects of HIV in the brain. Neurology. 2009;73(9):702–8.
8. Khoury MN, Gheuens S, Ngo L, et al. Hyperperfusion in progressive multifocal leukoencephalopathy is associated with disease progression and absence of immune reconstitution inflammatory syndrome. Brain. 2013;136(11):3441–50.
9. Rangarajan K, Das CJ, Kumar A, Gupta AK. MRI in central nervous system infections: a simplified patterned approach. World J Radiol. 2014;6(9):716–25.
10. Starkey J, Moritani T, Kirby P. MRI of CNS fungal infections: review of aspergillosis to histoplasmosis and everything in between. Clin Neuroradiol. 2014;24(3):217–30.

3 PET Imaging

Jie Lu

3.1 Positron Emission Tomography (PET)

PET is a kind of molecular and functional imaging technology that measures the emitting annihilation photons and analyzes the distribution of radiotracer labelled with positron emitters by a ring of detectors. The radiotracer is delivered to living system firstly, and the emitted positron generated from radiotracer physical decay travels a short distance in tissue (generally <1 mm for common PET nuclides) before it comes across an electron and then produces a pair of two 511 keV annihilation photons in opposite direction (180° angle). Those photon pairs are detected by PET detectors after attenuation in body. Once the examination is completed, the coincident detections of γ-rays are reconstructed into a set of time frames measuring the distribution of the radioligand during the data acquisition. The spatial resolution of PET detector is about 2 mm now.

3.2 Positron Emission Tomography/Computed Tomography (PET/CT)

PET is a medical research tool which is used for clinical diagnosis of some brain diseases. The conception of PET was initiated in 1970s. In 1961, James Robertson and his associates had built the first single-plane PET scan. The first instrument of PET was designed in 1969 and reported in 1972. The first commercial PET/CT scanner was introduced in early 2001. PET is used to depict and quantify physiological function by assessing the radiation emitted after intravenously injected tracer [1]. The CT scan provides anatomical information to locate the lesions on PET image [2, 3]. 2-Deoxy2-(18F) fluoro-d-glucose (^{18}F-FDG) is the mostly used tracer with PET for imaging the patients with chronic inflammatory diseases, cancers, and so on. The PET advances include some new technologies such as LSO for improvement of detector's sensitivity, and time of flight (TOF) for improvement of spatial resolution modeling in PET image reconstruction [4, 5].

3.3 Positron Emission Tomography/Magnetic Resonance Imaging (PET/MRI)

Today's PET systems are either constructed as hybrid PET/CT or, more recently, PET/MRI system. PET/MRI is a new technology with advantages both PET and MR imaging. Hybrid PET/MR imaging assembles excellent soft tissue resolution and functional imaging provided by MRI and high sensitivity and quantification of radiotracer metabolism provided by PET [6, 7]. Clinical applications of integrated PET/MRI in neurology, pediatric oncology, and cardiovascular disease are highlighted. Brain PET/MRI scan now is the modality imaging of best choice in all intracranial diseases. It is often superior to PET/CT imaging. The hybrid PET/MRI imaging workflow needs to be tailored for the clinical indication in maximizing diagnostic information and minimizing acquisition time. However, there are metallic objects/implants that may pose a hazard either to the patient (e.g., aneurysm clips) or to the function of the implant (e.g., pacemakers or cochlear implants) in PET/MRI examination.

There are several commonly used radionuclides in PET imaging of brain diseases, such as fluorine-18 (^{18}F, half-life = 109.7 min), carbon-11 (^{11}C, half-life = 20.4 min), nitrogen-13 (^{13}N, half-life = 10.0 min), oxygen-15 (^{15}O, physical half-life = 2.03 min), and so on, whereas ^{18}F of the relatively long half-life can permit enough time for transporting ^{18}F labelled tracers from a cyclotron position to a PET scanner. In PET scan, ^{18}F-FDG is generally used to evaluate cerebral glucose metabolism. ^{18}F-FDG is phosphorylated by hexokinase after uptake in brain tissue by specific glucose

J. Lu (✉)
Department of Radiology and Nuclear Medicine, Xuanwu Hospital, Capital Medical University, Beijing, China

B. Gao et al. (eds.), *Imaging of CNS Infections and Neuroimmunology*, https://doi.org/10.1007/978-981-13-6904-9_3

transporter. ^{18}F-FDG-6-P is not only a substrate for transport out of the cell but also cannot be metabolized further. That is to say, this process is irreversible, which would lead to its staying in the cell. ^{18}F-FDG will distribute stably in 30–60 mins after injection, and then reflects abnormal glucose metabolism in the brain tissue.

3.4 Biomarkers for Inflammation Imaging

Inflammation process has a couple of pro-inflammatory mediators, such as cytokines, chemokines, and leukotrienes. All of these inflammatory mediators and dominant inflammatory cells are potential targets, which can be used to investigate inflammatory diseases. As follows, the major treacer (^{18}F-FDG) of PET and the specific inflammation related targets for inflammation imaging are covered.

3.5 ^{18}F-FDG PET in CNS Infectious and Immune Diseases

Inflammation reaction plays a key role in the processes of infectious and immune disease. Some novel molecular imagings in recent years have provided a new insight into the diagnosis and treatment evaluation of inflammatory disease. The tracer of ^{18}F-FDG is the currently most extensively used and applied in brain diseases. As the key indicators and core participants in inflammatory process, inflammatory cells always employ glucose at a much higher level than non-inflammatory cells. Infectious lesions show intense uptake of ^{18}F-FDG due to active inflammation process (Fig. 3.1). Indeed, ^{18}F-FDG of PET treacer has been used vividly in a mount of inflammatory diseases and therapy evaluations, such as intracranial abscess [8], intracranial tuberculoma [9], HIV-related CNS infectious diseases [10], tuberculosis meningitis [11], and autoimmune encephalitis [12].

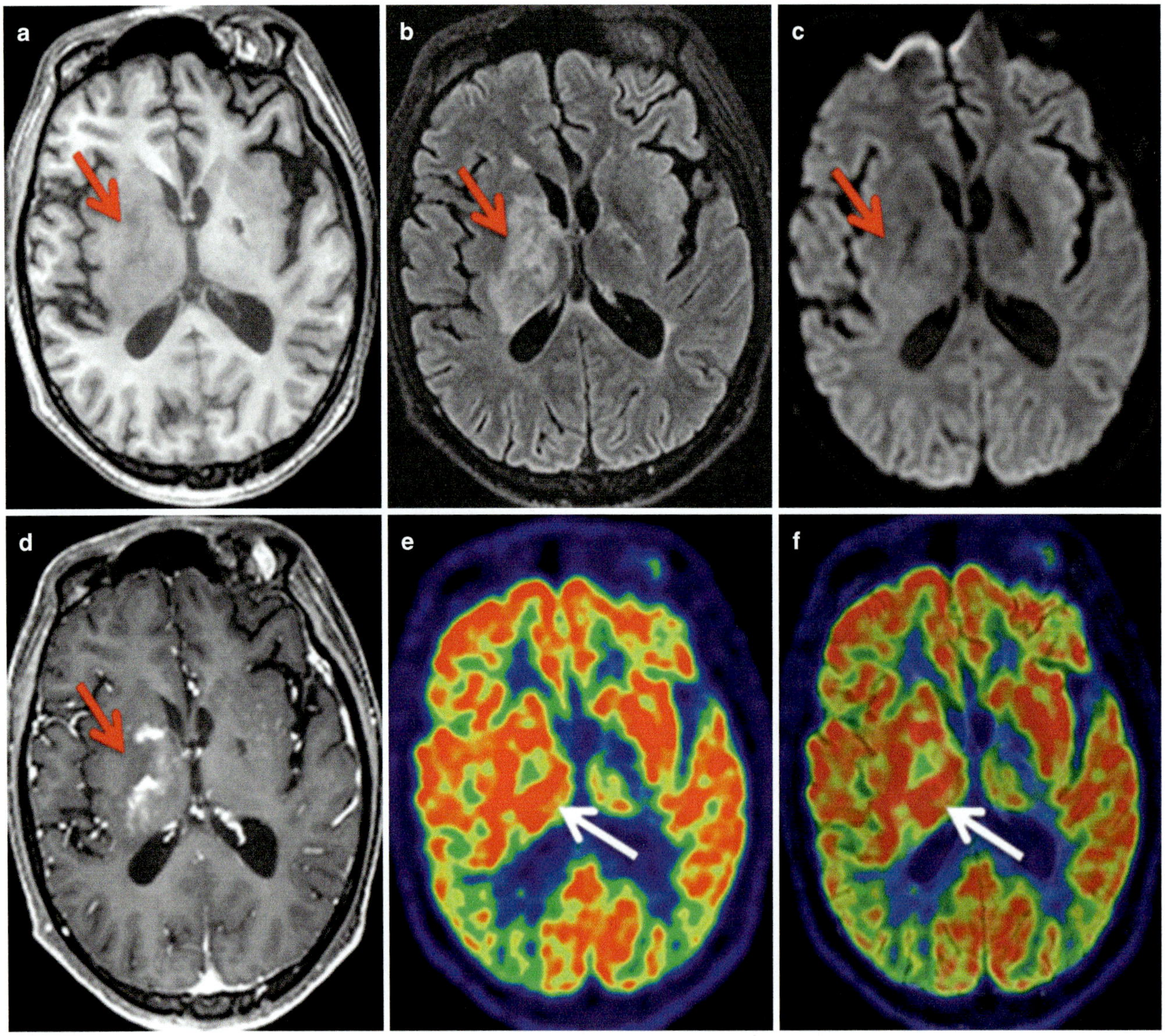

Fig. 3.1 A 28-year-old male patient with encephalitis of right basal ganglia and thalumus. (**a**) The lesion showed low intensity signal on T1WI (red arrow); (**b**) The lesion showed high intensity signal on T2-FLAIR (red arrow); (**c**) The lesion showed slightly high intensity signal on DWI (red arrow); (**d**) The lesion showed heterogeneous enhancement on T1WI+C (red arrow); (**e**) The lesion showed high metabolism on ^{18}F-FDG PET image (white arrow); (**f**) The lesion showed high metabolism on PET/MRI fusion image (white arrow)

3.6 Inflammation Imaging-Related Specific Targets

^{18}F-FDG PET Tracer accumulation in brain grey matter makes it difficult to detect inflammatory foci in brain tissue, which leads to false positive findings in the evaluation of intracranial inflammatory lesion. Therefore, some investigations utilized new PET tracers and targeted more specific inflammation reaction and for therapy evaluation. PET imaging with specific inflammation tracer will greatly enhance our understanding of the mechanism in inflammation process and increase clinical diagnostic specificity and accuracy on detection of brain inflammatory lesion. Translocator protein (TSPO) is an 18 kDa macromolecular protein with a structure of five alpha helices across the membrane lipid bilayer. TSPO was upregulated by the activation of microglia and astrocytes and measured different neural inflammatory conditions with PK11195 [13, 14]. TSPO is the most widely used target for PET imaging of neuroinflammation. Inflammatory progress has upregulated expression of TSPO due to immunomodulation, synthesis of steroid hormones, apoptosis, and cell proliferation [15]. TSPO is highly expressed in activated microglia, but it is always expressed at a lower level in the gray matter [16]. As a biomarker of microglial activation, TSPO's expression has been shown increased in many CNS pathological states, such as Huntington's disease (HD) [17], brain ischemia [18], and MS [19]. Nowadays, TSPO's upregulation in microglial cells is thought to be a sensitive biomarker of neuroinflammation, which mainly reflects microglial cells' activity [20, 21].

References

1. Ibrahim N, Kusmirek J, Struck AF, et al. The sensitivity and specificity of F-DOPA PET in a movement disorder clinic. Am J Nucl Med Mol Imaging. 2016;6(1):102–9.
2. Zhu Y, Du R, Zhu Y, et al. PET mapping of neurofunctional changes in a post-traumatic stress disorder model. J Nucl Med. 2016;57(9):1474–7.
3. Li CY, Klohr S, Sadick H, et al. Effect of time-of-flight technique on the diagnostic performance of 18F-FDG PET/CT for assessment of lymph node metastases in head and neck squamous cell carcinoma. J Nucl Med Technol. 2014;42(3):181–7.
4. Surti S, Karp JS. Application of a generalized scan statistic model to evaluate TOF PET images. IEEE Trans Nucl Sci. 2011;58(1):99–104.
5. Sacconi B, Raad RA, Lee J, et al. Concurrent functional and metabolic assessment of brain tumors using hybrid PET/MR imaging. J Neuro-Oncol. 2016;127(2):287–93.
6. Nabavizadeh SA, Nasrallah I, Dubroff J. Emerging PET/MRI applications in neuroradiology and neuroscience. Clin Transl Imaging. 2017;5(2):121–33.
7. Marner L, Henriksen OM, Lundemann M, et al. Clinical PET/MRI in neurooncology: opportunities and challenges from a single-institution perspective. Clin Transl Imaging. 2017;5(2):135–49.
8. Kang K, Lim I, Roh JK. Positron emission tomographic findings in a tuberculous brain abscess. Ann Nucl Med. 2007;21(5):303–6.
9. D'Souza MM, Sharma R, Jaimini A, et al. Metabolic assessment of intracranial tuberculomas using 11C-methionine and 18F-FDG PET/CT. Nucl Med Commun. 2012;33(4):408–14.
10. Tripathi M, Yadav S, Kumar V, et al. HIV encephalitis with subcortical tau deposition: imaging pathology in vivo using F-18 THK 5117. Eur J Nucl Med Mol Imaging. 2016;43(13):2456–7.
11. Rangan K, Ravina M, Yadav N, et al. 18F-FDG PET/CT of tuberculosis meningitis and carotid pseudoaneurysm. Clin Nucl Med. 2017;42(6):e304–5.
12. Newey CR, Sarwal A, Hantus S. [(18)F]-Fluoro-Deoxy-Glucose Positron Emission Tomography Scan Should Be Obtained Early in Cases of Autoimmune Encephalitis. Autoimmune Dis. 2016;2016:9450452.
13. Benavides J, Fage D, Carter C, et al. Peripheral type benzodiazepine binding sites are a sensitive indirect index of neuronal damage. Brain Res. 1987; 421(1-2):167–72.
14. Benavides J, Capdeville C, Dauphin F, et al. The quantification of brain LESIONS with an omega 3 site ligand: a critical analysis of animal models of cerebral ischaemia and neurodegeneration. Brain Res. 1990;522(2):275–89.
15. Papadopoulos V, Baraldi M, Guilarte TR, et al. Translocator protein (18kDa): new nomenclature for the peripheral-type benzodiazepine receptor based on its structure and molecular function. Trends Pharmacol Sci. 2006;27(8):402–9.
16. Doble A, Malgouris C, Daniel M, et al. Labelling of peripheral-type benzodiazepine binding sites in human brain with [3H]PK 11195: anatomical and subcellular distribution. Brain Res Bull. 1987; 18(1):49–61.
17. Schoemaker H, Morelli M, Deshmukh P, et al. [3H]Ro5-4864 benzodiazepine binding in the kainate lesioned striatum and Huntington's diseased basal ganglia. Brain Res. 1982;248(2):396-401.
18. Stephenson DT, Schober DA, Smalstig EB, et al. Peripheral benzodiazepine receptors are colocalized with activated microglia following transient global forebrain ischemia in the rat. J Neurosci. 1995;15(7 Pt 2):5263–74.
19. Vowinckel E, Reutens D, Becher B, et al. PK11195 binding to the peripheral benzodiazepine receptor as a marker of microglia activation in multiple sclerosis and experimental autoimmune encephalomyelitis. J Neurosci Res. 1997;50(2):345–53.
20. Cosenza-Nashat M, Zhao ML, Suh HS, et al. Expression of the translocator protein of 18 kDa by microglia, macrophages and astrocytes based on immunohistochemical localization in abnormal human brain. Neuropathol Appl Neurobiol. 2009;35(3):306–28.
21. Maeda J, Higuchi M, Inaji M, et al. Phase-dependent roles of reactive microglia and astrocytes in nervous system injury as delineated by imaging of peripheral benzodiazepine receptor. Brain Res. 2007;1157:100–11.

Imaging-Guided Brain Biopsies

4

Yubo Lyu

4.1 Introduction

CT can be limited used frequently with lesion suboptimal visualization and radiation expose for guidance of percutaneous brain biopsy. The choice and interest in the absence of ionizing radiation MRI guidance interventional continued to increase [1–3], with favorable advantages including true multi-planar imaging capabilities, high soft tissue contrast along with sufficient spatial resolution and good vessel depiction. Interventional MRI has the ability to lead to specimens with less necrosis and more chance of identification of the origin brain lesion, because MRI with contrast can easily identify cystic and necrotic inside a lesion with higher sensitivity than CT. At the same time, disadvantages of interventional MRI techniques, like restricted patient access inside closed-bore superconducting magnets and longer image acquisition times that precluded timely updates of device position during procedure [3], are hampering the enthusiasm of physicians to take advantage of MR imaging for interventional biopsy. Pulse sequence improvements and the introduction of open design systems, for example, low-field open-configuration MRI systems, provide improved patient access for interventional MRI guidance procedures [4], and the feasibility and potential benefits of this kind of MRI system were demonstrated by several groups. MRI guidance interventional technique will be gradually evolved into an effective minimally invasive procedure for brain biopsy with the availability of MRI-compatible instruments and open configuration.

Y. Lyu (✉)
Shanghai Jiahui International Hospital, Jiahui Health, Shanghai, China

Shandong Medical Imaging Research Institute, Shandong University, Jinan, China

4.2 Clinical Biopsy Under Open MR Imaging Guidance

MRI has several useful advantages [5, 6], like high conspicuity of anatomy and pathological abnormalities without ionizing radiation hazard, superior tissue contrast with or without intravenous contrast medium, good sensitivity particularly advantageous for lesions that are not visible on CT [7–9] or for lesions adjacent to critical structures which require better visualized or site-specific targeting by MRI, and real-time guidance sequences. The application and acceleration of MRI guidance interventional techniques depend on more creation of MR-compatible instruments and better access to patient scanner, in particular, the development of open magnetic resonance imaging (MRI) systems. The open low-field imaging systems began to be available in the late 1980s. Even though the system often required prolonged imaging time to obtain sufficient imaging, the better access to the patient provided by these open systems led to a lot of reports.

It's beneficial to combine needle tracking systems with MRI scanner. Open magnets can satisfy the need for moving the patient in and out repeatedly during the procedure guidance [10]. Our study and experience were based on our open-configuration MRI system (0.23-T, Outlook Proview, Philips Healthcare, Amsterdam, Netherlands) with optical tracking navigator (iPath 200, Panorama, Philips Healthcare) (Fig. 4.1). The C-arm design of the MRI scanner and the free-movable optical tracking system are flexible and convenient and allow the radiologists to puncture in an environment at different angles with very little limitation of patient access. The patient is positioned in the open system between flat magnetic poles allowing patient access from a range of side approaches with unrestricted horizontal access, but the vertical access is limited by the upper magnet pole.

B. Gao et al. (eds.), *Imaging of CNS Infections and Neuroimmunology*, https://doi.org/10.1007/978-981-13-6904-9_4

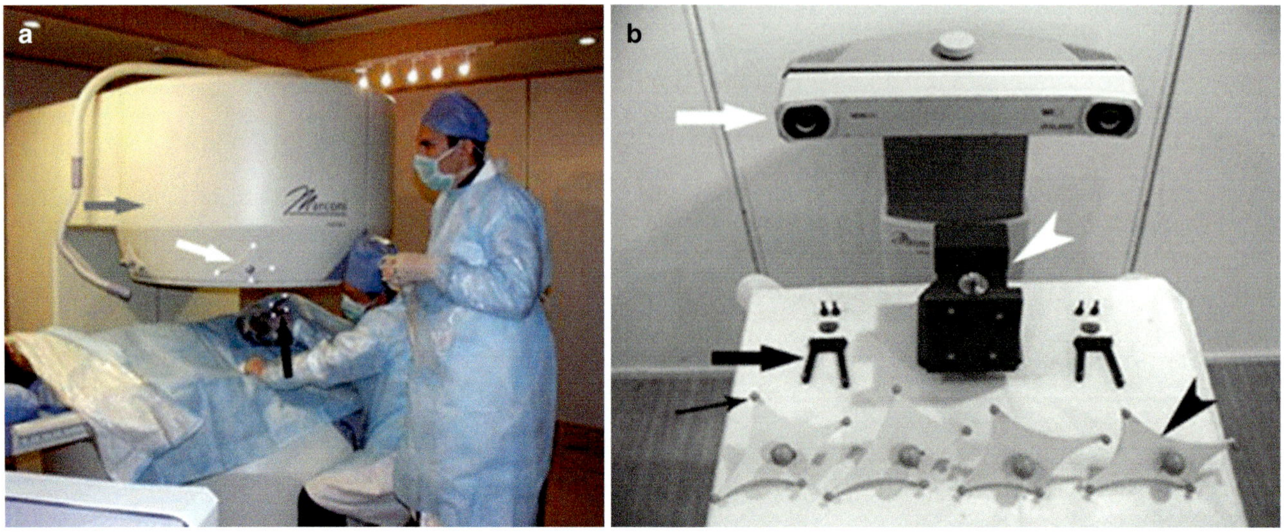

Fig. 4.1 (**a**) Interventional MRI suites with open MR imaging system (gray arrow), mounted magnetic body tracker (white arrow) with fixed reflective spheres and needle holder with four reflective spheres (black arrow). (**b**) The optical navigation suite (iPath 200) consisting of an infrared camera (white arrow), two instrument holder (black arrow), four magnet trackers (black arrowhead), reflective spheres (fine black arrow), MR-guided procedure (MRGP) calibration phantom and blocks (white arrowhead) (Reprint with permission from: Chengli Li, Yubo Lü, Ming Liu, et al. Magnetic resonance imaging-guided biopsy of musculoskeletal lesions using open low-field systems. Top Magn Reson Imaging. 2011 Aug;22(4):135–41)

If there are no contraindications or access to the lesion is considered to be safe, the open-configuration MRI is considered appropriate for the interventional procedure. Three magnet bore configurations used for interventional MRI were reported by Carrino [7]. The "cylinder" configuration is an adaptation of a short-bore high field system. The "clamshell" configuration is an adaptation and slight modification to the routine open low-field system. The third configuration is a midfield magnet specifically designed for intervention procedure, which has two cylinders separated by a gap for access. The open design of MR unit can provide sufficient and convenient access for the patients and operators. During the MRI guidance procedure, the instruments positioned parallel to the magnetic field may result in an artifact with only minimal apparent width on MRI limiting accurate instrument positioning and accuracy of the display of the instrument tip localization, because the low external magnetic field of the MRI system is horizontally oriented along the long axis of the magnet bore with instrument trajectories most often aligned in a no parallel fashion compared to the magnetic field. For the high field MRI systems, the scanning speed and imaging quality are usually better because of higher SNR, but the procedure, the patient has to be moved in and out of the magnet bore several time, comparing that procedure can be performed directly inside the in low field strength magnet.

4.3 Navigational Technique

Navigational system can enhance the operator's ability to take into account 2–3 dimensions according to the anatomy with needle location, and allow interactive manage and potentially more accurate needle actions. Three kinds of navigation systems such as externally referenced, self-referenced, and MR tracking were reported by the team of Carrino. The optical or radiofrequency guidance belongs to the externally referenced system or frameless stereotaxy methods. Anatomical landmarks or fiducial markers belong to self-referenced system. MRI hardware for guidance belongs to MR tracking system. Several navigational systems, for example, optically linked stereotaxy, freehand technique, frame-based stereotaxy, augmented reality techniques, nonoptical stereotaxy, and image fusion, were used as needle guidance navigation toward the target in MRI environment [8, 9]. Freehand technique requires a basic interventional skill experience and uses a set that is already familiar to regularly performing percutaneous procedures, which is the simplest and the most commonly used [11]. The radiologist can completely access to the patient and biopsy instruments during the procedure using the optical tracking stereotactic system with open MRI unit [8, 9]. This kind of technique depends on interactive coupling of the MR image plane to the orientation of the needle holder. The frameless stereotaxy technique requires localization and targeting using image guidance. The camera sensor of the navigator detects the orientation and location of the needle holder. This type of interactive guidance system also had been applied for MRI navigation in C-arm unit, was several described [12, 13]. The optical tracking system has a needle holder with two flashing infrared light-emitting diodes that can be detected by the magnet scanner mounted sensors. Using simple triangulation and the tracking system, the MRI interventional system console computer can detect continuous information about the position and angle of the instrument. One-step localization is selecting a right image plane as an interactive way to define trajectories, localize targets, and review alternative access routes from any image plane, which can be generated on the basis of the position of the instrument. In this interactive navigational system, the needle location and trajectory can be seen in the nearly real-time MR imaging during the interventional procedure on the in-room screen. Silverman et al. also reported this kind of optical tracking system to track the probe position. The spatial position in the system that describes the location of the light-emitting diodes can be used to extrapolate the path and the position of the instrument depending on the straight instrument length known. The best angle to the part of the lesion and skin entry point was determined by showing the needle icon projecting in the lesion on all three orthogonal imaging planes using the optical navigation system.

We frequently use an optical tracking navigation system (iPath 200, Panorama, Philips Healthcare) for the guidance of biopsy procedures. The optical tracking system includes a fixed magnetic body tracker with reflective spheres, a calibration phantom, a device holder with reflective spheres, and an infrared camera (Fig. 4.1). The tracking is performed using the infrared navigator camera during the procedure. The camera can detect two trackers simultaneously, one of which is attached to the housing of the upper magnet pole and another to the biopsy set which is attached providing a fixed frame of reference. The infrared camera system tracks the position of the needle holder in real time by comparing its space position to the point of reference indicated by the magnetic scanner tracker through the reflective spheres. The instrument and its trajectory are also real time shown as a graphic overlay in the procedure image set. The navigation system can provide multi-planar image acquisition to automatically track the instrument path. A graphic overlay blue line displayed on the in-room screen on the MR images shows the device position (Fig. 4.1). This overlay line can be used for determination of the skin entry point, preoperative lesion localization, procedural planning, and intraoperative guidance. Using this tracking system, which allows for dynamic adjustment of the image plane to the changing position of the needle during puncture, the needle is completely included in the image without the need of manual adjustments, which helps to achieve efficient and safe needle placement. The accuracy and practicability of this kind of optical tracking navigator system for device guidance have been proved previously [5, 6, 14, 15].

4.4 Monitoring Sequences

The interventional MRI scanning sequences, which are often different from those used in general MR imaging, should allow for accurate device position, fast imaging acquisition, and sufficient spatial resolution and soft tissue detail to meet the requirements of imaging guidance. Low field interventional MRI is frequently based on GRE sequences, which allow for short acquisition times. For device MR-guided, T1-weighted GRE with a useful compromise between temporal, spatial, and contrast resolution is preferred. High quality MR imaging including no image distortion, accurate device visualization and the optional ability to dynamically management the imaging plane is the challenging constraint for MR imaging guidance over x-ray based techniques especially the accurate visualization of instruments [16]. For lesion display and needle tracking, fast sequences such as balanced T1-weighted GRE techniques or single-shot T2-weighted spin-echo sequences can be used for the best.

Needle visualization in GRE images sequences is characterized by amplification of the metal artifact, which usually results in better needle visibility. Flip angle and TR are important protocols that affect the lesion conspicuity. Small flip angle is associated with lower T1 weighting, and a shorter TR results in diminished contrast imaging resolution. Instruments can be almost invisible in T2-weighted FSE sequences images depending on the orientation relative to the magnetic field. The lesion should be identified clearly and reliably on the images before initiation of the procedure using a variety of different scanning sequences.

We frequently use CBASS (completely balanced steady state, 3D 8 slices, TR 8.4 ms, TE 4.2 ms, flip angle 45°, slice thickness/slice interval 5.0/5.0 mm, FOV 300 × 300, matrix 180 × 216, acquisition time 45 s) sequence for the initial planning, which allows for quick high-resolution acquisition. Alternatively, a T2-weighted FSE sequence (9 slices, TR 150 ms, TE 3500 ms, slice thickness/slice interval 7.0 mm/8.0 mm, FOV 380 × 380, matrix 192 × 192, acquisition time 35 s) is used for lesions adjacent to vessels, which results in low signal of black blood. Three perpendicular imaging planes are obtained and used for lesion localization with surrounded anatomic relationships. A continuous, multi-planar field-echo T1-weighted (FE 5 slices,

Table 4.1 Interventional MRI sequences for localization and for monitoring needle position using a 0.23 Tesla open MR imaging system (Outlook Proview, Philips Healthcare, Amsterdam, Netherlands with permissions) (Reprint with permission from: Chengli Li, Yubo Lü, Ming Liu, et al. Magnetic resonance imaging-guided biopsy of musculoskeletal lesions using open low-field systems. Top Magn Reson Imaging. 2011 Aug;22(4):135–41)

	FSE (T1WI)	FSE (T2WI)	FSE	FE	CBASS
TR	380 ms	4250 ms	3500 ms	60 ms	8.4 ms
TE	18 ms	80 ms	150 ms	7.0 ms	4.2 ms
FA	90 deg	90 deg	90 deg	60 deg	45 deg
THK/SEP	7 mm	7 mm	7/8 mm	10/10 mm	5.0 mm
FOV	300 mm^2	300 mm^2	300 mm^2	300 mm^2	300 mm^2
MAT	169 × 256	169 × 256	180 × 180	270 × 270	216 × 216
Time	4 min 52 s	3 min 58 s	28 s	12 s	28 s

TR repeat time, *TE* echo time, *FA* flap angle, *THK* thickness, *SEP* separateness, *FOV* field of view, *MAT* matrix

TR 125 ms, TE 7.0 ms, flip angle 60°, slice thickness/slice interval 7.0 mm/7.0 mm, FOV 300 × 300, matrix 160 × 180, acquisition time 28 s) sequence or CBASS sequence can be used for intermittent instrument guidance, allowing for tracking and direction adjusting accordingly during placement or targeting. Black vessel conspicuity on FSE and CBASS sequences allows for safe without critical vessels or nerves injury. The optimization of pulse sequences and instruments results in high image quality with sharply demarcated device visualization, which ensures safety and accuracy (Table 4.1).

4.5 Procedure and Technique

4.5.1 Pre-procedure Preparation

Our interventional MRI system for brain biopsy includes an open C-arm MRI scanner, optical infrared tracking navigator, in-room console with monitor, and a flexible transmit-receive surface coil (diameter 20 cm). Mannitol (250 ml, 50 g) and ethamsylate (2.0 g) were administered preoperatively according to the clinical with local anesthesia using lidocaine (2%, 5 ml) and conscious sedation using diazepam (5 mg). Blood pressure, oxygen saturation, and heart and respiratory rates were monitored, and strict sterility was maintained throughout the procedure.

4.5.2 Procedure

Completely balanced steady state (CBASS 3D 8 slice, TR 8.4 ms, TE 4.2 ms, flip angle 45°, slice thickness/slice interval 5.0/5.0 mm, FOV 300 × 300, matrix 180 × 216, acquisition time 45 s) imaging was used for scanning. The CBASS is a really fast sequence with true-FISP that allows high-quality brain images. Axial, coronal, and sagittal imaging planes were used for localization. A ProbeView II (plane parallel to tool axis and instrument tracker plane) scan was first obtained, followed by a ProbeView III (plane parallel to tool axis, perpendicular to ProbeView II), and finally a ProbeView I (plane perpendicular to tool axis). Integrated optical frameless stereotaxy was used concomitantly with MRI for localization, planning, skin point, and navigation.

Once the skin entry route was determined, a 3 mm hole at the site of skin puncture was drilled in the skull bone. MR-compatible (16 gauge, 15 cm length) trocar neuroneedle (Invivo Germany GmbH, Germany) was used to initially puncture the scalp. A slight depression was made with the needle into the skin at the desired entry point without cutting into the skin or bending the needle. At this time, continuous multi-planar FE T1WI (FE 5 slice, TR 125 ms, TE 7.0 ms, flip angle 60°, slice thickness/slice interval 7.0/7.0 mm, FOV 300 × 300, matrix 160 × 180, acquisition time 25 s) scanning with MRI contrast (gadolinium-DTPA, 0.2 ml/kg) was used in order to visualize the wall of abscesses, the needle, and anatomic structure to verify that the needle artifact on the surface of the skin was at the appropriate entry point. After that, the needle was inserted toward the lesion under the guidance of a graphic overlay line on the screen of in-room monitor. The blue line is the automatic simulation of the tracking of needle position through the optical tracking suite (Fig. 4.2). The reflecting infrared light can trigger multi-planar scanning at any needed time. The near real-time three-dimensional images allowed to keep showing needle's location and to correct direction accordingly.

Aspiration procedure would be performed after the needle was rightly placed in the brain abscess. MR T1WI with contrast enhancement scanning was performed periodically to confirm the location of the tip and to monitor the changes of the abscess during the procedure (Fig. 4.3b–d). The fluid was sent to microbiological inspection, culture, and drug sensitivity testing (Fig. 4.3e, f). Subsequent abscess irrigation was performed in each patient using dioxogen (2–3%), physiological saline (0.9%), and metronidazole (10 ml, 50 mg). Abscess was drained and rinsed repeatedly until clear. Before

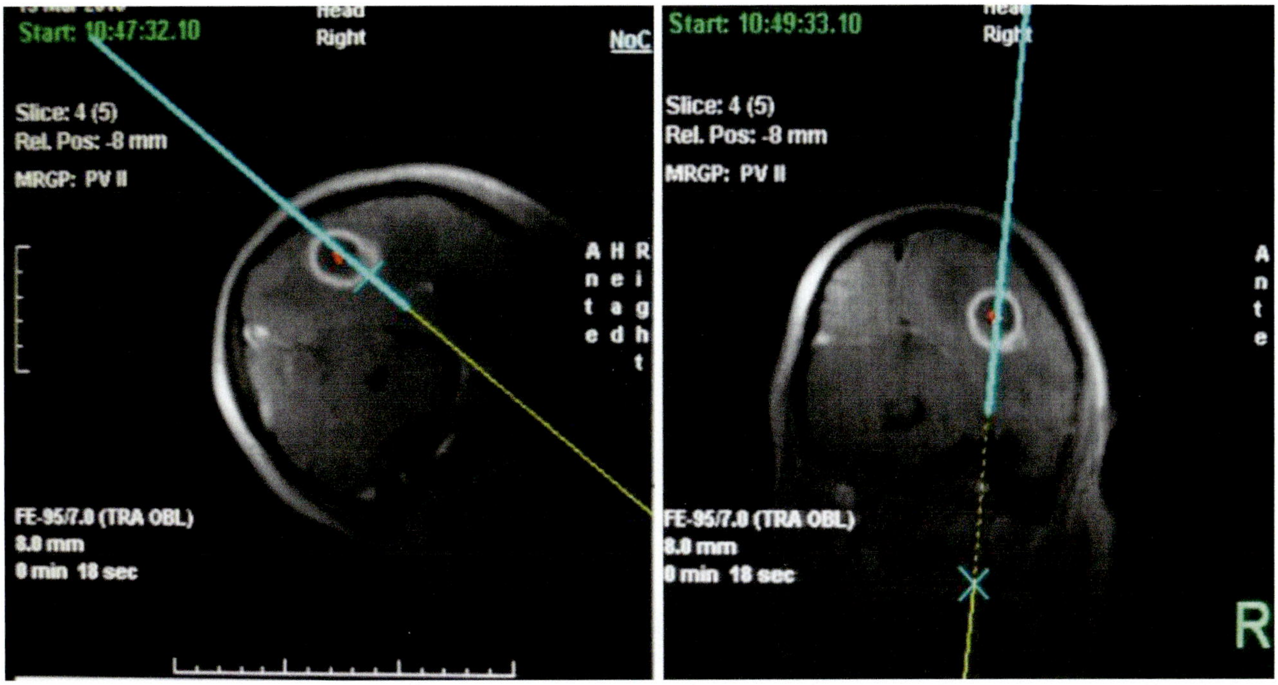

Fig. 4.2 The overlay blue line was shown on the screen to guide the procedure. The red point in the central of the abscess was the target

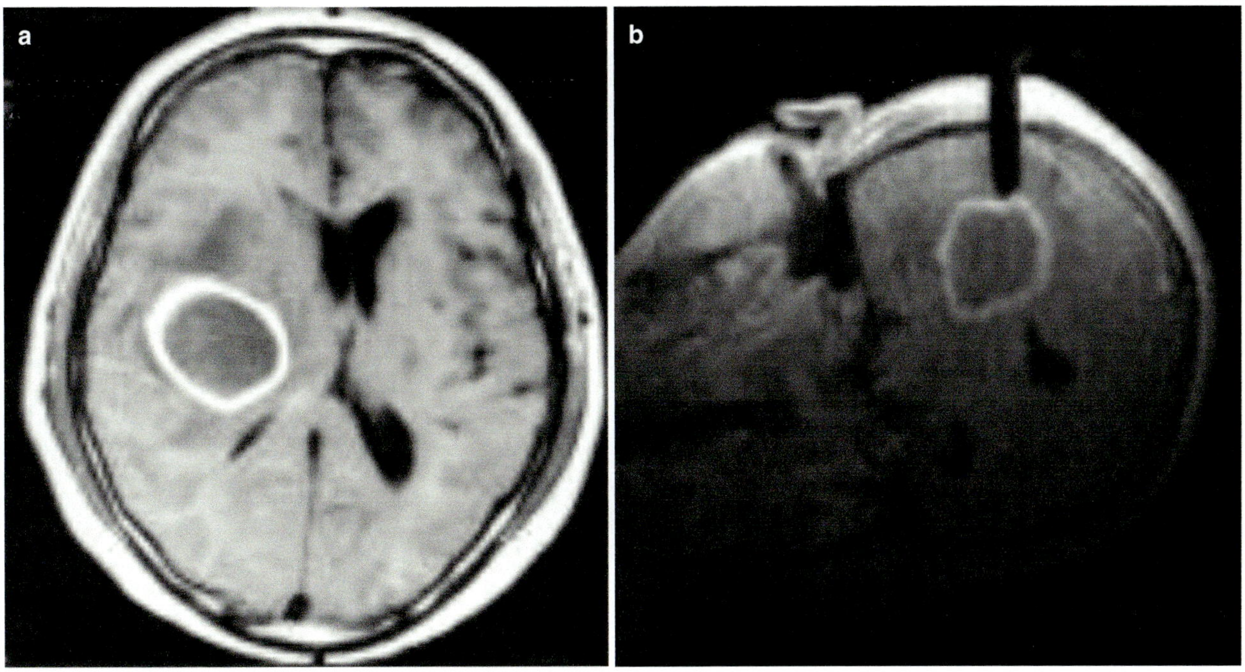

Fig. 4.3 A 42-year old male was admitted to hospital due to fever, headache and vomiting. Enhanced T1 Weighted Imaging shows "ring enhancement" of the abscess in the right basal ganglia regionin (**a**). Intraoperative enhanced FE scanning shows the magnetic compatible needle penetrating into the abscess accurately (**b**, **c**) and the reduction of the abscess after aspiration (**d**). The extractive thick pus shows yellowish gray (**e**). Cytological smear of the pus shows a large number of lobulated neutrophils (Wright's staining, amplification factor ×1000), which confirmed the diagnosis of the abscess (**f**). The abscess was resolved completely in MRI of 6 months follow-up, hemosiderin are visible (**g**, **h**)

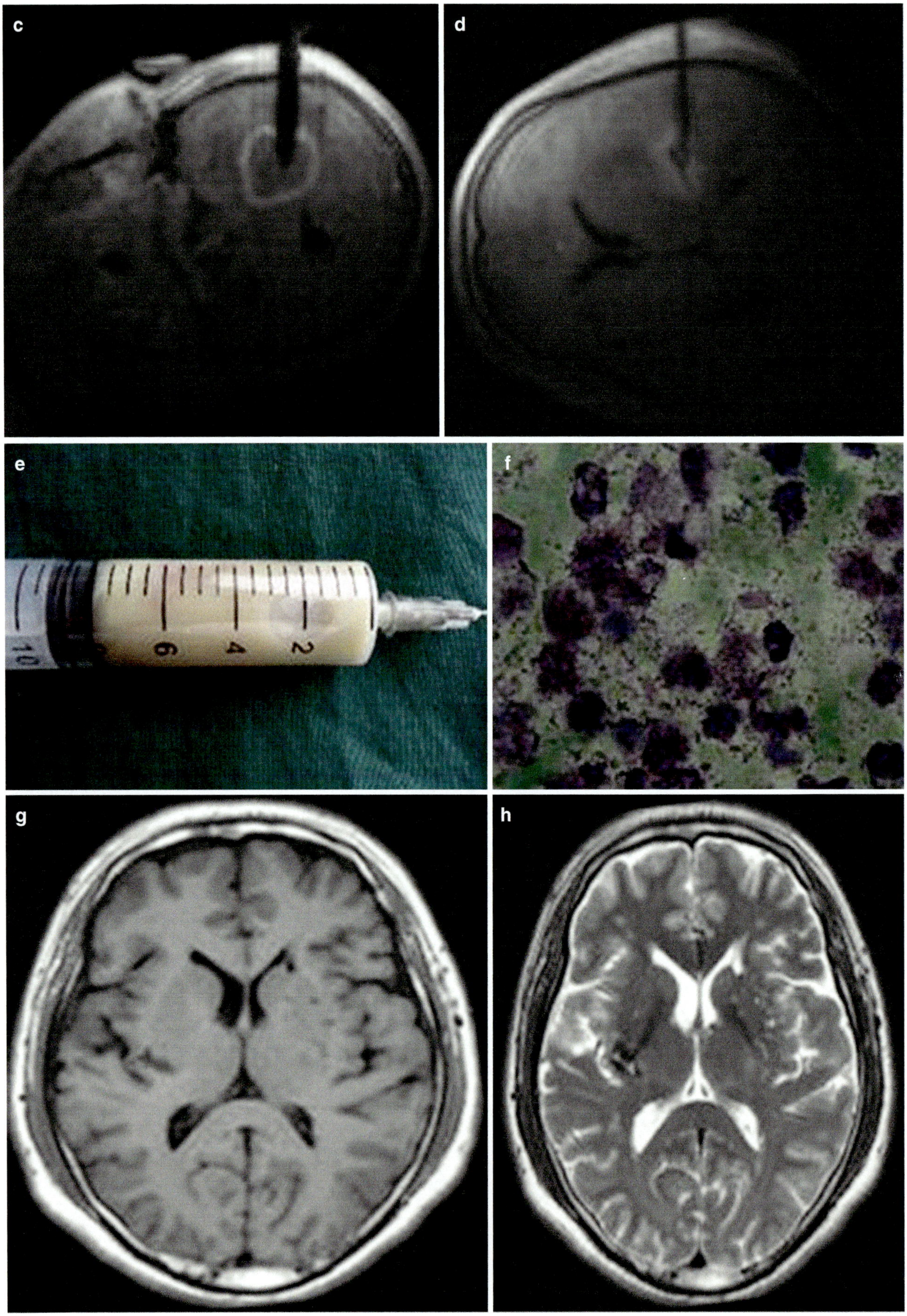

Fig. 4.3 (continued)

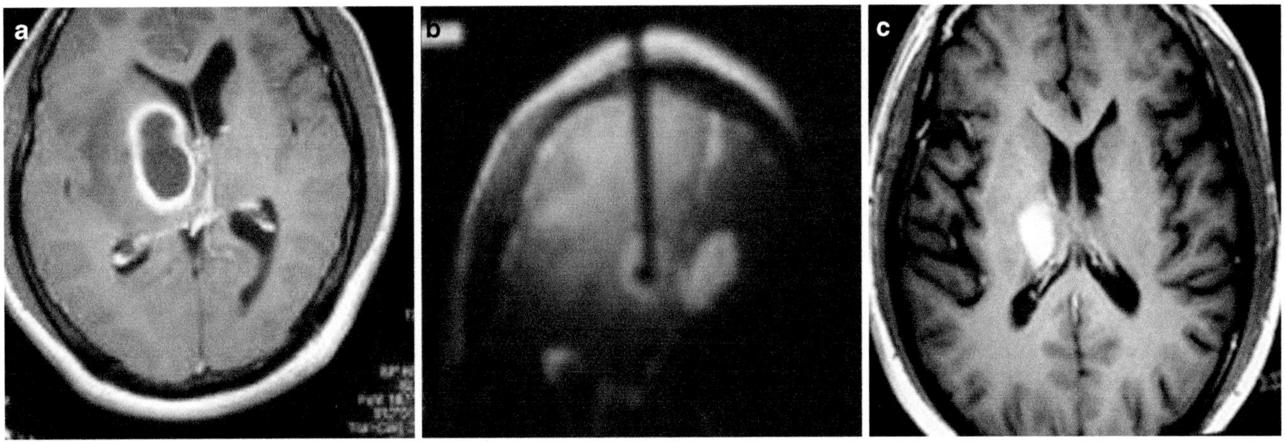

Fig. 4.4 A 35 years old male with fever and headache. Post-contrast T1WI (**a**) shows "ring enhancement". Intraoperative CBASS imaging shows the needle penetrating into the abscess accurately and the fluid in the cavity (**b**). The pus cavity disappeared in the MR imaging of 3 months follow-up, however, gliosis and glial scar formation are visible (**c**)

withdrawing the needle out, the abscess cavity should be cleared. MR CBASS imaging was performed to monitor the fluid content in the abscess (Fig. 4.4b). A soft plastic drainage catheter (16 gauge) was implanted inside the residual abscess for external drainage and irrigation with normal saline, dioxogen, or metronidazole in three larger abscesses (diameter greater than 4.5 cm) for 3 days under the guidance of a MRI visible straight tip guide wire. Nine patients with single brain abscess underwent single operation, and the two patients with two lesions underwent a second operation.

4.5.3 Postoperative Care

Patients were observed for 30–60 min in the radiology suite and sent to the neurosurgical ward to be monitored using electrocardiogram for 24 h. Intravenous drip of mannitol (250 ml/day) and corticosteroid (dexamethasone, 10 mg/day) was performed after the procedure. A broad-spectrum antibiotic was administered according to culture of the aspirated material. The course of intravenous antibiotics was 7 weeks.

4.6 Result Evaluation

In this study, 11 patients (9 men, 2 women; mean age 37 years) with clinical and previous imaging findings (CT or MRI) suggesting brain abscess underwent transcranial aspiration under the guidance of an open-configuration MRI scanner (0.23-T, Outlook Proview, Philips Medical Systems, Finland) with an optical navigator (iPath 200, Panorama, Philips Medical Systems, Finland) from January 2007 to November 2009. The diagnosis of 13 brain abscesses (9 had solitary abscess and 2 had double lesions) in 11 patients were made by a radiologist and a neurologist jointly through the clinical symptoms and imaging features. Only mature abscesses with capsule formation were included in this study (Figs. 4.3a and 4.4a). Normal hemostasis values, no contraindications to MRI, and no history of serious cardiopulmonary diseases were regarded as eligible for interventional therapy. Informed consent was acquired from each patient. The study protocol was approved in the institutional ethics board of our hospital. The schedule of follow-up was 1 week, 1 month, 3 months, and 6 months. MR follow-up scanning and subsequently analyses were done in each patient. The diameter of abscess was measured by a radiologist. The CNS signs and symptoms, including fever, headache, vomiting, epilepsy, papilledema, meningismus, hemiparesis, and altered sensorium, were evaluated and recorded by a neurologist through detailed history and physical examination at each follow-up visit. Descriptive statistics were applied to the MRI features and clinical signs and symptoms. The abscess diameters ranged from 1.6 to 5.7 cm with a mean of 3.5 cm before aspiration. They were located within the basal ganglia region in four cases, temporal lobe in three, frontal lobe in two, parietal-occipital lobe in two, external capsule region in one, and cerebellum in one. Punctures of all these abscesses with aspiration were performed successfully using interventional MRI by monitoring and navigating the procedure (Figs.4.3b–d and 4.4b). The outer drainage tubes were successfully placed in three larger abscesses and removed in post-procedure day 3. The fast imaging sequences used in this study provided a reliable visualization of all the brain abscesses and met the need of near real-time monitoring. MRI contrast-enhanced examination using gadolinium-DTPA made the wall of all abscesses more conspicuous during procedure (Fig. 4.3b, c). The mean operating time was 70 min (range 45–100 min), including intraoperative MR scanning and drainage tube placement. All patients tolerated the procedure without serious complications.

Staphylococcus aureus infections were identified in seven patients (including one with double lesions), *Streptococcus hemolyticus* in two, anaerobic streptococci in one, and *Pseudomonas aeruginosa* in one (the other double lesion) and verified by microbiological inspection and culture. MR scanning at 1 week follow-up showed that the mean diameter of abscesses was 1.4 cm (range 0.4–2.6 cm) and the average reduction rate of the abscess size was 60% (2.1/3.5). The abscesses showed the greatest reduction within the first month and decreased by up to 89.7% (mean 0.36 cm, range 0–1.0 cm, 3.14/3.5). Later follow-up MRI showed gradual diameter diminution of the enhancing ring structure until resolution (Figs. 4.3g, h and 4.4c). At the end of 6 months, all patients treated with stereotactic aspiration combined with 7 weeks' intravenous sensitive antibiotic treatment had a good outcome without new sequelae. This treatment modality allowed infection control and healing for all 11 patients with 0% recurrence rate. One patient with epilepsy and one with hemiparesis did not recover during follow-up, but their conditions improved obviously. The rate of recovery was 100% with fever, headache, vomiting, papilledema, meningism, and altered sensorium, 75% (3/4) in hemiparesis, and 83.3% (5/6) in epilepsy.

Histologically, there are four stages in brain abscess formation: early cerebritis (days 1–3), late cerebritis (days 4–9), early encapsulation (days 10–13), and late capsule stage (days 14 onward) [17]. About 2 weeks is required for encapsulation. Characteristic ring enhancement, which can be seen with contrast-enhanced MRI, shows uniform thick wall and smooth contour on its inner surface especially in the late encapsulation (Figs. 4.3a and 4.4a). Image guidance stereotactic aspiration as a minimally invasive approach to cure brain abscesses with good outcomes had been reported [18–20]. By applying interventional magnetic resonance imaging tracking systems for guidance of stereotactic evacuation of 13 brain abscesses, we found that the minimally invasive approach allows accurate performance of the procedure and provides good clinical results for the management. Follow-up MRI demonstrated gradual resolution of the abscesses and a successful return to nearly normal function in all the cases.

With the development of image-guided technology, percutaneous stereotactic evacuation approach has been applied widely in clinical practice (Lunsford 1987; [17, 21–23]). CT-guided stereotactic aspiration of brain abscesses could help achieve the treatment goals, draining the contents of the abscess, reducing mass effect, and confirming diagnosis [24]. However, the inferior imaging and the radiation hazard are a restriction for the CT-guided approach. With the capability of high-resolution and multi-planar imaging, the development of fast sequences, and the application of navigation technology, interventional MRI-guided system can be used. Punctures of cystic or necrotic intracranial lesions with subsequent aspiration and management of hydrocephalus or intracerebral hematomas can be performed safely and accurately by monitoring the procedure using interventional MR scanning to obtain immediate feedback on associated dynamic tissue changes [25, 26].

Our results are in accordance with other reports using image guidance to perform stereotactic interventional procedure of brain abscesses as a feasible and safe method. Brain MRI provides exact localization and accurate characterization and determination of number, size, and staging of the abscess. MRI can also detect associated complications such as hydrocephalus, cerebral edema, and infections like subdural empyema and ventriculitis thus helping in treatment planning. Compared with CT, MRI-guided technique has some advantages. High-quality MR imaging demonstrates the wall of the abscess clearly and its fast sequence offers near real-time monitoring of the operative procedure. Lack of exposure to ionizing radiation with magnetic resonance scanning ensures the safety of patients and operators in the operating room. Applying MRI as a guidance modality, the procedure can be more accurate and reliable [27].

Open magnetic resonance imaging (MRI) technology introduces new features that, in combination with navigation, seem particularly valuable for performing these interventional operations [28, 29]. In our study we used optical navigator suite for instrument guidance. Its practicability and accuracy have been shown in previous work [5, 6, 30–33]. The optical camera can be moved freely around the magnet, which is very convenient for the operator to complete the puncture at any point or angle. High-quality scanning in optional plane orientation and location, which is realized by changing the position of the needle tracker using this suite, was exact and practical in the process of guidance and monitoring. The near real-time scanning and navigation capabilities of the system can also eliminate the inaccuracies that may result from brain shift during evacuation procedure.

The choice of initial antimicrobial therapy depends on the suspected pathogen(s) and ability of antibiotics to penetrate the blood-brain barrier and abscess wall [29]. Prescription of intravenous sensitive antibiotic treatment is an effective auxiliary means for the cerebral abscess after stereotactic aspiration. Followed lavaging with dioxogen and metronidazole alternately was effective local disinfection and sterilization for each abscess. Three large abscesses needed drainage catheter for 3 days' outer drainage, which helped to shorten the absorbed period.

There were some limitations. We did not directly compare magnetic resonance imaging with computed tomography as the guiding modality or compare to craniotomy. Our sample size and selective group were small that need larger random. Even though the low-field MR scanner can offer clear images to demonstrate the brain anatomical structure and the lesion, pre- or intraoperative functional MRI and DTI are not possible on these platforms. Brain functional MRI is valuable and may be helpful for safer procedure planning. MRI-guided percutaneous aspiration and drainage of brain abscess is safe and effective. This procedure can be accomplished without general anesthesia. This technique can be a valuable therapeutic option in the practice of neurosurgery for the management of intracranial abscess.

4.7 Summary

Interventional MRI guidance is a helpful tool for the management of brain diagnostic procedures. MRI guidance percutaneous brain biopsy was proved safe. Inherent disadvantages of MRI interventional require consideration, for example, the cost and availability low-filed MR scanner with navigational system and MRI compatible instruments are frequently higher. Specific contraindications of MR imaging, such as certain cerebral aneurysm clips, the presence of pacemakers, cochlear implants, or other strongly ferromagnetic material near critical locations also need to be considered as disadvantages. Anyway, low-field open-configuration MR system really broadens the scope of MRI interventional procedures using its navigation systems, which actually contributed to high accuracy and to optimization of brain lesion management.

References

1. Lü Y, Liu M, Li C, et al. MRI-guided biopsy and aspiration in the head and neck: evaluation of 77 patients. Eur Radiol. 2012;22(2):404–10.
2. Lewin JS, Nour SG, Duerk JL. Magnetic resonance image-guided biopsy and aspiration. Top Magn Reson Imaging. 2000;11(3):173–83.
3. Weiss CR, Nour SG, Lewin JS. MR-guided biopsy: a review of current techniques and applications. J Magn Reson Imaging. 2008;27(2):311–25.
4. Silverman SG, Collick BD, Figueira MR, et al. Interactive MR-guided biopsy in an open-configuration MR imaging system. Radiology. 1995;197(1):175–81.
5. Sequeiros RB, Rauli Klemola MD, Risto Ojala MD, et al. Percutaneous MR-guided discography in a low-field system using optical instrument tracking: A feasibility study. J Magn Reson Imaging. 2003;17(2):214–9.
6. Sequeiros RB, Hyvönen P, Sequeiros AB, et al. MR imaging-guided laser ablation of osteoid osteomas with use of optical instrument guidance at 0.23 T. Eur Radiol. 2003;13(10):2309–14.
7. Carrino JA, Khurana B, Ready JE, et al. Magnetic resonance imaging-guided percutaneous biopsy of musculoskeletal lesions. J Bone Joint Surg Am. 2007;89(10):2179–87.
8. Fritz J, Tzaribachev N, Thomas C, et al. Magnetic resonance imaging-guided osseous biopsy in children with chronic recurrent multifocal osteomyelitis. Cardiovasc Intervent Radiol. 2012;35(1):146–53.
9. Fritz J, Uthainual P, Ungi T, et al. Augmented reality visualization with image overlay for MRI-guided intervention: accuracy for lumbar spinal procedures with a 1.5-T MRI system. AJR Am J Roentgenol. 2012;198(3):W266–73.
10. Daniel BL. Intraprocedural magnetic resonance imaging-guided interventions in the breast. Top Magn Reson Imaging. 2000;11(3):184–90.
11. Fritz J, Clasen S, Boss A, et al. Real-time MR fluoroscopy-navigated lumbar facet joint injections: feasibility and technical properties. Eur Radiol. 2008;18(7):1513–8.
12. Jolesz FA, Kikinis R, Talos IF. Neuronavigation in interventional MR imaging. Frameless stereotaxy. Neuroimaging Clin N Am. 2001;11(4):685–93.
13. Schneider JP, Dietrich J, Lieberenz S, et al. Preliminary experience with interactive guided brain biopsies using a vertically opened 0.5-T MR system. Eur Radiol. 1999;9(2):230–6.
14. Li C, Wu L, Song J, et al. MR imaging-guided cryoablation of metastatic brain tumours: initial experience in six patients. Eur Radiol. 2010;20(2):404–9.
15. Sequeiros RB, Reinikainen H, Sequeiros AM, et al. MR-guided breast biopsy and hook wire marking using a low-field (0.23 T) scanner with optical instrument tracking. Eur Radiol. 2007;17(3):813–9.
16. Duerk JL, Butts K, Hwang KP, et al. Pulse sequences for interventional magnetic resonance imaging. Top Magn Reson Imaging. 2000;11(3):147–62.
17. Stranjalis G, Protopapa D, Sakas DE, et al. Stereotactic biopsy in the era of advanced neuroimaging. Does the minimal therapeutic gain justify its current wide use? Minim Invasive Neurosurg. 2003;46(2):90–3.
18. Boviatsis EJ, Kouyialis AT, Stranjalis G, et al. CT-guided stereotactic aspiration of brain abscesses. Neurosurg Rev. 2003;26(3):206–9.
19. Hsieh PC, Pan HC, Chung WY, et al. Computerized tomography-guided stereotactic aspiration of brain abscesses: experience with 28 cases. Zhonghua Yi Xue Za Zhi (Taipei). 1999;62(6):341–9.
20. Bernays RL, Kollias SS, Yonekawa Y. Dynamic changes during evacuation of a left temporal abscess in open MRI: technical case report. Neuroradiology. 2002;44(5):438–42.
21. Strowitzki M, Schwerdtfeger K, Steudel W. Ultrasound-guided aspiration of brain abscesses through a single burr hole. Minim Invas Neurosur. 2001;44(3):135–40.
22. Lee SH, Tomlinson C, Temple M, et al. Imaging-guided percutaneous needle aspiration or catheter drainage of neonatal liver abscesses: 14-year experience. Am J Roentgenol. 2008;190(3):616–22.
23. Savitz MH. CT-guided needle procedures for brain lesions: 20 years' experience. Mt Sinai J Med. 2000;67(4):318–21.
24. Mehendiratta V, Mccarty BC, Gomez L, et al. Computerized tomography (CT)-guided aspiration of abscesses: outcome of therapy at a tertiary care hospital. J Infect. 2007;54(2):122–8.
25. Tyler D, Mandybur G. Interventional MRI-guided stereotactic aspiration of acute/subacute intracerebral hematomas. Stereotact Funct Neurosurg. 1999;72(204):129–35.
26. Kollias SS, Bernays RL. Interactive magnetic resonance imaging-guided management of intracranial cystic lesions by using an open magnetic resonance imaging system. J Neurosurg. 2001;95(1):15–23.
27. Unal O, Sakarya ME, Kiymaz N, et al. Brain abscess drainage by use of MR fluoroscopic guidance. AJNR Am J Neuroradiol. 2005;26(4):839–42.
28. Wu L, Li C, Chen L, et al. Magnetic resonance imaging guided bone biopsies in the iPath-200 system. Chin Med J. 2003;116:937–40.
29. Cavuşoglu H, Kaya RA, Türkmenoglu ON, et al. Brain abscess: analysis of results in a series of 51 patients with a combined surgical and medical approach during an 11-year period. Neurosurgl focus. 2008;24(6):E9.

30. Balmer B, Bernays RL, Kollias SS, et al. Interventional MR-guided neuroendoscopy: A new therapeutic option for children. J Pediatr Surg. 2002;37(4):668–72.
31. Blanco RT, Ojala R, Kariniemi J, et al. Interventional and intra-operative MRI at low field scanner – a review. Eur J Radiol. 2005;56(2):130–42.
32. Kariniemi J, Sequeiros RB, Ojala R, et al. MRI-guided percutaneous nephrostomy: a feasibility study. Eur Radiol. 2009;19(5):1296–301.
33. Moche M, Trampel R, Kahn T, Busse H. Navigation concepts for MR image-guided interventions. J Magn Reson Imaging. 2008;27(2):276–91.

Imaging Pattern-Based Diagnostic Algorithm

5

Ke Ding, Jiali Wang, Hui Dai, Zhiming Xiang, and Chi S. Zee

5.1 Overview of Imaging Pattern-Based Diagnostic Algorithm

It is called radiomics today [1]. As a new research field, radiomics apply a large number of automated data characteristic algorithms in the region of interest of the image data and transformed them to exploring the characteristics of spatial data with high resolution. Data analysis is a quantitative and high-throughput analysis of a large number of image data, and high-fidelity target information is used to evaluate the various phenotypes of the disease, including the morphological, molecular, gene, and other levels [2]. Therefore, medical image processing can be extremely important. In order to achieve this goal, people study the relation to medical image algorithm, the algorithm of structure constructing model and data structure of the software system, database, integration algorithm and other aspects of the platform has been developing rapidly. And, it is widely used in clinical medicine and other areas.

K. Ding (✉)
Department of Radiology, Third Affiliated Hospital of Guangxi Medical University, Nanning, China

J. Wang
Department of Radiology, Affiliated Hospital of Xuzhou Medical University, Xuzhou, China

H. Dai
Department of Radiology, First Affiliated Hospital of Soochow University, Suzhou, China

Z. Xiang
Department of Radiology, Guangzhou Panyu Center Hospital, Guangzhou, China

C. S. Zee
Department of Radiology, Keck School of Medicine, University of Southern California, Los Angeles, CA, USA

At present, 3D visualization technology and image matching algorithm have been an important research direction of computer image processing in recent years. The 3D visualization algorithm can be divided into two categories: surface rendering and volume rendering.

Surface rendering is the geometric primitives which are reconstructed from the original 3D medical image data, and then it was used to illumination calculated and drawn by the techniques of the realistic graphics. In the 1970s of the last century, there have been studies on the surface rendering. Until Herman successfully proposed a Cuberille algorithm in 1979, surface rendering began to gain its popularity [3]. Over the years, the results of surface rendering have evolved into a new field in recent years: digital geometry processing. The application of digital geometry processing technology can deal with surface rendering effectively.

Volume rendering does not need to extract the intermediate geometric primitives, but mapped the original three-dimensional medical image data directly to the two-dimensional projection plane according to the transmission equation of light to produce the final rendering results [4]. The study on volume rendering appeared in the end of the last century of the 1980s. The traditional algorithm can be divided into three categories: image space of rendering algorithm, object space of rendering algorithm, and image and object space mixed of rendering algorithm (hybrid). Though the hardware volume rendering algorithm has many advantages, it is restricted by many factors, and one of the biggest problems is the limited texture memory capacity, for a particularly large three-dimensional data sets, which cannot be loaded into the texture memory for processing; another one is the calculation accuracy. Because the graphics rendering engine is generally used in the fixed-point operation, the final accuracy will be affected. But with the updated graphics, the problem of calculation accuracy will certainly be solved [5].

In addition to the research of medical algorithm, the construction of medical image algorithm platform is also an important part of the development of medical image

B. Gao et al. (eds.), *Imaging of CNS Infections and Neuroimmunology*, https://doi.org/10.1007/978-981-13-6904-9_5

algorithm. In order to avoid duplication of labor and facilitate for the field of peers, some research organizations have developed a number of Algorithms Toolkit. There are two algorithm platforms in the most authoritative areas which are VTK and ITK. VTK and ITK provide convenience for researchers in the field, but both of them still have flaws. First of all, VTK is a development platform for general visualization and is not specifically for the medical field. The scale of VTK is quite huge, and there are many algorithms inside, so it is widely used. Researchers in different fields use it. But on the other hand, its complexity increased greatly. Secondly, although ITK is developed for the field of medical imaging, it is designed by many modern C++ language features, so there are some compilers that cannot be compiled by ITK fully [6].

In summary, the birth of radiomics is a product of rapid development of big data technology and the medical image-aided diagnosis technology and integration. The emergence of medical image changes the traditional image into the data, so that people can explore all kinds of hidden, unknown information. It has an important influence on the development of medical imaging.

5.2 Imaging Pattern-Based Diagnostic Algorithm in CNS Infections

It's a huge challenge for neuroradiologists to make an accurate diagnosis of central nervous system (CNS) infections, not only because of the large extensive types and series of CNS infections themselves but also the likelihood for confusion of tumors and infections for resemblance in imaging performances. As we know, conventional computed tomography (CT) and magnetic resonance (MR) imaging are most frequently used in obtaining structural cross-sectional images to basically provide anatomic information. MR has a great superiority to demonstrate the features and details of the abnormal imaging changes pertained to CNS infection, especially minor details, in spite of less sensitivity in calcification detection.

Nowadays, most of CNS infections are potentially treatable, with the availability of excellent antimicrobials and the development of new treatment strategies [7, 8]. Early recognition and diagnosis, facilitating early treatment and then minimizing the long-term complications of the disease and its treatment, is an urgent and necessary task. To access an accurate diagnosis, the radiologists should consider clinical history, symptoms, laboratory findings, and sometimes even pathological results. MR is the most useful and indispensable way and a noninvasive imaging modality to discern CNS infections. With advanced molecular and functional sequences of MR, an abundance of information was available from the images, which are useful in diagnosis of CNS infections. Therefore, imaging plays an important role in CNS infections.

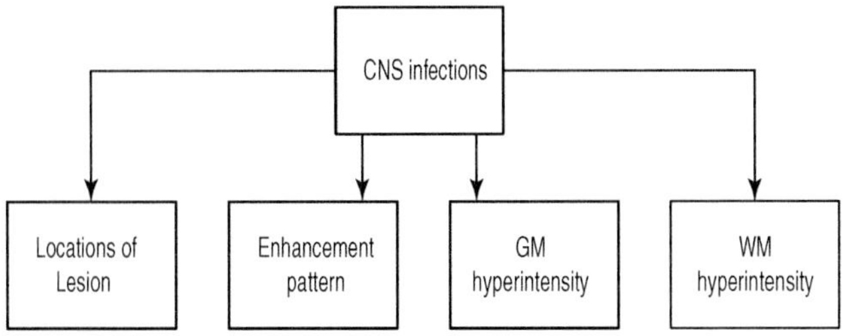

Fig. 5.1 Four components of contents

Generally, there are some diagnostic rules formed and repetitively trained in the image analysis, such as looking for image asymmetry, incorporating a structured report to reduce errors of omission, and so on. However, in this chapter, we will concentrate on how to apply imaging pattern-based diagnostic algorithm in CNS infections. Imaging modality contains basic MR sequences (T1, T2, and enhancement pattern with gadolinium) and more advanced molecular and functional sequences (diffusion-weighted imaging (DWI), perfusion-weighted imaging (PWI), susceptibility-weighted imaging (SWI), and MR spectroscopy (MRS)). A patterned approach, based on T1, T2, and contrast enhancement characteristics, will be elucidated by a classification in the following categories (locations of the lesion, enhancement pattern, gray matter (GM) hyperintensities, and white matter (WM) hyperintensities) (Fig. 5.1), to guide the radiologists narrowing the list of differentials when faced with a diagnostic challenge.

5.2.1 Location of the Lesion

As a neuroradiologist, the anatomy of brain and skull is an essential knowledge that one must master. Each radiologist may have different analytic/interpretive skills, but each diagnosis should refer a precise anatomic location to an abnormality. Some differential diagnostic clues can be added, by reporting the location of the lesions, combined with morphologic changes (will be discussed in the following couple of sections).

To be easily available, we list the common locations for some types of CNS infections (pyogenic infections, viral infections, granulomatous infections, and parasitic infections) in the table (common infections of neonates are not included) (Table 5.1).

Table 5.1 The infection type and common anatomical locations

Infection type	Locations
Pyogenic	*Infratentorial and/or supratentorial infections*
Meningitis	Leptomeningeal and dural
Subdural/epidural empyema	Subdural/epidural
Cerebritis/abscess	Gray-white junction, anywhere but most common in frontal lobes
Viral	*Infratentorial and/or supratentorial infections*
Meningitis	Leptomeningeal and dural
Encephalitis	
Herpes simplex encephalitis (HSE) (type 1)	Neurons and glial cells in the limbic system with involvement of the temporal lobes, orbital frontal gyri, insular cortex, and cingulate gyrus, with the tendency to spare the putamen; bilateral involvement
Creutzfeldt-Jakob disease (CJD)	Cerebral cortex, basal ganglia
Poliomyelitis viral encephalitis	Motor cortex, cerebellum, and spinal motor neurons
Rabies viral encephalitis	GM of the brain and spinal cord (neurons and to a lesser degree oligodendrocytes)
Arboviruses St. Louis encephalitis	Substantia nigra
John Cunningham viral encephalitis	Oligodendrocytes
West Nile viral encephalitis	Deep thalamic regions
Japanese encephalitis (JE)	Basal ganglia, brain stem, cerebellum, and cortical areas
HIV encephalitis	Cerebral atrophy, WM lesions
Rhombencephalitis	Brain stem and cerebellum
Noninfectious encephalitis	
Acute disseminated encephalomyelitis (ADEM)	Posterior fossa and the cerebral hemispheres (subcortical and deep WM)
Rasmussen's encephalitis	Ipsilateral hemisphere with progressive hemispheric atrophy
Granulomatous	*Meningeal (more commonly basal) or parenchymal (infratentorial and/or supratentorial)*
Tuberculosis	Basal meninges
Sarcoid	Basilar cisterns (dural/leptomeningeal and vascular involvement); brain parenchyma; cranial nerve
Fungal	Basal ganglia and deep WM
Single yeast cell form	Leptomeningitis or granuloma formation
Hyphal forms	Brain parenchyma
Large mycelia forms	Vasculitis, leading to septic infarction and mycotic aneurysms
Parasitic	*More commonly supratentorial than infratentorial*
Cysticercosis	Parenchymal (near the cortex and in the basal ganglia), leptomeningeal (subarachnoid/basal cistern), or intraventricular (fourth ventricle; attached to the ventricular wall or free floating)
Cerebral schistosomiasis	Cortical or subcortical

5.2.2 Contrast Enhancement Patterns

Meningitis-Leptomeningeal Enhancement

Enhancement patterns combined with the location of the lesion, meningitis, and subdural/epidural empyema are easily discerned. There are two patterns of meningeal enhancement: leptomeningeal (seen as a thin layer of continuous enhancement along the surface of the brain, which extends into the depths of the sulci) and dural (thicker and follows the inner margin of the calvarium). Leptomeningeal enhancement pattern is more common in inflammatory disease, while dural enhancement is more common in neoplastic disease (especially when meningeal nodular enhancement exists). T2-weighted fluid-attenuated inversion recovery (FLAIR) images may demonstrate hyperintense signal within the cerebral sulci as inflammatory exudates change the inversion time of cerebrospinal fluid. Post-contrast T1-weighted imaging may be more sensitive than FLAIR to demonstrate leptomeningeal enhancement [9]. Contrast-enhanced FLAIR images may further increase the diagnostic capability. However, abnormal contrast enhancement on MRI has been reported to occur in only 55–70% of patients with clinically proven infectious meningitis [10].

Subdural/Epidural Empyema-Rim Enhancement

Subdural/epidural empyema presents as extracerebral collections of fluid. It may be related to an extradural infection (including mastoiditis, sinusitis, and otitis media), penetrating trauma or surgery which has breached the dura, or may be secondary to leptomeningitis with spread to the subdural space through arachnoid villi or bridging veins. The typical appearance on imaging is of a crescent-shaped collection with rim enhancement and internal restricted diffusion. DWI is used to discriminate between a sterile effusion and an empyema. However, as to differentiate between subdural/epidural empyema and hematoma, DWI works less effective than conventional MRI [11].

Parenchymal Infections: Ranging from Non-enhancement to Well-Defined Rim Enhancement

Early cerebritis is characterized by localized vasogenic edema (hyperintense signal on T2-weighted and FLAIR images) and mass effect without enhancement, which is ill-defined. In late cerebritis, there are patchy, irregular enhancement will be obiquefactive necrosis that develops a peripheral collagen capsule. This is the early abscess capsule stage served. With continued progression of the disease, the process becomes more localized with an area of land, and then it evolves and becomes more mature abscess with time, and it appears as a fluid-filled cavity (hypointense signal on precontrast T1-weighted images and hyperintense signal on T2-weighted and FLAIR images) with well-defined rim enhancement. Part of parenchymal infections may present with nodular enhancement. The presence of contrast enhancement (representing disruption of the blood-brain barrier) is easily determined by visual inspection of MR images. In this section, as demonstrated above, we use conventional MRI with gadolinium to differentiate the types of infection by location and enhancement pattern, decide the stages of inflammatory disease, and discriminate inflammatory disease from neoplasms (Fig. 5.2).

5.2.3 Functional MRI on Ringlike Enhancing Lesions

Rim enhancement is a very common finding in CNS imaging. There must be a very long list of differentials ranging from infectious processes to high-grade necrotic neoplasms. It's pretty important to differentiate the rim enhancement lesions. Abscesses are usually associated with a thin smooth rim, in contrast to the nodular irregular rim seen in glioblastoma multiforme. Abscesses are commonly associated with satellite lesions, unlike necrotic neoplasm [12].

Advanced molecular and functional MRI, including DWI, PWI, SWI, and MRS, plays a key role in the differentiation of brain abscesses from mass lesions. In a meta-analysis, it is proved that DWI has a high sensitivity and specificity for the differentiation of brain abscess from other intracranial cystic mass lesions [13]. Some researchers found that PWI and DWI can serve as useful tools to differentiate abscess from glioblastoma and metastasis. High relative cerebral blood volume (rCBV) values in the peripheral areas, high incidence of hyperintense fractional anisotropy rim, and high ADC values within the core appear to indicate the possibility of a necrotic tumor; otherwise, they tend to indicate an abscess [14, 15]. Additionally, some researchers suggested a role for SWI in this differentiation. They found that a more complete and smooth hypointense rim showed on SWI an abscess compared with incomplete irregular rims seen in necrotic neoplasm [16]. As to MRS, amino acids are sensitive markers of pyogenic abscess, which can differentiate intracranial bacterial abscesses from cystic brain tumors [17]. Choline was seen in neoplasms and in tuberculomas, but not in the abscesses [18]. One study obtained the discriminatory boundary for the Cho/Cr ratio between inflammatory lesions and tumors which was 1.97, and for the NAA/Cr ratio, it was 1.12 based on the receiver operating characteristic (ROC) curve [19].

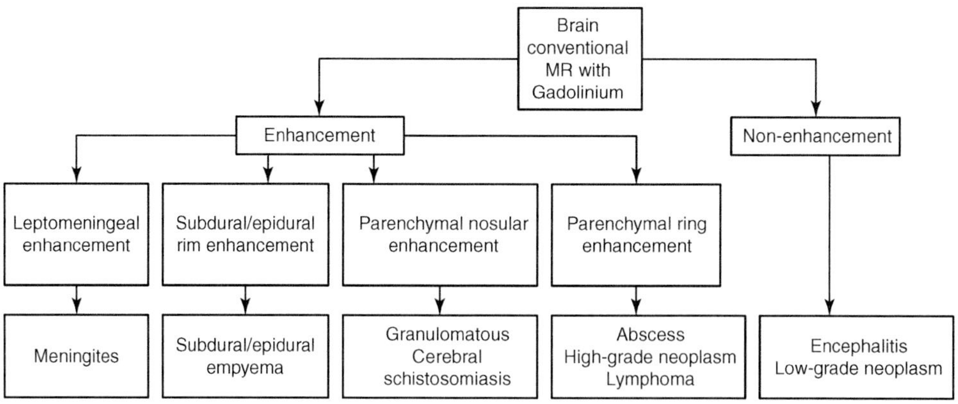

Fig. 5.2 The first step: conventional MRI with contrast medium in diagnosis and differentiation of CNS infections

Fig. 5.3 Flowchart for differentiation of abscess etiology

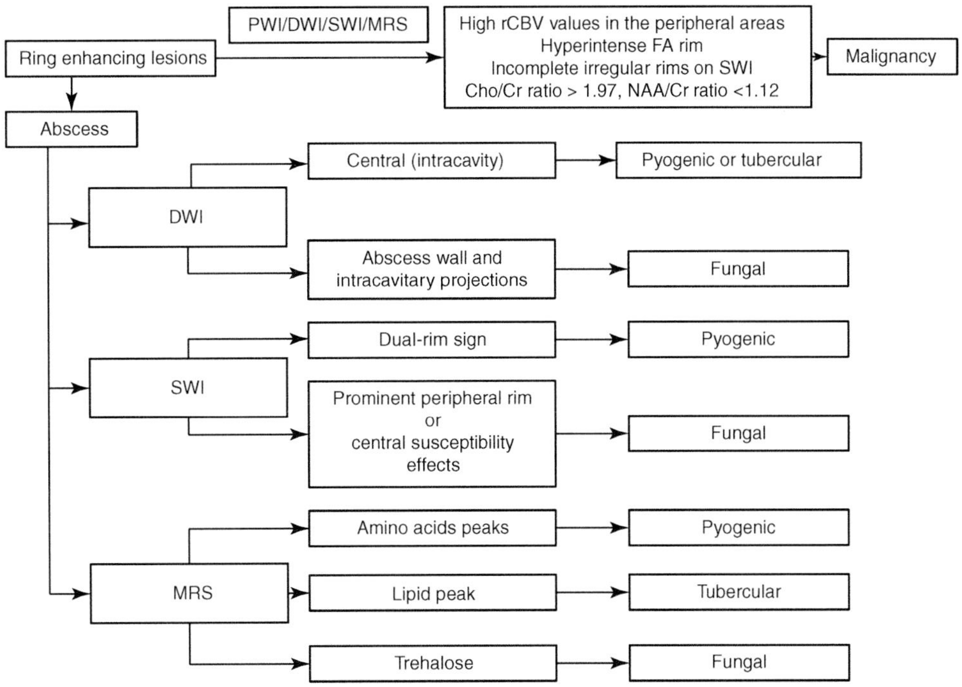

In the following sections, we will concentrate on differentiation for possible etiological cause (pyogenic, tubercular, or fungal) of abscess after ruling out the malignant lesions, as shown in Fig. 5.3, which may help to make early choice of targeted therapy.

DWI

The restricted diffusion brain regions are hyperintense on DWI, and the corresponding areas are hypointense on ADC maps. Bacterial abscesses generally present a low ADC (central diffusion restriction) due to intact inflammatory cells and bacteria that impede the microscopic motion of water molecules. Tubercular abscesses presenting with central low ADC as bacterial abscesses, ascribed to highly viscous necrotic tissue. Fungal abscesses showed restricted diffusion in the intracavitary projections and wall of the fungal abscess, but there is no restricted diffusion in the rest of the central part of the abscess [20].

SWI

SWI provides important additional information about a number of brain disorders, as well as intracranial hemorrhage, vascular malformations, amyloid angiopathy, traumatic brain injury, cerebral tumors, infections, and neurodegenerative disorders. In pyogenic abscesses, there is a specific feature of dual-rim sign shown on SWI, whereas in fungal abscesses, no dual-rim sign is present, but a prominent peripheral rim or central susceptibility effects on SWI will be seen [21].

MRS

Pyogenic brain abscesses contain large amounts of neutrophils and proteins in the viscous necrotic cavity. The neutrophils keep breakdown leading to plentiful releasement of proteolytic enzymes that hydrolyze the proteins into amino acids at 0.9 parts per million (ppm) which representing valine, leucine, and isoleucine [20]. The central necrotic area of pyogenic abscesses typically shows peaks of lipids (0.8–1.2 ppm), lactate (1.3 ppm), amino acids (0.9 ppm), succinate (2.4 ppm), and acetate (1.9 ppm). Acetate and succinate are seen only in pyogenic abscesses.

MRS feature of tubercular abscess is the lipids peaks at 0.9, 1.3, 2.0, and 2.8 ppm, without any other peak. Fungal abscesses show peaks of lipids, lactate, and amino acids, which are similar to pyogenic abscesses [22], and the special spectrum is the multiple signals between 3.6 and 3.8 ppm, assigned to the disaccharide trehalose which is present in the fungal wall [20]. In a recent study, some researchers applied multimodal (compared proton MRS with conventional culture and molecular methods (16S rRNA PCR and sequencing) to identify the microorganisms (aerobic and anaerobic) in the abscesses [23].

5.2.4 GM Hyperintensity

The most common causes of aseptic CNS infections are viruses [24], and HSE is the most common cause of infectious

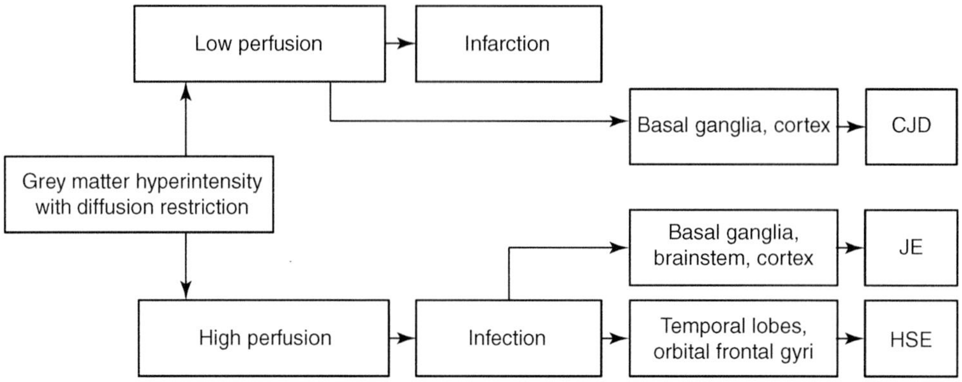

Fig. 5.4 Perfusion patterns in differentiation of GM hyperintense lesions with diffusion restriction

encephalitis [25]. GM hyperintensity on T2/FLAIR images is commonly seen in encephalitis, pertaining to cytotoxic and/or vasogenic edema. It is usually demonstrated as hyperintensity of corresponding areas on diffusion-weighted images. Some other lesions, like acute stroke, traumatic brain lesions, postoperative brain along the postsurgical bed, CJD and JE, demonstrating diffusion restriction should be further differentiated. Traumatic brain lesions and postoperative brain along the postsurgical bed are easily differentiated by clinical history. As for the rest, perfusion imaging patterns can be used in the differentiation, as shown in Fig. 5.4.

Reduced cerebral blood flow was found in CJD in an arterial spin labeling (ASL)-MRI study; ASL-MRI showed severe hypoperfusion in the cerebral cortex, basal ganglia, and thalami [26]. Low perfusion was shown in acute infarction. ASL study showed that HSV infection had a high perfusion on ASL-MRI. It is not easy to distinguish acute encephalitis such as HSE and JE on the clinical presentation because they are non-specific. Sometimes, even there is an overlap of imaging pattern among them on routine MRI sequences. Basal ganglia are the typical site involved in JE, which were not typically involved in HSE. The medial temporal is a typical site for the involvement of HSE [27].

5.2.5 WM Hyperintensity

CNS infections that involved WM, presenting with WM hyperintensity, mainly include acute disseminated encephalomyelitis (ADEM) [28], progressive multifocal leukoencephalopathy (PML) [29], HIV, and Rasmussen's encephalitis. Pattern recognition of MRI findings for Rasmussen's encephalitis, and the changes in serial MRI, might serve as a surrogate marker of the disease, namely, unihemispheric progressive focal cortical atrophy and signal changes predominantly in the perisylvian distribution and caudate followed by putamen involvement. This might assist in understanding and monitoring of the disease progression [30].

Most of WM hyperintensity lesions are immuno-relevant diseases. ADEM is an immune-mediated inflammatory demyelinating condition, and HIV is an acquired immune deficiency syndrome (AIDS). PML predominantly occurs in AIDS patients with impaired cell-mediated immune response. These diseases will be elucidated in the next section of autoimmune encephalitis.

5.3 Imaging Pattern-Based Diagnostic Algorithm in Neuroimmunology

Neuroimmunology is a scientific discipline that seeks to understand the importance of communication between the central nervous system (CNS) and immune system in both health and disease. Traditionally, the CNS was viewed as an immune-privileged site, since neurons are separated from the blood vessels by a physical barrier, the blood-brain barrier (BBB), which exerts both protective and homeostatic functions [31]. This statement set a clear separation between the nervous and immune systems. However, quite recently the concept of the brain as an immune-privileged site has been challenged by the following findings: (1) the regular passage of T and B lymphocytes through the BBB, (2) the existence of an extended lymph drainage of the CNS, and (3) the identification of the cerebrospinal space as an immunological compartment. Decades of researches have investigated the interaction between innate immunity and the CNS under conditions such as the immune response in infectious, autoimmune-mediated, ischemic, degenerative, traumatic, and neoplastic diseases of the nervous system [32] (Table 5.2).

Neuroimaging offers a wide array of non- or minimally invasive techniques to characterize neuroimmune processes. Imaging equipments are widely accessible, and the technologies afford a broad capability for different biological processes.

Table 5.2 Topics of classical neuroimmunology

Neuroinfections	Autoimmune diseases	Other diseases with accompanying immune reactions
Encephalitis, encephalomyelitis, meningitis, polyradiculitis, or polyneuritis caused by bacteria such as *Borrelia burgdorferi*, *Clostridium tetani*, *Clostridium botulinum*, and *Treponema pallidum* and various coccoid and rod bacteria,; viruses such as HIV, rabies, herpes, measles, mumps, coxsackie, JC, RS, and polio virus; prions and protozoa such as *Toxoplasma gondii*, *Trypanosoma brucei*, and plasmodia	Multiple sclerosis, acute demyelinating encephalomyelitis (ADEM), Guillain-Barré-Strohl syndrome, chronic immune-related demyelinating polyradiculoneuropathy (CIDP), myasthenia gravis pseudoparalytica, Lambert-Eaton myasthenic syndrome, dermatomyositis, polymyositis, inclusion body myositis, vasculitides, and collagenoses	Neurodegenerative diseases such as Parkinson's disease, Alzheimer's disease, Huntington's disease, and Lou Gehrig's disease (amyotrophic lateral sclerosis); cerebrovascular diseases such as stroke and intracerebral hemorrhage; neoplastic diseases such as primary brain tumors, leukemias, and lymphomas; paraneoplastic syndromes; traumata such as spinal cord injury; and psychic diseases such as schizophrenia, major depressive disorder, epilepsy, and narcolepsy

5.3.1 Multiple Sclerosis

Multiple sclerosis (MS) is the most frequent inflammatory demyelinating disease of the CNS, with a variety of neurological symptoms due to the distribution of time and space. There are four main morphologic features, demyelination, inflammation, axonal damage, and gliosis, while neuroinflammation and neurodegeneration are the two common components of its pathogenesis. MR imaging and PET are the common tools used for the diagnosis prognostic evaluation and treatment efficacy of MS. We focus on the MR imaging for the two reasons: firstly, MR imaging has a critical role in monitoring clinical course, and PET could only offer complementary support and, secondly, the costs of cyclotrons and radiochemical laboratories in the examination of PET are too high.

Brain MRI should be performed at a minimum magnetic field strength of 1.5T, while 3T MRI is recommended, since 3T MRI shows increased sensitivity to focal MS lesion due to better signal-to-noise ratio and image resolution. What's more, ultrahigh-field MR imaging (7T) has shown the presence of previously unseen small focal white matter lesions [33]. On MRI, MS plaques are commonly seen as multiple focal lesions with intermediate- to low-signal intensity on T1-weighted images (T1WI) and high-signal intensity on T2-weighted images (T2WI) and FLAIR images. T2WI (turbo/fast) spin echo sequences show higher detection rates in the posterior fossa, while FLAIR shows a higher lesion load in the periventricular white matter because of CSF attenuation. Gradient echo three-dimensional (3D) FLAIR is a recently developed sequence that has shown improved sensitivity in detecting white matter demyelinating plaques [34].

For the distinction between acute and chronic lesions, post-gadolinium T1-weighted imaging was allowed. Enhancement of lesions on post-contrast T1-weighted imaging is more often associated with subacute inflammation and increased BBB permeability. Contrast enhancement typically persists for 3 to 4 weeks on average. Enhancement patterns are variable but can be classified as nodular, punctate, or ringlike. Some lesions show an incomplete ring pattern, which may be helpful in discriminating a demyelinating lesion from the abscess or neoplasm.

Diffusion tensor imaging (DTI) may serve to evaluate the structural integrity of white matter and can also be used for tractography [35]. Three measures that can be derived from DTI are mean diffusivity (MD), apparent diffusion coefficient (ADC), and fractional anisotropy (FA). The overall diffusion of water molecules can be measured irrespective of the direction of motion, yielding maps of both MD and apparent ADC. FA is a measure of the nonrandomness of water diffusion in a particular region. Increases in MD and decreases in FA correlate with demyelination and axonal loss in patients with MS, and a multicenter validation study indicated that FA is the most comparable DTI measure across centers and supports its use in multicenter clinical trials.

Magnetic resonance spectroscopy (MRS) detects metabolites in the neural tissues. Alterations in various metabolites have been shown, including N-acetyl aspartate (NAA), choline, creatine, myoinositol, glutamate, and lactate [36]. In active enhancing MS white matter lesions, increases of choline, myoinositol, lactate, and glutamate and decreases of NAA have been identified. In non-enhancing MS lesions, NAA is markedly reduced, myoinositol remains increased, and glutamate levels are often normal. In chronic plaques, the further reductions in NAA are consistent with progression of neuronal loss.

Vascular inflammation plays an important role in the pathogenesis of MS. Various MR perfusion techniques have shown increased cerebral perfusion associated with acute enhancing MS plaques, while non-enhancing white matter plaques can show either increased or decreased perfusion, which suggests heterogeneity in the underlying pathophysiology of these lesions.

Spinal cord imaging should be performed routinely in the diagnostic workup of patients with suspected demyelination, and the clinical relevance of spinal cord imaging in the (differential) diagnosis of MS has conclusively been demonstrated. Spinal cord abnormalities are described in more than 80% of MS patients, with a proclivity for the cervical cord [37]. Due to the small tissue volume and the presence of artifacts caused by cerebrospinal fluid (CSF) flow and blood vessel pulsation, the acquisition of spinal cord images is more challenging in contrast to brain MRI. The value of contrast administration in spinal cord MRI is still under discussion, since only a small fraction of spinal cord lesions show contrast enhancement.

PET is a noninvasive, quantitative imaging technique that enables molecular and neuroreceptor imaging in vivo and can even provide functional information of molecular biology ahead of morphologic changes. There are various possible radioligands, such as choline tracers, glucose metabolism, γ-aminobutyric acid tracers, can be used as targets with high selectivity in PET imaging. Imaging of different PET tracers could enable better understanding of the pathologic MS processes (inflammation, neuronal damage, demyelination, or astrocyte activation) they stand for. 2′-[^{18}F]Fluoro-2′-deoxyglucose (^{18}F-FDG) PET has been applied as a marker for inflammation; in the activated inflammatory cells, there is higher uptake of ^{18}F-FDG, and the regions with ongoing inflammation can be discovered. This can also be used to differentiate acute (hypermetabolism) lesion from chronic (hypometabolism) lesion based on local glucose metabolism. However, the normal brain physiologic glucose high consumption always weakens the ability of finding small active lesions [38]. Translocator protein (TSPO) is an 18 kDa protein located on the outer membrane of mitochondria and upregulated obviously in activated microglial cells. Microglial cells widely distribute in the active inflammatory rim of MS plaques; using this TSPO radiotracer might detect the lesions. TSPO radioligands can also monitor the progression and its severity, which is not overexpressed in resting microglia cells [39].

5.3.2 Acute Disseminated Encephalomyelitis

Acute disseminated encephalomyelitis (ADEM) is an immune-mediated acute disease resulting in multifocal demyelination both in the brain and spinal cord. ADEM can occur at any age but is particularly common in children and young adults. Its clinical course in most cases is monophasic, typically transitory and self-limiting, and always resulting from para- or postinfectious complications. The clinical course often begins within 2 days to 1 month after a viral infection or vaccination; initial symptoms include a rapid-onset encephalopathy (behavioral change or altered consciousness) and multifocal deficits. Compared to adults, children present better in the prognosis for recovery from ADEM [40].

MR imaging plays a crucial role both in diagnosis of ADEM and in differentiation from other mimics. The most typical ADEM lesions show T2WI/FLAIR hyperintense, distributing asymmetric bilaterally in the deep and juxtacortical white matter regions without involving the periventricular white matter. Lesions confined to the corpus callosum are less common compared to MS. Four patterns of cerebral involvement have been proposed to describe the MRI findings in ADEM [41]: (1) ADEM with small lesions (less than 5 mm); (2) ADEM with large, confluent, or tumefactive lesions, with extensive perilesional edema and mass effect; (3) ADEM with additional symmetric bithalamic involvement; and (4) acute hemorrhagic encephalomyelitis (AHEM), when some evidence of hemorrhage can be identified in the large demyelinating lesions.

Advanced neuroimaging techniques can capture more pathological characteristics of the demyelinating process. For example, during the acute stage of ADEM, the lesions show restricted diffusion using DWI or DTI; however, in the subacute stage, the lesions present free diffusion. Researches in children with ADEM using MRS have shown increase of lipids and reduction in myoinositol/creatine ratio during the acute phase, and during the chronic phase, there is a decrease in lipid peak and increase in myoinositol/creatine ratio [42].

Spinal cord lesions accompanied with brain lesions are more frequent. The pattern of spinal cord lesions are various; can be focal, multifocal, or longitudinally extensive; and are partially or completely involved in the transverse cord. Only a small fraction of lesions show enhancement on post-contrast T1WI, and the most common enhanced pattern is incomplete ringlike enhancement, while nodular and complete ring enhancement can also be shown occasionally.

5.3.3 Neuromyelitis Optica

According to the 2006 criteria with further modifications to the criteria in 2015, neuromyelitis optica (NMO) requires the presence of both optic neuritis (ON) and acute myelitis along with supportive criteria for diagnosis [43]. NMO spectrum disorder (NMOSD), which includes typical NMO, is a newly emerging disease spectrum with or without anti-aquaporin-4-autoantibody (anti-AQP4-Ab).

The clinical presentation varies with transverse myelitis as the first clinical manifestation in up to a third of the cases and optic neuritis as well in 10% of the cases; the time gap between spinal and visual symptoms varies from days to years. NMO has a female predominance (4:1) and a peak presentation in the fourth decade. The discovery of the presence of aquaporin-4 (AQP4) antibodies has confirmed NMO as a distinct entity separate from multiple sclerosis. MRI is a major tool in diagnosis and classification, and some MRI patterns are highly suggestive of NMO, distinct from classic MS patterns.

Spine Cord MR Imaging: The cervical cord is most commonly involved and extends to the lower medulla. Longitudinally extensive spinal cord lesion (LESCL) characterized by long-segment (≧3 vertebral lengths) cord swelling and hyperintensity involving a large (>50%) area of cross section of the cord is the most common and characteristic finding [44]. LESCLs in NMO are T2 hyperintense and frequently T1 hypointense. Linear or patchy enhancement can be seen in active phase. Cord atrophy is the prominent findings in chronic phase, reflecting the severity of tissue injury and a propensity for recurrent bouts of inflammatory activity.

Optic Nerve MR Imaging: Long-segment involvement of the optic nerve associated with acute swelling and enhancement, particularly when bilateral or extending posteriorly into the optic chiasm, should raise the suspicion of NMO [45]. Follow-up imaging may show persistent hyperintensity and/or atrophy of the nerves.

Conventional Brain MR Imaging: Majority of brain "typical" NMO lesions mirror the distribution of AQP4 around the ventricle and aqueduct involving the hypothalamus, thalamus, midbrain, brain stem, and long segments of the callosum and periventricular white matter. Brain lesions in NMO have a variable appearance but are often of heterogeneous signal intensity with blurred margins [46]. While most reported NMO brain lesions do not show gadolinium enhancement, cloud-like enhancement has been described as specific feature of NMO as compared to more well-defined enhancement seen in MS.

5.3.4 Autoimmune Encephalitis

Autoimmune encephalitis (AE) is considered as one of the most common causes of noninfectious acute encephalitis. According to the different location of the antigen, AE is classified into AE with anti-*N*-methyl-D-aspartate receptor antibodies (NMDAR-Abs), AE with anti-α-amino-3-hydroxy-5-methyl-4-isoxazolepropionic acid receptor antibodies (AMPAR-Abs), AE with anti-leucine-rich glioma-inactivated protein 1 antibodies (LGI1-Abs), AE with anti-contactin-associated protein-like 2 antibodies (CASPR2-Abs), and AE with other autoantibodies. Both male and female can suffer from AE without significant age priority. The most common symptom in patients with AE is seizures, and a variety of movement disorders are also very common.

At present, the existing diagnostic criteria for AE is mostly relying on antibody testing and response to immunotherapy, because the only characterization of autoantibodies is the biomarker of disease, so the diagnosis of AE is very difficult clinically. Neuroimaging findings are variable, and at an early stage of disease, brain MR imaging is often normal without anatomy change, and even in a subset of AE patients who suffer profound neuropsychiatric dysfunction, the neuroimaging finding is negative. Clinically, the intracerebral lesions often involve the limbic structures [47], usually showing hyperintense signal on both T2 and FLAIR sequences in the medial of temporal lobes, which is often asymmetric or unilateral. Limbic encephalitis is a rare paraneoplastic disorder most commonly associated with lung cancer. In addition, limbic encephalitis is characterized by rapid development of mood changes, confusion, and memory deficit.

^{18}F-FDG PET imaging has been reported to show hypermetabolism characteristically in medial temporal lobe in limbic encephalitis, even in MRI-negative or controversial cases [48]. ^{18}F-FDG PET may possess better sensitivity than MRI in the diagnosis of AE. So in the near future, brain MR imaging combined with ^{18}F-FDG PET/CT would provide both morphological and metabolic information resulting in the improvement of diagnostic accuracy.

References

1. Lambin P, Rios-Velazquez E, Leijenaar R, et al. Radiomics: extracting more information from medical images using advanced feature analysis. Eur J Cancer. 2012;48(4):441–6.
2. Gillies RJ, Kinahan PE, Hricak H. Radiomics: images are more than pictures, they are data. Radiology. 2016;278(2):563–77.
3. Herman GT, Liu HK. Three-dimensional display of human organs from computed tomograms. Comp Graph Image Process. 1979;9(1):1–21.
4. Ranjan S, Ibanez L, Wood B, et al. Segmentation of liver tumors using the insight segmentation and registration toolkit. Int Congr. 2004;1268:1316.
5. Austern MH. Generic programming and the STL: using and extending the C++ Standard Template Library. Beijing: China Electric Power Press; 2003.
6. Ibanez L, Schroeder WJ, Ng L, et al. The ITK software guide: the insight segmentation and registration toolkit. Comput Stat Data Anal. 2003;21:231–56.
7. Tan YC, Gill AK, Kim KS. Treatment strategies for central nervous system infections: an update. Expert Opin Pharmacother. 2015;16(2):187–203.
8. Yang F, Wen W, Qin W. Bispecific antibodies as a development platform for new concepts and treatment strategies. Int J Mol Sci. 2016;18(1):E48.
9. Kamran S, Bener AB, Alper D, Bakshi R. Role of fluid-attenuated inversion recovery in the diagnosis of meningitis: comparison with contrast-enhanced magnetic resonance imaging. J Comput Assist Tomogr. 2004;28(1):68–72.
10. Borden NM, Forseen SE. Pattern recognition neuroradiology. Cambridge: Cambridge University Press; 2011.
11. Tsuchiya K, Osawa A, Katase S, Fujikawa A, Hachiya J, Aoki S. Diffusion-weighted MRI of subdural and epidural empyemas. Neuroradiology. 2003;45(4):220–3.
12. Aiken AH. Central nervous system infection. Neuroimaging Clin N Am. 2010;20(4):557–80.

13. Xu XX, Li B, Yang HF, et al. Can diffusion-weighted imaging be used to differentiate brain abscess from other ring-enhancing brain lesions? A meta-analysis. Clin Radiol. 2014;69(9):909–15.
14. Muccio CF, Esposito G, Bartolini A, et al. Cerebral abscesses and necrotic cerebral tumours: differential diagnosis by perfusion-weighted magnetic resonance imaging. Radiol Med. 2008;113(5):747–57.
15. Toh CH, Wei KC, Ng SH, et al. Differentiation of brain abscesses from necrotic glioblastomas and cystic metastatic brain tumors with diffusion tensor imaging. AJNR Am J Neuroradiol. 2011;32(9):1646–51.
16. Toh CH, Wei KC, Chang CN, et al. Differentiation of pyogenic brain abscesses from necrotic glioblastomas with use of susceptibility-weighted imaging. AJNR Am J Neuroradiol. 2012;33(8):1534–8.
17. Hsu SH, Chou MC, Ko CW, et al. Proton MR spectroscopy in patients with pyogenic brain abscess: MR spectroscopic imaging versus single-voxel spectroscopy. Eur J Radiol. 2013;82(8):1299–307.
18. Mohan S, Verma A, Lim CC, et al. Lipid resonance on in vivo proton MR spectroscopy: value of other metabolites in differential diagnosis. Neuroradiol J. 2010;23(3):269–78.
19. Ferraz-Filho JR, Santana-Netto PV, Rocha-Filho JA, et al. Application of magnetic resonance spectroscopy in the differentiation of high-grade brain neoplasm and inflammatory brain lesions. Arq Neuropsiquiatr. 2009;67(2A):250–3.
20. Luthra G, Parihar A, Nath K, et al. Comparative evaluation of fungal, tubercular, and pyogenic brain abscesses with conventional and diffusion MR imaging and proton MR spectroscopy. AJNR Am J Neuroradiol. 2007;28(7):1332–8.
21. Antulov R, Dolic K, Fruehwald-Pallamar J, et al. Differentiation of pyogenic and fungal brain abscesses with susceptibility-weighted MR sequences. Neuroradiology. 2014;56(11):937–45.
22. Muccio CF, Caranci F, D'Arco F, et al. Magnetic resonance features of pyogenic brain abscesses and differential diagnosis using morphological and functional imaging studies: a pictorial essay. J Neuroradiol. 2014;41(3):153–67.
23. Bajpai A, Prasad KN, Mishra P, et al. Multimodal approach for diagnosis of bacterial etiology in brain abscess. Magn Reson Imaging. 2014;32(5):491–6.
24. Calleri G, Libanore V, Corcione S, et al. A retrospective study of viral central nervous system infections: relationship amongst aetiology, clinical course and outcome. Infection. 2017;45(2):227–31.
25. Bertrand A, Leclercq D, Martinez-Almoyna L, et al. MR imaging of adult acute infectious encephalitis. Med Mal Infect. 2017;47(3):195–205.
26. Chen S, Guan M, Shang JK, et al. Reduced cerebral blood flow in genetic prion disease with PRNP D178N-129M mutation: an arterial spin labeling MRI study. J Clin Neurosci. 2015;22(1):204–6.
27. Sawlani V. Diffusion-weighted imaging and apparent diffusion coefficient evaluation of herpes simplex encephalitis and Japanese encephalitis. J Neurol Sci. 2009;287(1–2):221–6.
28. Zuccoli G, Panigrahy A, Sreedher G, et al. Vasogenic edema characterizes pediatric acute disseminated encephalomyelitis. Neuroradiology. 2014;56(8):679–84.
29. Cuvinciuc V, Martin-Blondel G, Marchou B, et al. Proton MR spectroscopy of progressive multifocal leukoencephalopathy-immune reconstitution inflammatory syndrome. AJNR Am J Neuroradiol. 2010;31(8):E69–70.
30. Pradeep K, Sinha S, Saini J, et al. Evolution of MRI changes in Rasmussen's encephalitis. Acta Neurol Scand. 2014;130(4):253–9.
31. Selmi C, Barin JG, Rose NR. Current trends in autoimmunity and the nervous system. J Autoimmun. 2016;75:20–9. https://doi.org/10.1016/j.jaut.2016.08.005.
32. Mix E, Goertsches R, Zettl UK. Immunology and neurology. J Neurol. 2007;254:112–7. https://doi.org/10.1007/s00415-007-2002-9.
33. Wattjes MP, Steenwijk MD, Stangel M. MRI in the diagnosis and monitoring of multiple sclerosis: an update. Clin Neuroradiol. 2015;25(Suppl 2):157–65.
34. Aliaga ES, Barkhof F. MRI mimics of multiple sclerosis. Handb Clin Neurol. 2014;122(3rd):291–316.
35. Fox RJ, Sakaie K, Lee JC, et al. A validation study of multicenter diffusion tensor imaging: reliability of fractional anisotropy and diffusivity values. AJNR Am J Neuroradiol. 2012;33(4):695–700.
36. Klawiter EC. Current and new directions in MRI in multiple sclerosis. Continuum. 2013;19(19):1058–73.
37. Sudhakar SV, Muthusamy K, Mani S, et al. Imaging in pediatric demyelinating and inflammatory diseases of the brain—part 1. Indian J Pediatr. 2015;83(9):952–64. https://doi.org/10.1007/s12098-015-1916-y.
38. Faria DDP, Copray S, Buchpiguel C, et al. PET imaging in multiple sclerosis. J Neuroimmune Pharmacol. 2014;9(4):468–82.
39. Doorduin J, de Vries EF, Dierckx RA, et al. PET imaging of the peripheral benzodiazepine receptor: monitoring disease progression and therapy response in neurodegenerative disorders. Curr Pharm Des. 2008;14(31):3297–315.
40. Krupp LB, Tardieu M, Amato MP, et al. International pediatric multiple sclerosis study group criteria for pediatric multiple sclerosis and immune-mediated central nervous system demyelinating disorders: revisions to the 2007 definitions. Mult Scler. 2013;19(10):1261–7.
41. Tenembaum S, Chamoles N, Fejerman N. Acute disseminated encephalomyelitis: a long-term follow-up study of 84 pediatric patients. Neurology. 2002;59(8):1224–31.
42. Tenemaum SN. Acute disseminated encephalomyelitis. Handb Clin Neurol. 2014;122(3rd):1253–62.
43. Akaishi T, Nakashima I, Sato DK, et al. Neuromyelitis optica spectrum disorders. Neuroimag Clin N Am. 2017;27:251–65. https://doi.org/10.1016/j.nic.2016.12.010.1052-5149/17.
44. Sudhakar SV, Muthusamy K, Mani S, et al. Imaging in pediatric demyelinating and inflammatory diseases of brain—part 2. Indian J Pediatr. 2016;83(9):965–82. https://doi.org/10.1007/s12098-016-2052-z.
45. Barnett Y, Sutton IJ, Ghadiri M, et al. Conventional and advanced imaging in neuromyelitis optica. AJNR Am J Neuroradiol. 2014;35(8):1458–66.
46. Kim HJ, Paul F, Lanapeixoto MA, et al. MRI characteristics of neuromyelitis optica spectrum disorder an international update. Neurology. 2015;84(11):1165–73.
47. Kelley BP, Patel SC, Marin HL, et al. Autoimmune encephalitis: pathophysiology and imaging review of an overlooked diagnosis. AJNR Am J Neuroradiol. 2017;38(6):1070–8.
48. Morbelli S, Djekidel M, Hesse S, et al. Role of ^{18}F-FDG-PET imaging in the diagnosis of autoimmune encephalitis. Lancet Neurol. 2016;15(10):1009–10.

Part II

Infections of CNS

Emerging Infectious Diseases

6

Bo Gao

6.1 Introduction

During the last several years, some novel avian influenza A viruses or even recently reported Zika virus (ZIKV), for their fatal attack to CNS, have drawn great attentions all over the world [1–3]. Emerging infectious diseases (EIDs) are usually defined as diseases that have infected new hosts or have spread into new geographic area or have changed their pathogenic features or are caused by pathogenic agents not previously recognized. The outbreaks of these diseases frequently occur starting from viruses mutated from an animal host and obtained the ability of infecting humans [4]. Viruses may invade the brain or spinal cord, causing acute or chronic neurologic durations. Emerging infections affecting the CNS often present as encephalitis with substantial morbidity and mortality [5, 6]. Despite notable improvements in disease prevention and treatment, infectious diseases of the CNS remain an important source of morbidity and mortality, particularly in less-developed countries and in immunocompromised individuals [5, 6]. These emerging and challenging CNS infections are still increasing. The upcoming decades are sure to provide us with an ever-evolving landscape of infection. We are encountering more opportunities and facing more challenges in the future.

6.2 Emerging Viral Pathogens

The number of EIDs and their threat to global health are increasing. It is reported that over 100 viral pathogens can affect the nervous system [5, 6]. Neurological infections from EIDs are attributed to the particular sensitivity of the CNS to pathogens from dysregulated inflammatory responses [7]. Special attention was given to the neurological complications seen in many patients with Ebola virus disease, West Nile virus (WNV), Eastern equine encephalitis virus, and Zika virus (ZIKV) [8, 9]. The outbreak of swine influenza virus H1N1 began in early 2009, and radiology could assist in the early diagnosis of severe cases [1]. Middle East respiratory syndrome (MERS) is caused by the Middle East respiratory syndrome coronavirus (MERS-CoV), CT scans showing ground-glass opacities preferably in peripheral lower lobe [10]. Ebola infections in West Africa have been a major threat in the past 3 years, whereas radiology workup could not provide any specific diagnosis [11]. Since the outbreak of October 2015, about 1.5 million cases of Zika mosquito-borne virus and 4000 suspected cases of microcephaly with over 40 deaths have been reported [9]. The evidence of Zika virus infection of aborted fetuses associated with microcephaly has been confirmed. The imaging features of microcephaly secondary to Zika virus infection include calcifications, cortical abnormalities, diminution of white matter, large ventricles with or without hydrocephalus, cortical malformations, hypoplasia of the cerebellum and brain stem, and enlargement of the cerebellar cistern (Fig. 6.1). CT and US could show a consistent pattern of widespread brain calcifications (Fig. 6.2) [3]. Radiology plays a key role on the monitoring of patients with ZIKV infection [10, 11].

Combining with the clinical data and imaging findings, it is necessary to optimize the decision of treatment and ultimately improve patient outcomes. Preoperative imaging examination plays a critical role on planning the procedure and prognosis assessment in patients with CNS infection [8]. Early neurosurgical intervention is advocated to prevent the ongoing risk of fatal complications [12]. CT is probably useful in the specific patients with calcification and hemorrhage, typically in the acute stage or in the early stages of *Paragonimus* migration [13]. Routine MRI generally could show its great advantages over CT. Advanced MRI, such as MR spectroscopy (MRS) have provided a surrogate marker of tissue chemical components, thereby could differentiate parasitic infections from other infections and also possibly monitor therapeutic response.

B. Gao (✉)
Department of Radiology, Affiliated Hospital of Guizhou Medical University, Guiyang, Guizhou, China

B. Gao et al. (eds.), *Imaging of CNS Infections and Neuroimmunology*, https://doi.org/10.1007/978-981-13-6904-9_6

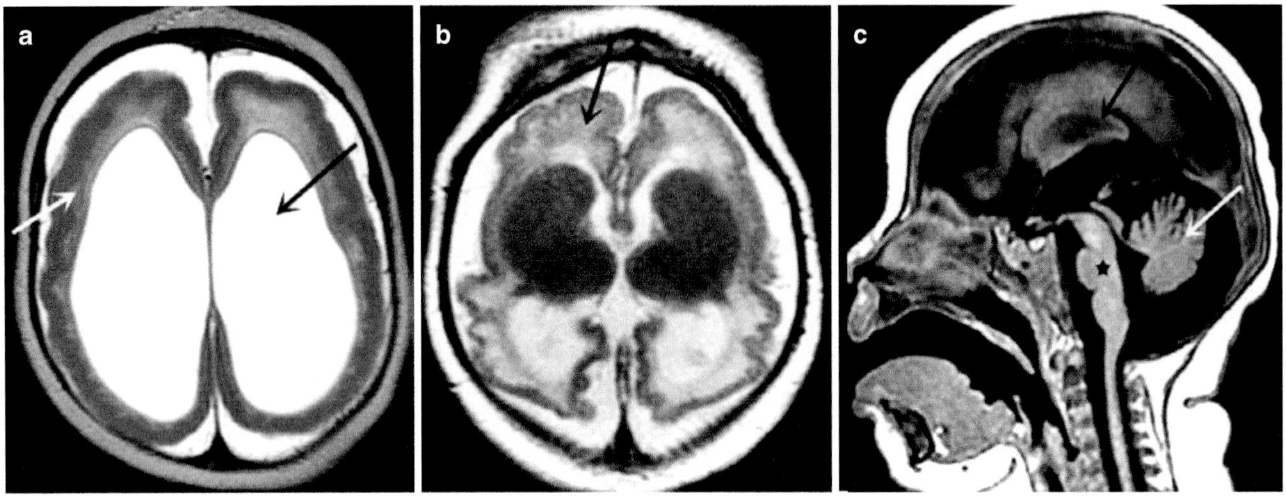

Fig. 6.1 (**a**) Axial T2-weighted MR image shows a thickened cortex (white arrow) and ventriculomegaly (black arrow). (**b**) Axial T2-weighted MR image shows cortical malformations (black arrow). (**c**) Sagittal T1-weighted MR image shows cerebellar atrophy (white arrow), corpus callosum abnormalities (black arrow), and brain stem dysplasia (black star) (Courtesy of Lara Brandão MD, Rio De Janeiro, Brasil)

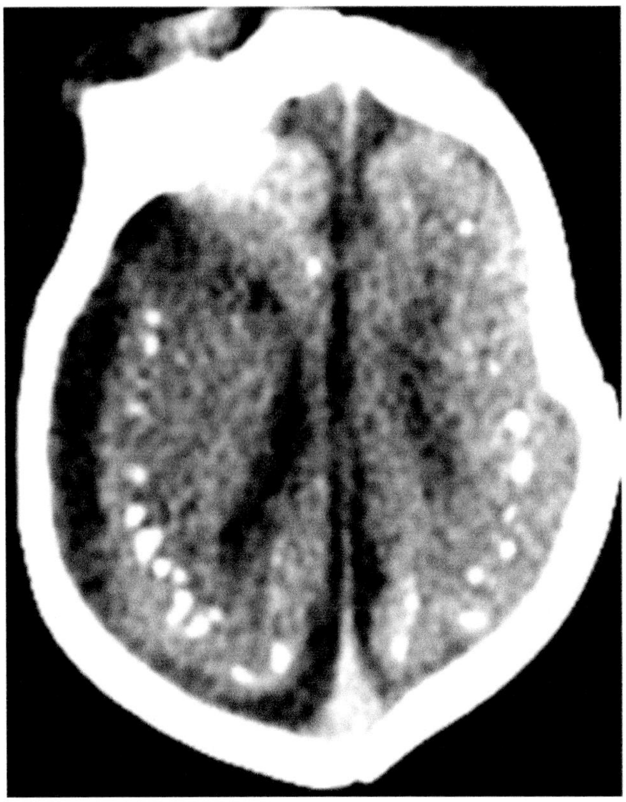

Fig. 6.2 Axial CT image shows diffuse calcifications in cortical/subcortical white matter junction and parenchymal atrophy (Courtesy of Lara Brandão MD, Rio De Janeiro, Brasil)

6.3 New Detecting Techniques and Diagnosing Strategies

It is essential to make early and accurate etiological diagnosis for patient's life and public healthcare. During the past 30 years, though the prevention of infections is by vaccine and antimicrobial agents, infections remain to be the major killer of permanent neurologic disability globally [14]. Diagnosis requires not only careful inquiring history but also applying newly developed diagnostic tests. It is still a major challenge to confirm the etiology of inflammatory disorders in the clinical setting, as over 50% cases would be undiagnosed [15]. Next-generation sequencing (NGS) is able to discover the transcriptome of host tissue and capture microbial genomes (i.e., bacteria, fungi, and viruses) that reside in the tissue niche. Deep sequencing of total DNA or RNA provides an unbiased approach that can detect even rare components of the microbiome [16]. Unbiased metagenomic next-generation sequencing (mNGS) represents a wholly different approach using random hexamer primers to amplify all the nucleic acids in a biological sample like cerebrospinal fluid or brain biopsy samples. Using bioinformatic pipelines, it also can analyze enormous sequencing data sets to identify the microbial source in samples promptly [17]. Moreover, diagnostic decision-making of viral CNS infections demands a global knowledge of epidemiology, including the foci and spread of arboviruses worldwide [18].

The global health and biodefense communities are focused on the threat of emerging pathogens, many of which have severe neurologic sequelae. With the globalization and time change, we would have to confront a changing landscape of neurological infections.

References

1. Ussel IV, Boer W, Parizel P, et al. Encephalitis related to a H1N1 vaccination: case report and review of the literature. Clin Neurol Neurosurg. 2014;124(9):8–15.
2. Gao R, Cao B, Hu Y, et al. Human infection with a novel avian-origin influenza A (H7N9) virus. N Engl J Med. 2013;368(20):1888–97.
3. Carod-Artal FJ. Epidemiology and neurological complications of infection by the Zika virus: a new emerging neurotropic virus. Rev Neurol. 2016;62(7):317–28.
4. Marošová L, Neradil P, Zilka N. How can viruses influence the neuroinflammation and neurodegeneration in the aged human brain. Acta Virol. 2013;57(3):273–81.
5. Tyler KL. Emerging viral infections of the central nervous system: part 1. Arch Neurol. 2009;66(8):939–48.
6. Tyler KL. Emerging viral infections of the central nervous system: part 2. Arch Neurol. 2009;66(9):1065–74.
7. Lyons J, McArthur J. Emerging infections of the central nervous system. Curr Infect Dis Rep. 2013;15(6):576–82.
8. Shih RY, Koeller KK. Bacterial, fungal, and parasitic infections of the central nervous system: radiologic-pathologic correlation and historical perspectives. Radiographics. 2015;35(4):1141–69.
9. de Oliveira WK, Carmo EH, Henriques CM, et al. Zika virus infection and associated neurologic disorders in Brazil. N Engl J Med. 2017;376(16):1591–3.
10. Das KM, Lee EY, Langer RD, et al. Middle east respiratory syndrome coronavirus: what does a radiologist need to know? AJR Am J Roentgenol. 2016;206(6):1193–201.
11. Bluemke DA, Meltzer CC. Ebola virus disease: radiology preparedness. Radiology. 2015;274(2):527–31.
12. Cornett CA, Vincent SA, Crow J, et al. Bacterial spine infections in adults: evaluation and management. J Am Acad Orthop Surg. 2016;24(1):11–8.
13. Xia Y, Ju Y, Chen J, You C. Hemorrhagic stroke and cerebral paragonimiasis. Stroke. 2014;45(11):3420–2.
14. Millichap JJ, Epstein LG. Emerging subspecialties in neurology: neuroinfectious diseases. Neurology. 2009;73(4):e14–e15.
15. Wilson M, Tyler KL. Emerging diagnostic and therapeutic tools for central nervous system infections. JAMA Neurol. 2016;73(12):1389–90.
16. Salzberg SL, Breitwieser FP, Kumar A, et al. Next-generation sequencing in neuropathologic diagnosis of infections of the nervous system. Neurol Neuroimmunol Neuroinflamm. 2016;3(4):e251.
17. Wilson MR, Naccache SN, Samayoa E, et al. Actionable diagnosis of neuroleptospirosis by next-generation sequencing. N Engl J Med. 2014;370(25):2408–17.
18. Papa A, Kotrotsiou T, Papadopoulou E, et al. Challenges in laboratory diagnosis of acute viral central nervous system infections in the era of emerging infectious diseases: the syndromic approach. Expert Rev Anti-Infect Ther. 2016;14(9):829–36.

Viral Encephalitis

7

Yan Ren

7.1 Herpes Simplex Encephalitis (HSE)

7.1.1 Introduction

HSV includes type 1 (HSV-1) and type 2 (HSV-2). Both are DNA viruses from the alphaherpesvirus subfamily. HSV-1 is common in children and adults, and the less common HSV-2 mainly infects neonates via maternal transmission. HSV-1 accounts for 95% of cases of HSE and is a common cause of mucocutaneous infections, in which it causes the direct destruction of neurons or induces immune-mediated injury of the central nervous system (CNS) [1]. Primary HSV infection accounts for 30% via the trigeminal or olfactory tracts or from hematogenous spread, while 70% of cases are attributed to HSV reactivation from prior viral latency within the ganglia or CNS.

HSE can cause a life-threatening brain parenchymal infection, with an estimated incidence of one case per 2.5–5.0 million throughout the world. In most studies of infectious encephalitis, HSV is the most frequently identified sporadic pathogen, causing 13.8% of all encephalitis cases [2], which, if left untreated, can lead to death. HSE has no seasonal variation and shows equal incidence in males and females. The age of onset of HSE presents a bimodal distribution, with one third of patients aged less than 20 years and one half of patients aged over 50 years.

7.1.2 Pathology

In HSE, pathological changes result from the combination of viral replication and immune injury. In the early stage of viral infection, a vigorous initial immune response is necessary to inhibit viral replication and reactivation from long-term pathological changes [3].

Hemorrhagic and necrotizing encephalitis are the basic histopathological changes and are characterized by frequent involvement of the temporal lobe, insular cortex, and orbital surface of the frontal lobes. Unilateral involvement of the temporal lobe is described commonly, with occasional subsequent extension to the contralateral side. The cingulate gyrus and occipital cortex are involved less frequently. Microscopic examination demonstrates intense perivascular cuffing, interstitial lymphocytic inflammation, and intranuclear inclusion bodies (typically eosinophilic Cowdry A intranuclear inclusion) in infected cells (e.g., neurons, astrocytes, and oligodendrocytes). Immunohistochemical staining may identify antibodies to HSV-1.

7.1.3 Clinical Presentation

HSE is often an acute (or sometimes subacute) course of encephalitis: over 50% of cases typically present as fever, headache, and seizures; less than 50% of cases present with focal or diffuse neurological deficit, behavioral changes, and altered mental status. As the disease progresses, symptoms associated with increasing intracranial pressure become prominent (e.g., lethargy and altered sensorium). However, clinical presentations of infectious encephalitis frequently overlap and are often indistinguishable from other etiological encephalitides. For those patients with immunodeficiency or who are receiving immunosuppressive therapy, the clinical manifestations of HSE are more atypical. Relapses of HSE are uncommon and mostly occur within 4 months of acute HSE episode [4].

7.1.4 Laboratory Examination

Once a patient is suspected of having HSE, lumbar acupuncture should be performed as soon as possible. CSF often shows elevated protein and lymphocytic pleocytosis, with a predominance of lymphocytes (median of approximately

Y. Ren (✉)
Department of Radiology, Huashan Hospital, Fudan University, Shanghai, China

B. Gao et al. (eds.), *Imaging of CNS Infections and Neuroimmunology*, https://doi.org/10.1007/978-981-13-6904-9_7

80%; range: 60–98%) [2]. Red blood cells and glucose values are usually non-diagnostic. Polymerase chain reaction (PCR) of cerebrospinal fluid (CSF) is the most accurate diagnosis, with sensitivity and specificity of 95–100%. However, false-negative PCR is also possible if the CSF is obtained in the first 3 days of HSE.

7.1.5 Imaging Findings

Imaging is a key tool that can provide essential diagnostic clues to identify acute encephalitis. Brain computed tomography (CT) helps to identify promptly those intracranial lesions with a mass effect that would contraindicate a lumbar puncture. Brain magnetic resonance imaging (MRI) plays a crucial role in suggesting a diagnosis of HSE, especially when the CSF HSV PCR assay is negative [5]. Delay in brain imaging has been reported as an independent factor for delayed treatment [6].

Brain CT scans are often normal within the first 72 h of HSE. With the further development of HSE, there appears to be low attenuation, with a mild mass effect in the frequently affected limbic system, which is most common in the medial temporal lobes, followed by the insular, cingulate, and frontobasal cortex. Some cases also demonstrate hemorrhagic lesions in the affected areas. In more than 60% of cases, the unilateral temporal lobe is involved, occasionally bilaterally. Contrast-enhanced CT (CECT) can show patchy or gyriform enhancement and sulcal effacements of the temporal lobes in the late acute and/or subacute stage of HSE.

Brain MRI typically shows a swollen area involving both the cortex and the white matter, with hypointense lesions on T1WI and hyperintense lesions on T2WI and FLAIR. Meanwhile, the junction of cortex and white matter becomes invisible, especially on T1WI. In the acute phase of HSE, DWI is the most sensitive sequence for detecting an abnormal hyperintense cortex, with a decrease in ADC compared with T1WI, T2WI, and FLAIR sequences. However, in the subacute phase of HSE, T2 and FLAIR show more sensitive hyperintense lesions than DWI. If hemorrhage occurs with HSE, T1WI also shows hyperintense lesions in acute/subacute HSE. Basal ganglia are often spared, which is suggestive of encephalitis, but not temporal glioma. Extensive lesions on MRI are associated with poor prognosis. In the late acute and/or chronic stage of HSE, the involved area also shows encephalomalacia. Gyral enhancement along the brain surface can also be present (Fig. 7.1).

Susceptibility weighted imaging (SWI) is a specific sequence to detect microbleeding lesions, with a remarkable blooming dark signal in amplitude image and bright signal in phase image (Fig. 7.2). In perfusion sequence, the involved temporal lobes may demonstrate high perfusion with increased measurement of relative cerebral blood volume (rCBV) and/or relative cerebral blood flow (rCBF) (Fig. 7.3), which represents the congestive status of inflammatory reaction. MR spectroscopy on the involved area may show a decreased *N*-acetyl aspartate peak and/or increased lactate peak.

7.1.6 Differential Diagnosis (DDX)

Top DDX for HSE includes acute ischemia infarction, status epilepticus, autoimmune limbic encephalitis, and diffuse infiltrating glioma. For acute ischemia infarction, the involved area also presents restricted diffusion with or without occasional hemorrhage, which is difficult to differentiate from HSE. But the ischemia infarction is often hyperacute with intracranial lesion which is consistent with the cerebrovascular distribution. There are similar signal changes with HSE for status epilepticus, but almost no hemorrhagic change has been reported in status epilepticus. Autoimmune encephalitis manifests as a normal brain MRI more frequently (40%) than HSE (5%) and often involves bilateral temporal lobes [5]. Diffuse infiltrating glioma with insular and/or temporal lobe involvement is hard to distinguish when HSE shows no hemorrhagic change, but bilateral distribution and increased perfusion for HSE may help to differentiate from low-grade diffuse infiltrating glioma. And in MRS, the low-grade glioma usually demonstrates no increased lactate peak, which usually represents necrotic components in malignant tumors or infectious lesions.

7.1.7 Summary

Recent studies suggest the initiation of acyclovir management as soon as possible contributes to a good prognosis for those patients with HSE. Initially extensive lesions of the bilateral and extra-temporal lobes on MRI are associated with a lower risk of HSE than other etiologies [7]. Early identification of HSE for physician is the key to successful treatment. In early stage of HSE, brain CT is often normal, and brain MRI is the best choice in early defining cortical lesions and evaluating the extent of brain damage. Advanced MRI can provide more diagnostic clues than conventional MRI.

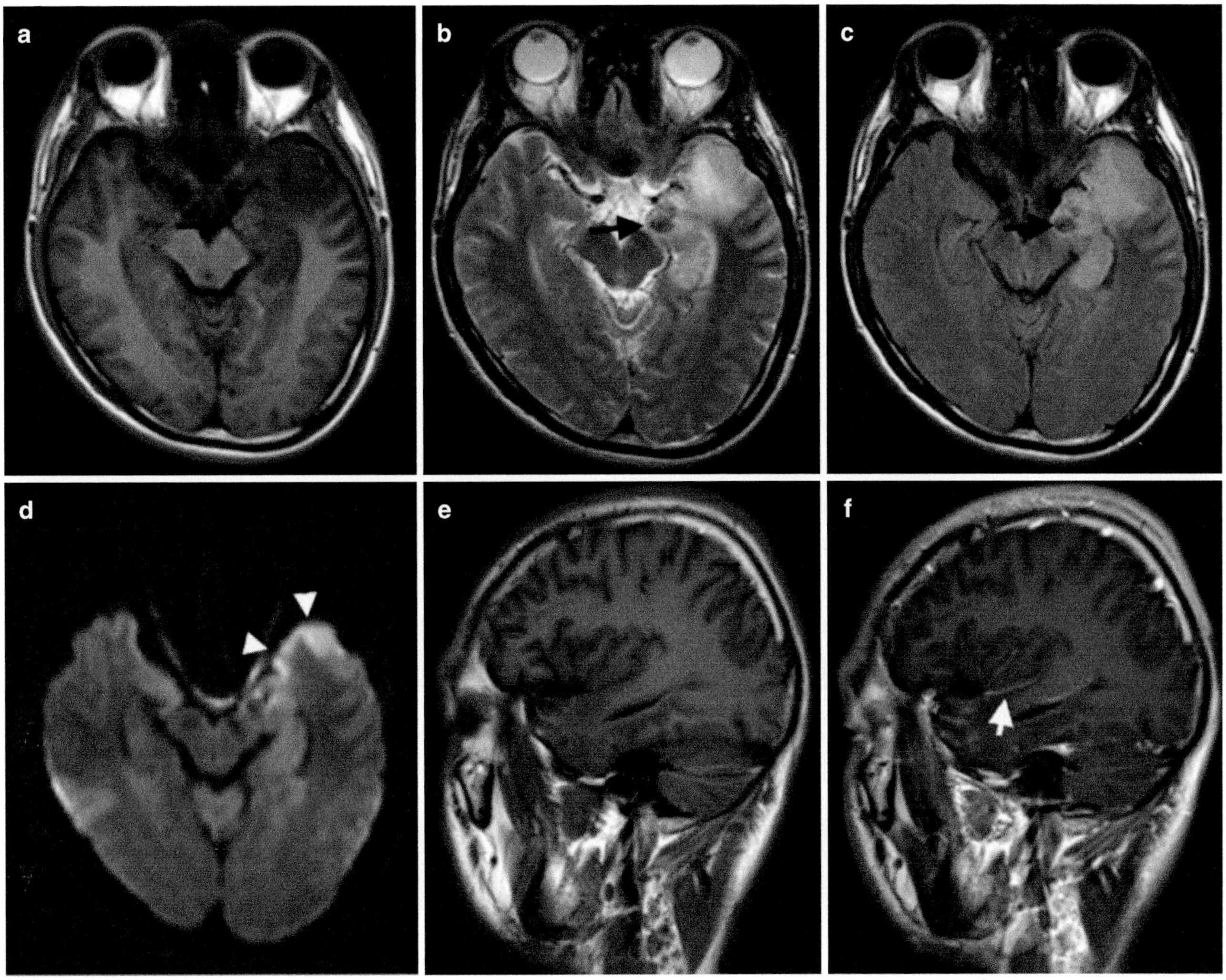

Fig. 7.1 A 24-year-old man with left temporal involvement due to HSV infection. (**a–c**) A patchy area with T1WI hypointense and T2/Flair hyperintense was shown in the left temporal lobe, which is typical in HSE; meanwhile, suspected hemorrhagic change also was seen (black arrow). (**d**) The remarkable cortical hyperintense was noted on axial DWI (arrow head). (**e, f**) On sagittal T1WI and contrast-enhanced T1WI, meningeal enhancement along the sulcus was shown (white arrow) (Courtesy of Chong Li MD., Department of Radiology, Huashan Hospital, Fudan University)

7.2 EV71 Encephalitis

7.2.1 Introduction

Enterovirus 71 (EV71) was first identified in California in 1969. It is a single-stranded RNA virus that belongs to the human enterovirus A species of the *Picornaviridae* family. EV71 is one of the main causative pathogens of hand, foot, and mouth disease (HFMD). Although coxsackie virus was the first pathogen to be identified as a cause of HFMD, the disease is now more commonly caused by EV71. Neurological complications are more common in HFMD caused by EV71 [8]. Generally, enterovirus does not cause life-threatening disease. Complications such as brainstem encephalitis, aseptic meningitis, and acute flaccid paralysis are rarely seen in only <1% children with HFMD due to EV71. However, EV71 can cause severe brainstem encephalitis, and many children and infants have died of neurological complications during epidemics.

7.2.2 Pathology

EV71 encephalitis characteristically affects the gray nuclei in the posterior part of the medulla oblongata, pon, and midbrain [9]. Pathological examination reveals neural cell degeneration or necrosis inside the lesion, with infiltration by neutrophils and glial cells. A large number of lymphocytes appear in the involved pia mater, and a sleeve shape formed by monocytes around vessels may be visible.

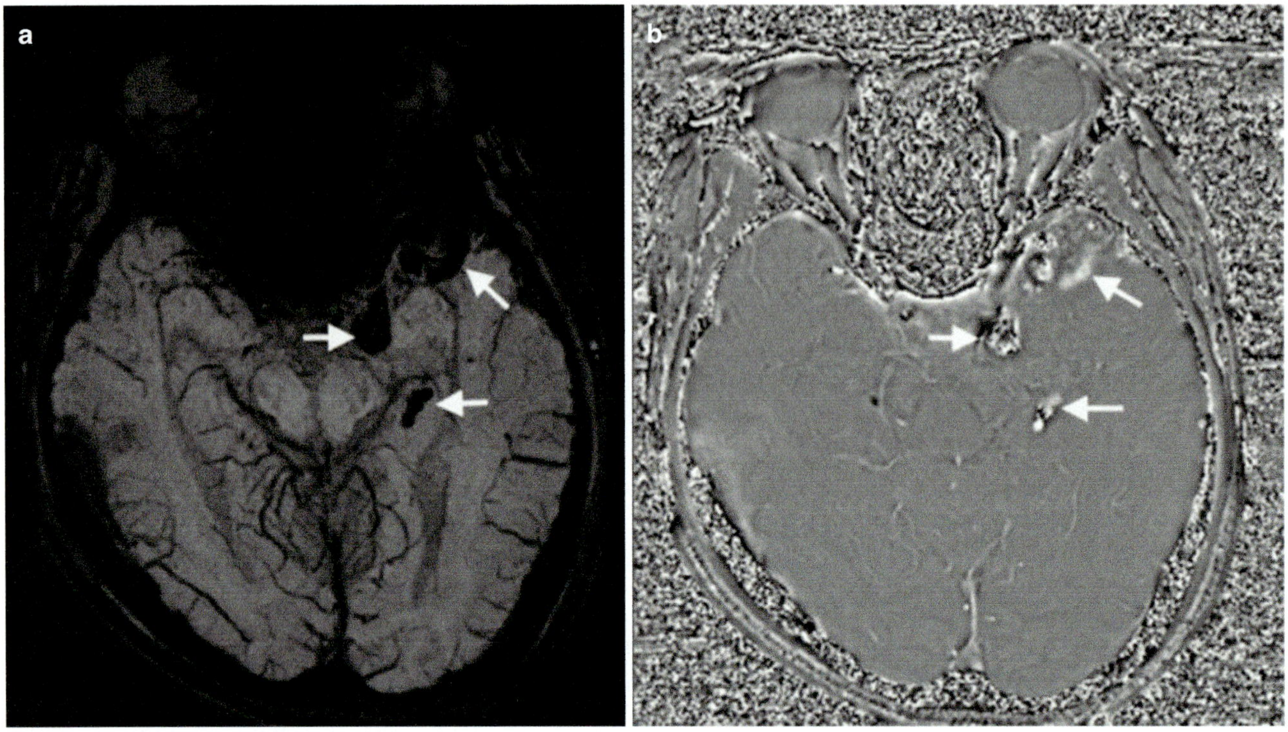

Fig. 7.2 Two weeks later, axial SWI in the same patient with Fig. 7.1 shows hemorrhagic lesions in the left temporal lobe, note remarkable blooming dark signals on amplitude image (**a**: white arrow) and hyperintensity on phase image (**b**: white arrow)

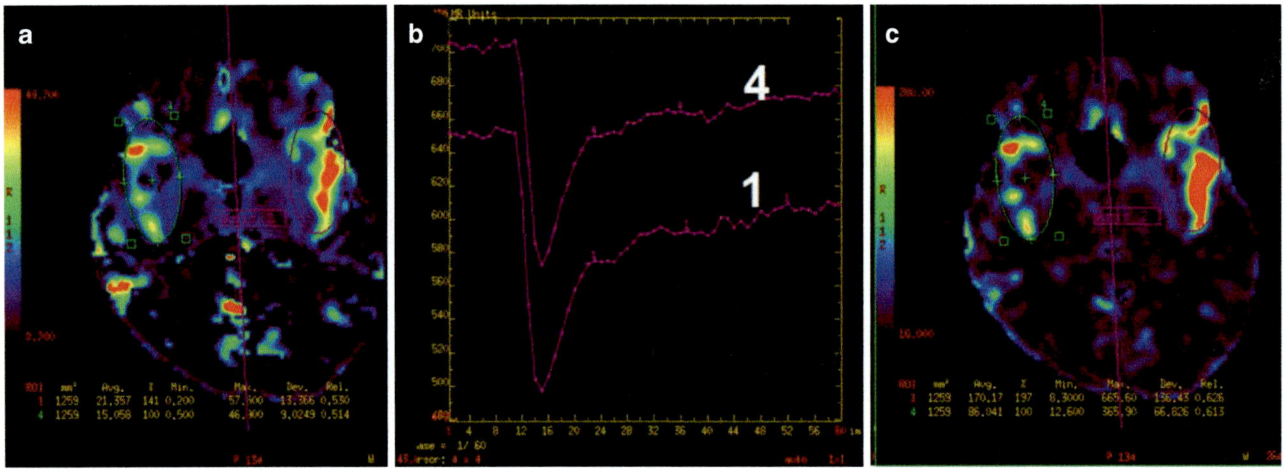

Fig. 7.3 Two weeks later, perfusion MRI in the same patient as Fig. 7.1 showing higher rCBV on color map (**a**) with relatively increased AUC in the left temporal lobe (**b**: curve 1) than the contralateral side (**b**: curve 4). Also note higher signal in the left temporal lobe on rCBF map (**c**). (Note: rCBV, relative cerebral blood volume; AUC, area under the curve; rCBF, relative cerebral blood flow)

The reason for EV71 neurotropism to the brainstem is still unknown; a probable mechanism may be via active retrograde axonal transport [10].

7.2.3 Clinical Presentation

EV71 can be transmitted via contaminated hands. The transmission rate between siblings and cousins is approximately 80%. The disease peaks in late spring to summer, although infections occur with high incidence through the year in tropical areas [11]. Although 50% of infected adults present no symptoms, they can transmit the disease to children.

Clinically, EV71 infection passes through four stages: (1) HFMD, (2) CNS involvement, (3) cardiopulmonary failure, and (4) convalescence. Most EV71 infections remain at stage 1, some progress to stage 2, and only a few advanced to the most severe stage 3. Some survivors of stage 3 have long-term sequelae [12, 13]. A fairly large proportion of patients have CNS involvement. In one previous

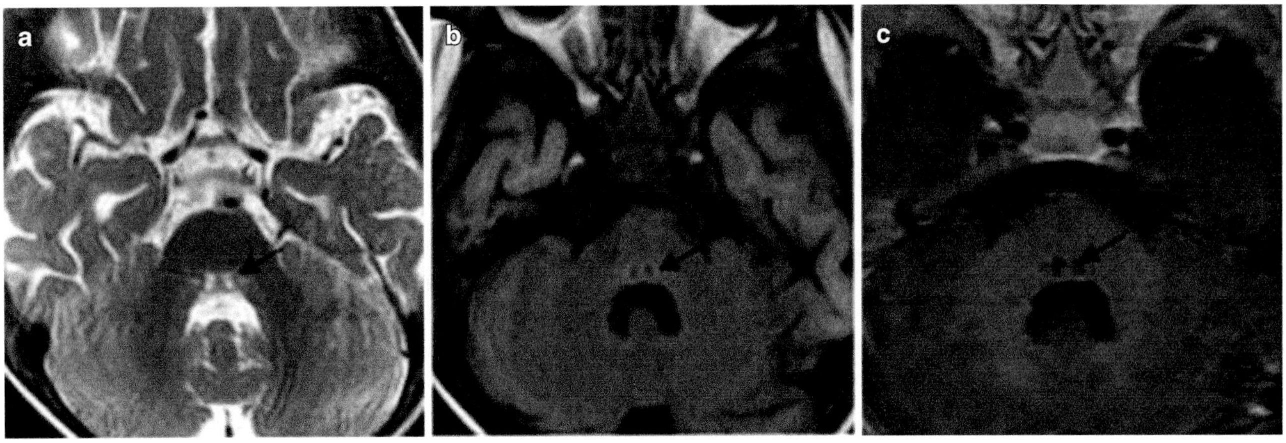

Fig. 7.4 A 7-month-old boy with brainstem encephalitis due to EV71 infection presented with fever, headache, and herpangina. On MRI of brain, axial T2WI (**a**) shows bilateral hyperintensity (*arrow*) in the posterior region of the pons; a central hypointensity surrounded by hyperintensity (*arrow*) also is seen on axial FLAIR (**b**). Axial T1WI (**c**) shows no enhancement in the lesion located in the posterior pons after contrast agent administration. (Courtesy of Qun Lao MD, Department of Radiology, Hangzhou Municipal Children's Hospital)

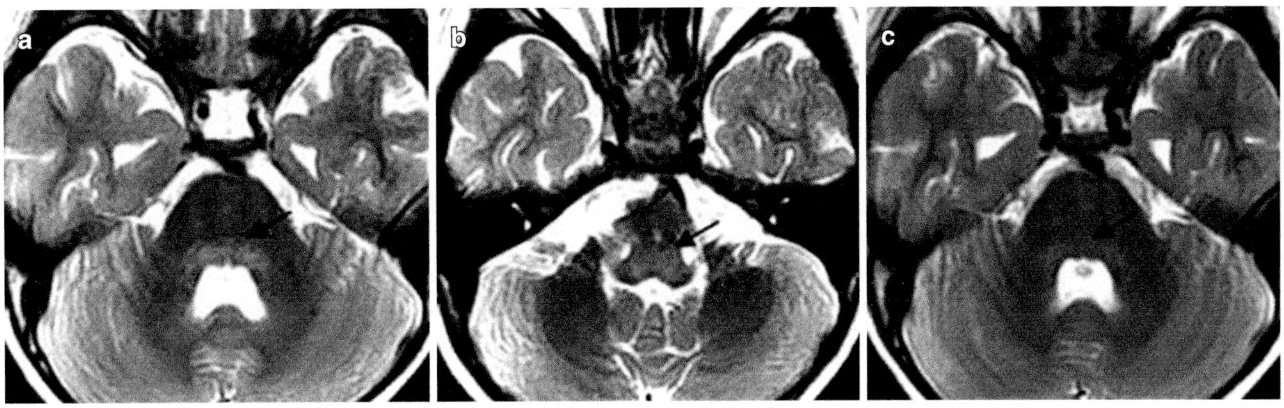

Fig. 7.5 A 36-month-old girl with brainstem encephalitis due to EV71 infection presented with fever, headache, and herpangina. On brain MRI, axial T2WI (**a**, **b**) shows bilateral hyperintensity in the posterior region of the pons and medulla oblongata (*arrow*). At follow-up after treatment, the bilateral patchy hyperintensity on T2WI (**c**) has almost disappeared in the posterior region of the pons. (Courtesy of Qun Lao MD, Department of Radiology, Hangzhou Municipal Children's Hospital)

report, 38 of 154 (24.7%) patients with EV71 infection developed CNS complications; of these, one died and four had sequelae [12].

Neurological complications of HFMD are more frequent in children under the age of 5 years. Neurological symptoms and signs occur within 3–5 days of the onset of fever or skin lesions. Myoclonus and ataxia are characteristic of brainstem involvement. Brainstem encephalitis is a major presentation with a high morbidity of 33.8% (24/71) from a local report related to HFMD in China [8], accounting for 58% of neurological complications. And 4% of brainstem encephalitis has cardiorespiratory dysfunction [11]. Neurogenic pulmonary edema and hemorrhage induced by brainstem encephalitis are the main causes of death.

7.2.4 Laboratory Examination

The gold standard for the diagnosis of EV71 infection is viral culture and isolation of the virus. However, this usually takes more than 7 days. Nowadays, PCR and sequencing of VP1 gene are more frequently employed for diagnosis of EV71. For patients with neurological complications, the detection rate by CSF PCR is very low (0–5%), and diagnosis is usually based on isolation of EV71 from throat and stool specimens.

7.2.5 Imaging Findings

Brain CT may demonstrate morphological changes such as widened subdural space and/or enlarged ventricular system and help exclude hemorrhagic lesions. In EV71 brainstem encephalitis, brain MRI typically shows hyperintensity in the posterior regions of the pons, medulla oblongata, midbrain, and the bilateral dentate nuclei of the cerebellum on T2WI/FLAIR sequences, with no abnormal enhancement on T1 contrast-enhanced images (Figs. 7.4 and 7.5). There have been some reports of the cerebral cortex, subcortical white matter, and thalamus being affected, but this is unusual for EV71 encephalitis and was probably caused by coinfection by other viruses or bacteria [8]. It should be noted that brain MRI may also sometimes be normal. When the anterior horns of spinal cord are invaded by EV71, spinal MRI may also demonstrate abnormal hyperintensity on T2WI and obvious enhancement of the anterior roots of spinal nerves in the EV71-infected cases [8]. There is good correlation between clinical features and MRI findings, which makes MRI a valuable modality for evaluating disease and predicting prognosis. Most patients with serious illness will have neurologic sequelae. The brainstem lesions present encephalomalacia (Fig. 7.4) or vanish after treatment (Fig. 7.5). In one study, most lesions located in the anterior horn regions of spinal cord became smaller and vanished during follow-up as muscle strength improved [14].

7.2.6 Summary

Since the outbreak of EV71 infection in Malaysia in 1997, HFMD has come to be recognized as a serious public health problem. Brainstem encephalitis, the most serious CNS complication of HFMD, can cause neurogenic pulmonary hemorrhage and/or edema, leading to death. It is still unknown why EV71 mainly involves the brainstem. T2/FLAIR hyperintensity in the posterior brainstem is characteristic of EV71 encephalitis. MRI findings, in conjunction with the isolation of EV71 from stool, throat swab, or CSF sample, can confirm the diagnosis of EV71 encephalitis. Early diagnosis followed by prompt management can improve prognosis.

7.3 HIV Encephalitis

7.3.1 Introduction

The human immunodeficiency virus (HIV) is a member of lentivirus (part of the retrovirus family) that causes long-duration HIV infection and, over time, acquired immunodeficiency syndrome (AIDS). HIV infection causes few or no symptoms for up to 10 years or more, after which the symptoms of AIDS develop. There is no cure for HIV/AIDS, but treatment is available. The brain is a major target for HIV infection [15], and HIV encephalitis (HIVE) is the most common manifestation of AIDS. HIVE is seen in 33–67% of adult AIDS patients and 30–50% of pediatric AIDS patients. Both sexes are equally affected. Recent studies suggest that the central nervous system (CNS) can act as a reservoir for the HIV and has the potential to reseed the systemic compartment [15]. Neurologic involvement in AIDS patients is related either to direct CNS invasion by the HIV or to opportunistic infection by other organisms.

In AIDS-associated CNS invasion, neuroimaging can reveal white matter disease, meningoencephalitis, intracranial mass lesions, and hydrocephalus. Though different diseases can produce similar imaging findings, certain characteristic patterns may suggest a particular pathogen and thus help guide decisions related to treatment.

7.3.2 Pathology

Brain biopsy has shown that CNS involvement is present in 80–90% of AIDS patients. Despite the use of highly active antiretroviral therapy (HAART), approximately 70% of HIV-infected patients develop neurologic complications [16]. HIV can directly invade the brain mater and parenchyma and cause nonsuppurative encephalitis and/or meningitis. HIV initially invades the white matter and then the basal ganglia, cortex, brainstem, cerebellum, spinal cord, and meninges. Pathologically, HIV encephalitis is characterized by the presence of many glial nodules and brain edema, with infiltration by multinuclear giant cells and noninflammatory cells.

7.3.3 Clinical Presentation

HIV encephalitis mainly manifests with altered sensorium, behavioral abnormalities, and motor decline – the so-called AIDS dementia syndrome. In children the clinical characteristics include microcephaly, cognitive defects, muscle weakness, pyramidal signs, ataxia, and seizures. Systemic HIV infection can cause suppression of immunity, leading to multiple complications such as HSE, multifocal white matter encephalopathy, cryptococcal encephalitis, toxoplasmosis, and primary CNS lymphoma.

7.3.4 Laboratory Examination

HIV enters the CNS in the first weeks after infection and can be detected throughout the course of untreated illness. Cell-associated HIV DNA in peripheral blood mononuclear cells (PBMCs) and CSF cell pellets can be measured by digital droplet polymerase chain reaction (PCR) test.

7.3.5 Imaging Findings

Neuroimaging provides a noninvasive means to evaluate progressive changes in the brain due to HIV infection. Initial changes include decreases in cortical and subcortical volumes. HIV-infected children also show substantial abnormalities in brain structure, especially within the corpus callosum [15].

Brain CT scans may present a normal appearance. Most HIV-infected patients demonstrate diffuse cerebral atrophy. Multiple or diffuse low densities can be seen in the bilateral periventricular white matter, basal ganglia, cerebellum, and brainstem. In in utero HIV infection, plain CT scan demonstrates the characteristic findings of bilateral and symmetrical calcifications in the basal ganglia and frontal white matter. Brain conventional MRI typically shows periventricular spotty and "hazy" hyperintensity on T2/FLAIR sequences (Fig. 7.6). Nonenhanced lesions without mass effect are typical of HIV encephalitis. Enhanced lesions usually suggest an opportunistic infection, such as toxoplasmosis (Fig. 7.7).

Multiple advanced modalities, including metabolic, structural, and functional neuroimaging, have been used in HIVE, mostly in the research setting. MR spectroscopy

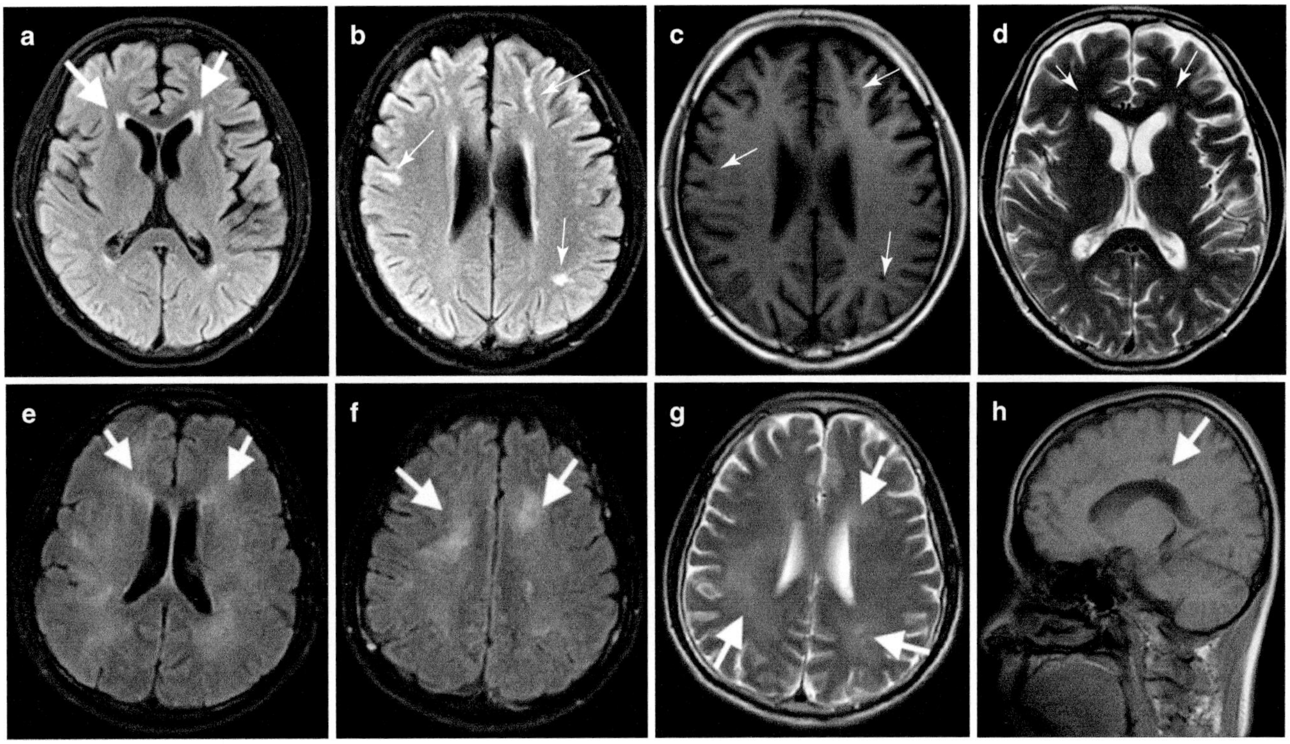

Fig. 7.6 A 45-year-old HIV-positive male patient (**a**–**d**). On MRI axial FLAIR images show spotty hyperintensity (arrow) in the periventricular (**a**) and subcortical (**b**) regions. Widened and deepened sulci in bilateral frontal and parietal lobes are seen on FLAIR (**a**, **b**), T1WI (**c**), and T2WI (**d**). A 45-year-old HIV-positive male (**e**–**h**). On axial FLAIR (**e**, **f**) and T2WI (**g**) of brain MRI, spotty and "hazy" hyperintensity are seen in the periventricular regions (*arrow*). Spotty hypointensity is seen on sagittal T1WI (**h**). (Courtesy of Jielan Li MD., Department of Radiology, Zhongnan Hospital, Wuhan University)

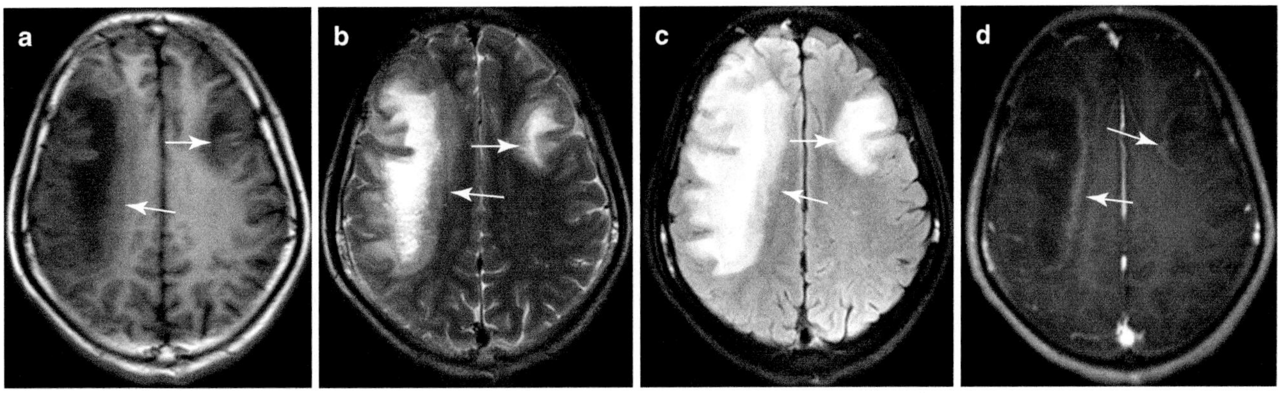

Fig. 7.7 A 22-year-old man who has been HIV positive for 10 years and also has suspected toxoplasmosis. (**a**–**c**) MRI pre-contrast axial images demonstrate abnormal signal intensity with mass effect (*arrows*) in the left frontal lobe and right frontal and parietal lobes; (**d**) Marked enhancement (*arrow*) is seen on axial ce-T1WI (Courtesy of Haopeng Pang MD., Department of Radiology, Huashan Hospital, Fudan University)

(MRS) shows elevated choline peak and myoinositol peak and a decreased *N*-acetylaspartate (NAA) peak [17]. Structural neuroimaging and volumetric analysis have demonstrated HIV-associated volumetric reductions within the amygdala, caudate nuclei, and corpus callosum [18], as well as in cortical areas [19]. Diffusion tensor imaging has been used to measure diffusion of water molecules in white matter tracts, specifically within the corpus callosum; decrease in mean diffusivity and increase in fractional anisotropy are typically associated with HIV. These measures can be used to track the effect of combination antiretroviral therapy [20, 21]. Functional MRI (fMRI) has been found to be a sensitive modality for detecting the subtle changes in brain activation associated with cognitive changes in HIV patients [22].

7.3.6 Summary

Recent studies suggest that the CNS acts as an HIV reservoir in AIDS patients. Imaging findings of "cerebral atrophy" do not necessarily indicate AIDS dementia complex in the HIV-positive patient; other diagnosis should be considered first, including dehydration, malnutrition, protein depletion, and alcoholism [17]. A combination of neuroimaging, CSF analysis, and neuropsychologic performance testing is necessary for a complete understanding of the brain changes caused by HIV infection.

7.4 Prion Encephalopathy

7.4.1 Introduction

Creutzfeldt-Jakob disease (CJD), also known as subacute spongiform encephalopathy, is the most common human prion disease (HPD). It is caused by a misfolded human prion protein [23]. CJD is a rare disease with a rapidly progressive course and a mortality rate of almost 100%. CJD occurs in three forms: an inherited familial form, a sporadically occurring form (sCJD), and an acquired form; the acquired form includes kuru, iatrogenic CJD (iCJD), and variant CJD (vCJD) (Table 7.1) [24]. The most common type is sCJD; with an incidence of 1 in 1,000,000 per year, it accounts for 85% of CJD cases. The vCJD form is thought to be the result of the spread of bovine spongiform encephalopathy to humans [25].

Brain biopsy is the gold standard for diagnosis of CJD. However, because of the potential risk of infectious transmission, noninvasive methods are preferred in clinical practice, and diagnosis is usually made using a combination of clinical features and electroencephalography (EEG) and imaging findings. For diagnosis of CJD, imaging is reported

Table 7.1 Classification and molecular subtypes of human prion diseases

Sporadic prion disease	Acquired (infected) prion disease	Familial (inherited or genetic) prion disease
Sporadic Creutzfeldt-Jakob disease (sCJD) (Molecular subtypes: MM1, MM2, MV1, MV2, VV1, and VV2) Sporadic fatal insomnia (sFI) Variably protease-sensitive prionopathy	Human origin Iatrogenic CJD (due to medical procedures) Kuru Bovine origin Variant CJD (vCJD)	Genetic CJD Gerstmann-Straussler-Scheinker syndrome (GSS) Fatal familial insomnia (FFI)

Modified from recent report [24]

to be much more sensitive and specific than CSF analysis for protein 14-3-3 or EEG findings of periodic sharp waves complexes (PSWCs) [25, 26]. Currently, MRI has been included in the diagnostic workup for sCJD.

7.4.2 Pathology

CJD mainly involves the cerebral cortex; it also affects the basal ganglia, thalamus, and cerebellum. Macroscopically, cerebral atrophy is the main pathological change. Microscopic changes include neuronal loss, astrocyte hyperplasia, and spongiform degeneration (cytoplasmic vacuolization). In the damaged brain tissues, abnormal PrP amyloid plaque can be found, without any inflammatory response [24]. Spongiform degeneration is more frequent in the thalamus in vCJD than in other types of CJD.

7.4.3 Clinical Presentation

Classically, CJD presents as rapidly progressive dementia of unknown origin with a higher mortality rate than human cancers. The most common form, sCJD, can be classified into several subtypes according to the molecular phenotype; these include MM1/MV1, VV2, MV2, MM2, and VV1 (Table 7.1) [27]. The age of onset of CJD ranges from 25 to 78 years (mean, 58 years). Both sexes are equally affected. CJD patients survive for only 5 months to 1 year from onset of the disease.

Typical CJD cases present with a "classic triad" of rapidly progressive cognitive dysfunction, myoclonus, and PSWCs on EEG [28]. However, clinical features can vary between the different CJD forms and between the different molecular subtypes of sCJD. Myoclonus is related to cortical damage and is characteristic of sCJD; it is generally accompanied by periodic discharges in the EEG. Cerebral cortex damage manifests as progressive dementia; once memory begins to decline, the disease will progress quickly until death. In vCJD, ataxia and behavioral abnormalities are the major clinical manifestations, which help differentiate it from sCJD. Clinically, typical CJD passes through three stages: In the early stage, nonspecific symptoms such as psychiatric symptoms, visual disorder, and memory disturbance are observed; in the second stage, the classic triad is seen; and in the late stage, the patient deteriorates into akinetic mutism. The cause of death is generally infection, aspiration pneumonia, respiratory failure, or general prostration.

7.4.4 Laboratory Examination

Several protein biomarkers, such as 14-3-3, t-tau, and p-tau (and the t-tau/p-tau ratio), have shown promising sensitivity and specificity for identification of CJD. In sCJD, the VV2 and MV2K subtypes demonstrate higher CSF levels of p-tau than the other subtypes. Recently, real-time quaking-induced prion conversion (RT-QuIC) assay has been shown to have high sensitivity (82.1%) and specificity (99.4%) for early diagnosis of HPDs. The combination of RT-QuIC and t-tau assays has been suggested as the first line laboratory investigation for clinical diagnosis of CJD [29].

7.4.5 Imaging Findings

Imaging findings, especially for MRI, are essential for diagnosis of CJD. Brain CT has a limited role in HPD. In fact, 80% of HPD patients have normal brain CT at the onset; the other 20% may show brain atrophy and/or ventricular dilatation [30]. Brain MRI is of great importance as a noninvasive examination for CJD patients. Generally, diagnosis of CJD at an early stage can be made on the basis of the findings on T2WI, proton density (PD)-weighted imaging, FLAIR, and diffusion-weighted imaging (DWI) sequences (Fig. 7.8). FLAIR and DWI sequences are more useful for evaluation of gyral changes as they provide higher contrast between gray and white matter and therefore display cortical hyperintensities better than T2WI sequences. FLAIR and DWI are also more sensitive than T2WI for assessment of basal ganglia abnormalities. Due to the impact of T2 shine-through on DWI signal, the apparent diffusion coefficient (ADC) map is indispensable.

DWI hyperintense lesions in the caudate nucleus and putamen (Fig. 7.8), and ribbon-like hyperintensities in the cerebral cortices (Fig. 7.9), are the essential clues for the diagnosis of sCJD. With disease progression, the signal abnormalities become more extensive—usually bilateral and

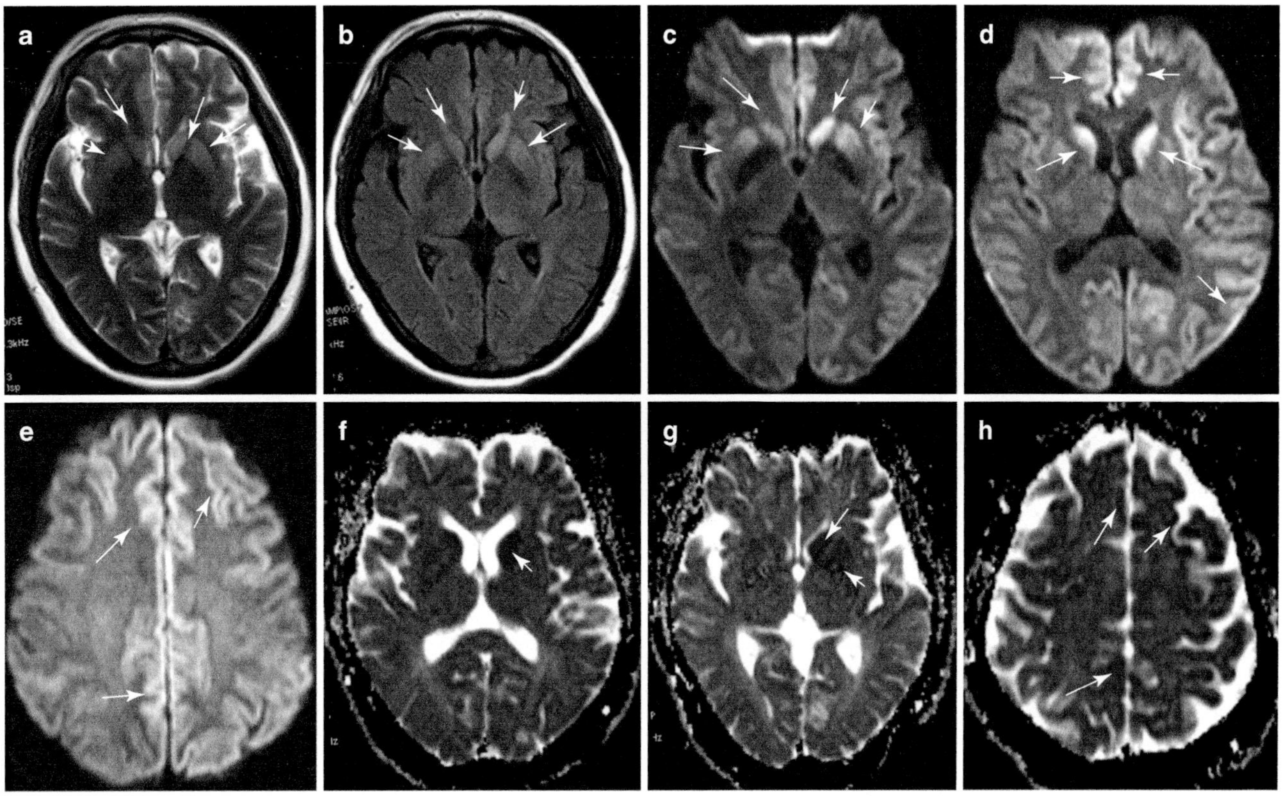

Fig. 7.8 A 53-year-old female with clinical diagnosis of CJD. (**a**, **b**). Brain MRI axial T2WI/FLAIR shows symmetrical hyperintense lesions (arrow) in bilateral caudate heads and putamens (**c**–**e**). Obviously diffusion-restricted areas of bilateral frontal lobes and basal ganglions on axial DWI (arrows) were also demonstrated; (**f**–**h**). Decreased ADC was noted on corresponding ADC maps (arrows) (Courtesy of Rong Lu M.D., Department of Radiation Oncology, Shanghai Proton and Heavy Ion Center)

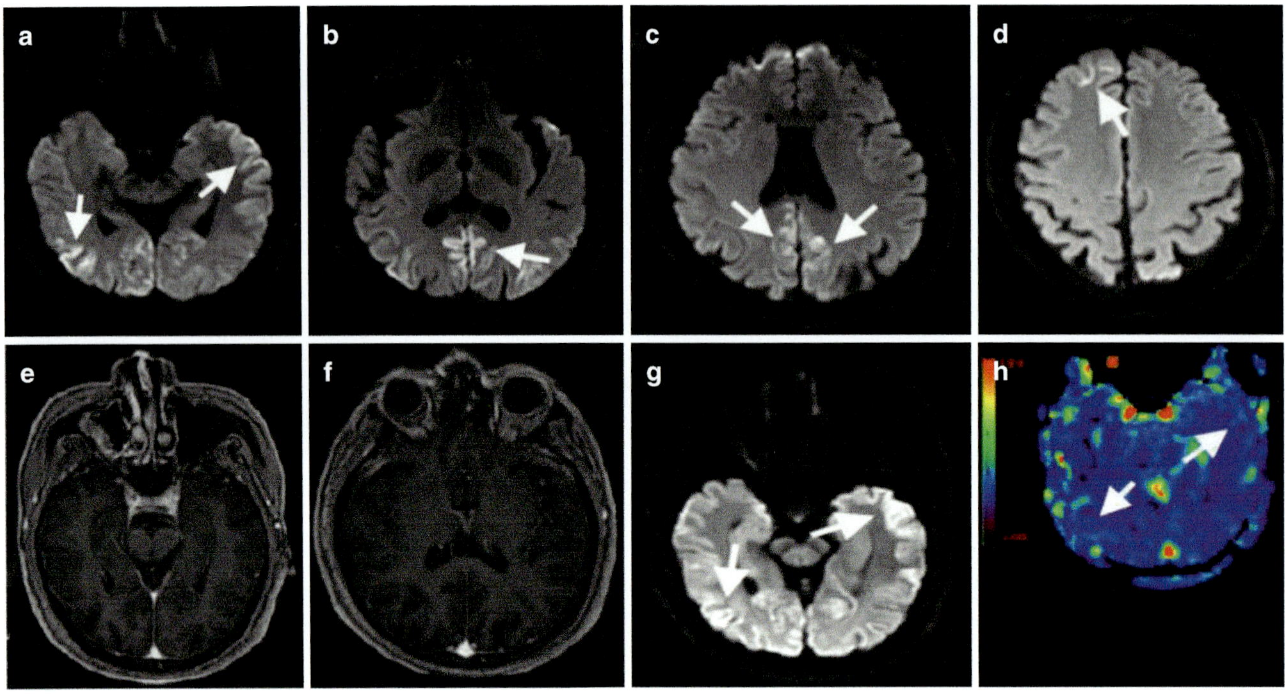

Fig. 7.9 A 54-year-old male with clinical diagnosis of CJD (**a**–**d**). Brain MRI with axial DWI demonstrates abnormal cortical "ribbon"-like hyperintensity (arrows) on the bilateral of temporal and occipital lobes and the right frontal lobe; (**e**, **f**). Where no abnormal contrast enhancement was noted on the CE-T1WI (**g**, **h**). In the cortical regions with DWI hyperintensity (arrows), no obviously increased perfusion was demonstrated on CBV map (arrows)

asymmetric—but show no mass effect or contrast enhancement. White matter involvement is rare and is only visible in the late stages, when it is secondary to brain atrophy and thickening of the cerebral cortex. Some associations between MRI findings and the clinical variants of CJD have been described; for example, occipital involvement is indicative of the Heidenhain variant, and involvement of the cerebellum and hippocampus is indicative of the Brownell-Oppenheimer variant [31]. MRI may also help differentiate between the molecular subtypes of sCJD; for example, thalamic involvement is more frequently found in the MV2 and VV2 subtypes than in the MM1 subtype [33]. The so-called "hockey stick" or "pulvinar" sign within the dorsomedial thalamus and the posterior thalamus (pulvinar) is indicative of vCJD. The hockey stick sign denotes a high signal in both the pulvinar and the dorsomedial thalamic nuclei, with a symmetrical distribution, which is obviously different from the picture seen in sCJD (Simona et al. 2017). MRI findings in inherited and infectious HPD are similar to those seen in sCJD.

Arterial spin labeling (ASL)-perfusion MRI has demonstrated marked reduction of blood flow in the cerebral cortex and basal ganglia in a patient with fCJD [34]. MRS has indicated decrease in NAA, but the finding is nonspecific and has limited value for diagnosis of CJD [35].

7.4.6 Differential Diagnosis

Clinically, several diseases may mimic HPD; for example, paraneoplastic encephalitis, cerebral vasculitis, infectious encephalitis (HIV and JC virus), and some dementia-related diseases present with similar clinical symptoms and rapidly progressive dementia [33]. Paraneoplastic encephalitis is characterized by sparing of the basal ganglia, which helps differentiate it from CJD. Multiple subcortical hyperintense lesions on T2WI/FLAIR images and patchy contrast-enhanced areas are consistent with CNS vasculitis but not with CJD. Extensive involvement of subcortical white matter supports the diagnosis of infectious diseases, not CJD. Meanwhile, restricted diffusion in cortical areas is rarely seen in other neurodegenerative diseases such as Alzheimer disease, vascular dementia, and frontotemporal dementia.

There are many diseases that, like CJD, involve the cerebral cortex and/or basal ganglia; these include herpes simplex encephalitis (HSE); mitochondrial encephalomyopathy, lactic acidosis, and stroke-like episodes (MELAS); Wilson's disease; acute disseminated encephalomyelitis (ADEM); and arterial or venous infarct [33]. Despite similar cortical changes on T2/FLAIR in both HSE and CJD, the MR findings of sparing of the basal ganglia, petechial hemorrhage, and patchy enhancement in the subacute stage help differentiate HSE from CJD. Multifocal and bilateral cortical hyperintensities in MELAS sometimes appear similar to CJD, but the increased cerebral blood flow (CBF) seen in MELAS is in contrast with the reduced CBF seen in CJD. Moreover, MRS may show an elevated lactate peak, which suggests a diagnosis of MELAS, not CJD. Typical hyperintensity on T1 in the affected basal ganglia and the involvement of subcortical areas, mesencephalon, pons, vermis, and dentate nuclei are key features that help differentiate Wilson's disease from CJD. Generally, lack of restricted diffusion and extensive involvement of white matter helps differentiate ADEM from CJD. In addition, T2 shine-through effects are more frequently seen in ADEM with contrast-enhanced lesions than in CJD. In the cases of arterial infarct, the lesions often lie along the vascular distribution, and MR angiography may show the arterial occlusion. In venous infarct, MR venography readily demonstrates the sinus thrombosis.

7.4.7 Summary

CJD is characterized by rapidly progressive cognitive dysfunction, myoclonus, and akinetic mutism state, along with DWI hyperintensity on MRI and PSWCs on EEG. Clinical and neuroimaging findings correlate well with neuropathologic observations in both typical and atypical cases in CJD. MR imaging has come to play a prominent role in the diagnosis of CJD, and MRI findings have now been included in the diagnostic criteria for sCJD. As in any disease, imaging cannot replace thorough physical examination and history; nevertheless, MRI contributes greatly in the diagnosis of patients presenting with a rapidly progressive dementia, as it can help differentiate between CJD and non-CJD diseases.

References

1. Boucher A, Herrmann JL, Morand P, et al. Epidemiology of infectious encephalitis causes in 2016. Med Mal Infect. 2017;47(3):221–35.
2. Gnann JW Jr, Whitley RJ. Herpes simplex encephalitis: an Update. Curr Infect Dis Rep. 2017;19(3):13.
3. Conrady CD, Drevets DA, Carr DJ. Herpes simplex type I (HSV-1) infection of the nervous system: is an immune response a good thing? J Neuroimmunol. 2010;220(1–2):1–9.
4. Skoldenberg B, Aurelius E, Hjalmarsson A, et al. Incidence and pathogenesis of clinical relapse after herpes simplex encephalitis in adults. J Neurol. 2006;253(2):163–70.
5. Bertrand A, Leclercq D, Martinez-Almoyna L, et al. MR imaging of adult acute infectious encephalitis. Med Mal Infect. 2017;47(3):195–205.
6. Poissy J, Wolff M, Dewilde A, et al. Factors associated with delay to acyclovir administration in 184 patients with herpes simplex virus encephalitis. Clin Microbiol Infect. 2009;15(6):560–4.
7. Chow FC, Glaser CA, Sheriff H, et al. Use of clinical and neuroimaging characteristics to distinguish temporal lobe herpes simplex encephalitis from its mimics. Clin Infect Dis. 2015;60(9):1377–83.
8. Li J, Chen F, Liu T, et al. MRI findings of neurological complications in hand-foot-mouth disease by enterovirus 71 infection. Int J Neurosci. 2012;122(7):338–44.
9. Shen WC, Chiu HH, Chow KC, et al. MR imaging findings of enteroviral encephalomyelitis: an outbreak in Taiwan. AJNR Am J Neuroradiol. 1999;20(10):1889–95.
10. Chen YC, Yu CK, Wang YF, et al. A murine oral enterovirus 71 infection model with central nervous system involvement. J Gen Virol. 2004;85(Pt 1):69–77.
11. Lee KY. Enterovirus 71 infection and neurological complications. Korean J Pediatr. 2016;59(10):395–401.
12. Chang LY, Lin TY, Hsu KH, et al. Clinical features and risk factors of pulmonary oedema after enterovirus-71-related hand, foot, and mouth disease. Lancet. 1999;354(9191):1682–6.
13. Chang LY, Hsia SH, Wu CT, et al. Outcome of enterovirus 71 infections with or without stage-based management: 1998 to 2002. Pediatr Infect Dis J. 2004;23(4):327–32.
14. Liu K, Ma YX, Zhang CB, et al. Neurologic complications in children with enterovirus 71-infected hand-foot-mouth disease: clinical features, MRI findings and follow-up study. Zhonghua Yi Xue Za Zhi. 2012;92(25):1742–6.
15. Spudich SS, Ances BM. CROI 2016: neurologic complications of HIV infection. Top Antivir Med. 2016;24(1):29–37.
16. Bilgrami M, O'Keefe P. Neurologic diseases in HIV-infected patients. Handb Clin Neurol. 2014;121:1321–44.
17. Osborn AG, Jhaveri MD, Salzman KL. Diagnostic imaging brain. Philadelphia: Elsevier; 2015.
18. Ances BM, Ortega M, Vaida F, et al. Independent effects of HIV, aging, and HAART on brain volumetric measures. J Acquir Immune Defic Syndr. 2012;59(5):469–77.
19. Thompson PM, Dutton RA, Hayashi KM, et al. Thinning of the cerebral cortex visualized in HIV/AIDS reflects CD4+ T lymphocyte decline. Proc Natl Acad Sci U S A. 2005;102(43):15647–52.
20. Nakamoto BK, Jahanshad N, McMurtray A, et al. Cerebrovascular risk factors and brain microstructural abnormalities on diffusion tensor images in HIV-infected individuals. J Neurovirol. 2012;18(4):303–12.
21. Wright PW, Heaps JM, Shimony JS, et al. The effects of HIV and combination antiretroviral therapy on white matter integrity. AIDS. 2012;26(12):1501–8.
22. Hakkers CS, Arends JE, Barth RE, et al. Review of functional MRI in HIV: effects of aging and medication. J Neurovirol. 2017;23(1):20–32.
23. Prusiner SB. Prions. Proc Natl Acad Sci U S A. 1998;95(23):13363–83.
24. Iwasaki Y. Creutzfeldt-Jakob disease. Neuropathology. 2017;37(2):174–88.
25. Geschwind MD, Shu H, Haman A, et al. Rapidly progressive dementia. Ann Neurol. 2008;64(1):97–108.
26. Vitali P, Maccagnano E, Caverzasi E, et al. Diffusion-weighted MRI hyperintensity patterns differentiate CJD from other rapid dementias. Neurology. 2011;76(20):1711–9.
27. Parchi P, Strammiello R, Giese A, et al. Phenotypic variability of sporadic human prion disease and its molecular basis: past, present, and future. Acta Neuropathol. 2011;121(1):91–112.
28. Manix M, Kalakoti P, Henry M, et al. Creutzfeldt-Jakob disease: updated diagnostic criteria, treatment algorithm, and the utility of brain biopsy. Neurosurg Focus. 2015;39(5):E2.
29. Lattanzio F, Abu-Rumeileh S, Franceschini A, et al. Prion-specific and surrogate CSF biomarkers in Creutzfeldt-Jakob disease: diagnostic accuracy in relation to molecular subtypes and analysis of neuropathological correlates of p-tau and Abeta42 levels. Acta Neuropathol. 2017;133(4):559–78.
30. Garcia Santos JM, Lopez Corbalan JA, Martinez-Lage JF, et al. CT and MRI in iatrogenic and sporadic Creutzfeldt-Jakob disease: as far as imaging perceives. Neuroradiology. 1996;38(3):226–31.

31. Poon MA, Stuckey S, Storey E. MRI evidence of cerebellar and hippocampal involvement in Creutzfeldt-Jakob disease. Neuroradiology. 2001;43(9):746–9.
32. Puoti G, Bizzi A, Forloni G, et al. Sporadic human prion diseases: molecular insights and diagnosis. Lancet Neurol. 2012;11(7):618–28.
33. Gaudino S, Gangemi E, Colantonio R, et al. Neuroradiology of human prion diseases, diagnosis and differential diagnosis. Radiol Med. 2017;122(5):369–85.
34. Chen S, Guan M, Shang JK, et al. Reduced cerebral blood flow in genetic prion disease with PRNP D178N-129M mutation: an arterial spin labeling MRI study. J Clin Neurosci. 2015;22(1):204–6.
35. Kim JH, Choi BS, Jung C, et al. Diffusion-weighted imaging and magnetic resonance spectroscopy of sporadic Creutzfeldt-Jakob disease: correlation with clinical course. Neuroradiology. 2011;53(12):939–45.

Bacterial and Mycoplasmal Infections

8

Yinfeng Qian

8.1 Pyogenic Bacterial Infections

8.1.1 Introduction

Pyogenic bacterial infections involve inflammation of the parenchyma or meninges covering the brain and spinal cord, and *N. meningitidis*, *S. pneumoniae*, and *H. influenzae* are the three main causes of acute pyogenic infections in the recent years; some gram-negative bacteria are responsible for non-epidemic cases of the infection. Pyogenic bacterial infections usually occur in male patients more than in female patients and most commonly occur among children and young people. According to Thigpen's research in the United States during the twenty-first century [1], pneumococcus accounted for 58% of annual incidence of pyogenic bacterial infections, *Streptococcus* species accounted for 86% of cases in infants, and the mortality was estimated to 12%.

8.1.2 Pathophysiology

The brain abscess is usually caused by the following sources: otomastoiditis (Fig. 8.1), sinusitis (Fig. 8.2), odontogenic abscess, hematogenous dissemination, and complication of neurosurgery [2]. Aggressive surgical management of otitis media is still the main source of brain abscess in developing countries although it has been rare in developed countries. Pathologically, pyogenic infections can be divided into four stages: diffuse stage (meningitis), focal stage (cerebritis and abscess), extra-axial stage (empyema and subdural effusions), and ventricular infections (ventriculitis). In 1983, Britt and Enzmann [1] firstly described the development of brain abscess as four different stages, including early cerebritis phase, late cerebritis phase, early capsule formation phase, and late capsule formation phase. During the first stage, the brain parenchyma becomes soft because the inflammatory response to bacterial invasion and histopathologically corresponding to perivascular inflammatory cuffing poorly delineate it from the surrounding normal brain. During the second stage, the central necrosis is formed, and fibroblasts deposit an early reticulin matrix around the periphery of necrosis. During the early and late capsule stage, the round, oval, or multiloculated central core is formed, which is filled with pus and surrounded with capsule. The immature capsule in the early stage is consisted of scant collagen and progresses to a mature collagen capsule containing gliosis during the late stage.

8.1.3 Clinical Features

Symptoms of pyogenic bacterial infections depend on the location and degree of the infection. The triad of fever, cervical rigidity, and altered mental status is the most classic symptom of meningitis although few patients present with it; other symptoms include headache, focal neurological damage, nausea, vomiting, and epilepsy. The white blood cell count in blood biochemical is variably elevated or normal; the CSF analysis can be normal; thus pyogenic bacterial infections should be diagnosed according to both clinical and laboratory features. CSF analysis and blood cultures are the reference standard for the diagnosis of pyogenic infection. However, because of nonspecific symptoms and high mortality, empirical antibiotic therapy should be started immediately and not be delayed for performance of blood culture or head computed tomography if meningitis or cerebritis is suspected [3]. Vancomycin and a third-generation cephalosporin have been proven effective in the treatment of *Haemophilus* species, meningococcus, and penicillin-resistant pneumococcus.

Y. Qian (✉)
Department of Radiology, The First Affiliated Hospital of Anhui Medical University, Hefei, China

B. Gao et al. (eds.), *Imaging of CNS Infections and Neuroimmunology*, https://doi.org/10.1007/978-981-13-6904-9_8

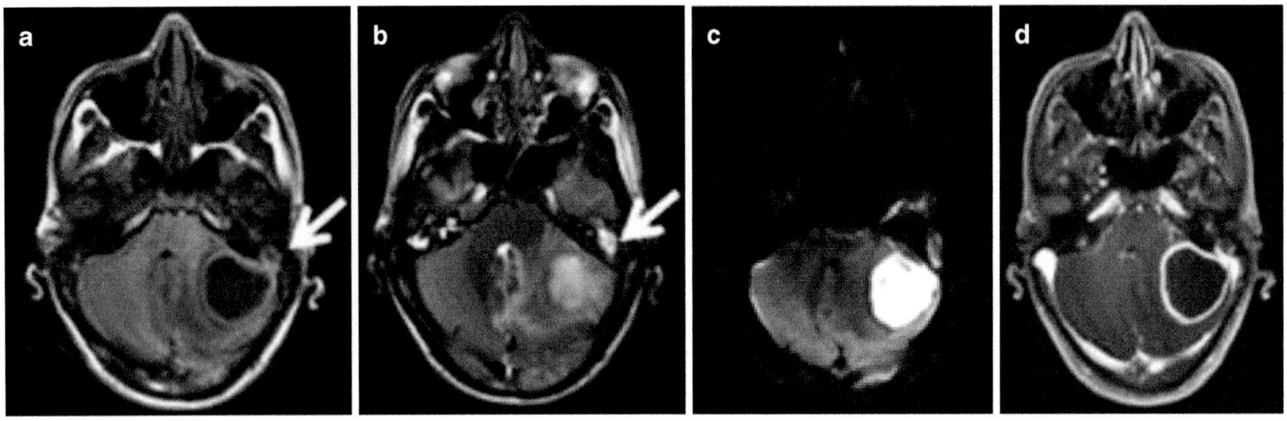

Fig. 8.1 Brain abscess from left mastoiditis. (**a**, **b**) Signal abnormalities are observed in the left mastoid (white arrow). An abscess is also noted in the left cerebellum, which has central hyperintense signal corresponding to the pus cavity and the characteristic surrounding T2 hypointense signal of the abscess capsule. The pus cavity is hypointense on axial T1WI sequence, and the wall of abscess is hypointense. (**c**) Diffusion-weighted sequence demonstrates central diffusion restriction as hyperintense signal intensity. (**d**) On axial post-contrast T1WI, the mature abscess demonstrates a ringlike enhancement

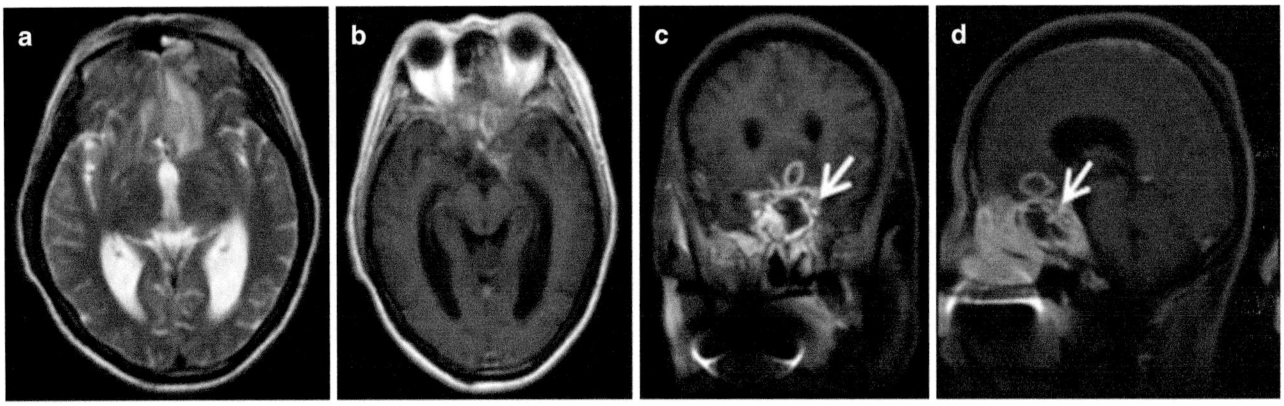

Fig. 8.2 Nasosinusitis and abscess. (**a**) On axial T2WI sequence, the abscess has central hypointense signal and edema surrounding the T2 hypointense signal of the abscess capsule. (**b–d**). On axial T1-weighted post-contrast image, the abscess demonstrates a ringlike enhancement. Nasosinusitis close to the abscess (white arrow) is also found in coronal and sagittal post-contrast T1WI

8.1.4 Radiologic Imaging

Diffuse Pyogenic Infections (Meningitis)

CT imaging is neither sensitive nor specific for detection of meningitis. Swelling and effacement of sulcus with slight hyperattenuation is typical but subtle on non-contrast CT images. MR imaging is the most sensitive neuroimaging method for detection of meningitis. Abnormal hyperintensity along cerebral sulci may be visible on both fluid-attenuated inversion recovery (FLAIR) images and diffusion-weighted images (DWI). Thin linear enhancement in the cerebral sulci is found after contrast material injection (Fig. 8.3), and the image characteristic is noted in about 55–70% of patients with clinically proven meningitis [4]. However, there is still a controversy whether enhanced T1-weighted imaging is more effective than FLAIR sequence in the diagnoses of meningeal diseases. Thin linear enhancement in the cerebral sulci is the typical pattern of acute bacterial and viral meningitis, while thick nodular enhancement in the basal cisterns is more typical for granulomatous or carcinomatous meningitis.

Focal Pyogenic Infections (Cerebritis and Abscess)

CT and MRI have important value in the diagnosis of focal pyogenic brain infections. The CT and MRI characteristics vary according to different phases of the brain infections and can be arbitrarily divided into four phases. In early cerebritis phase, CT image shows low attenuation with ill-defined margin and subtle mass effect, which is consistent with the neutrophilic response to the invasive organism mani-

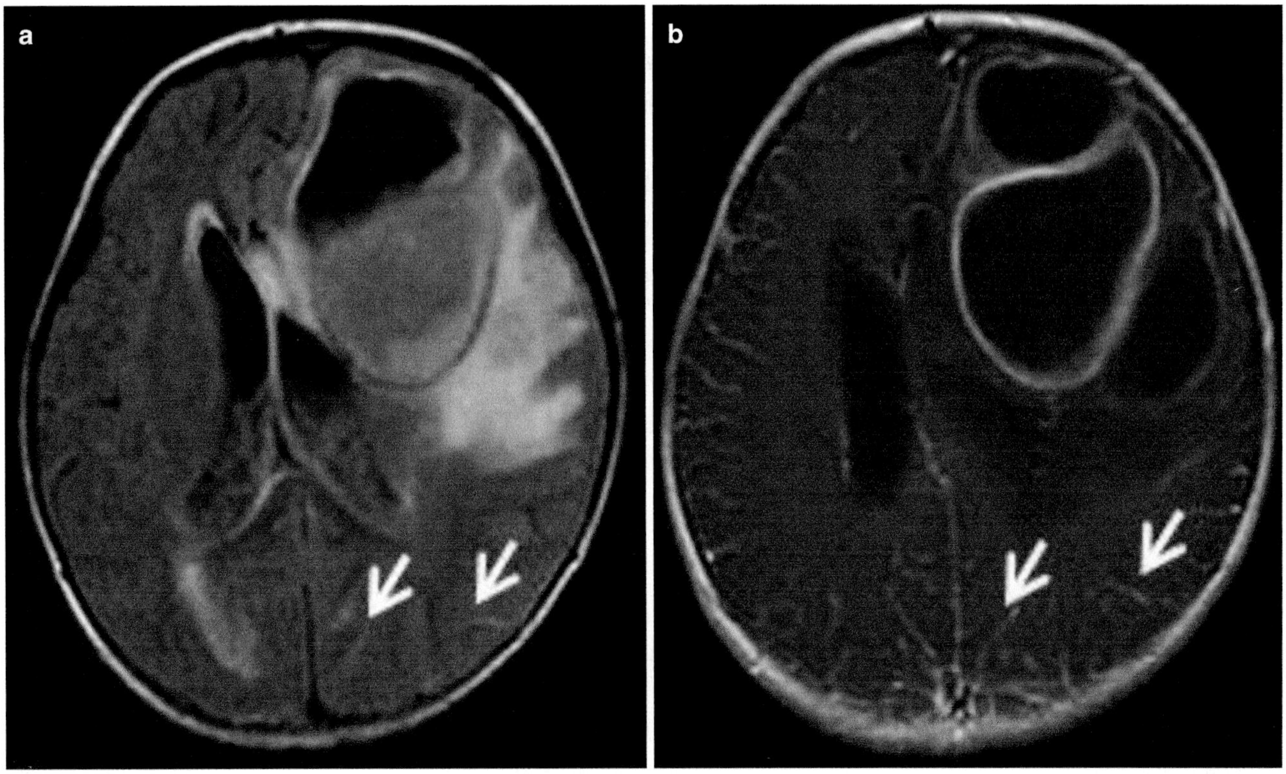

Fig. 8.3 Meningitis. (**a**) Axial T2-FLAIR image reveals linear hyperintensity (arrowheads) in left occipital sulci. (**b**) Corresponding thin linear enhancement is noted on axial T1-weighted post-contrast MR image (arrowheads)

fests. MR images show a hyperintense signal on T2WI and hypointense signal on T1WI, with indistinguishable edema around the lesion (Fig. 8.4). There is no purulent fluid in this phase; the critical diagnostic characteristic is that the DWI sequence presented as marked diffusion restriction. The enhancement of lesion is mild or absent on T1-weighted-enhanced images.

In late cerebritis phase, fibroblast accumulates at the margins; therefore irregular low-attenuation area of edema can be found on non-contrast CT images; the thick ringlike or nodular enhancement that is stable or increased can be found on delayed enhanced images. The periphery may demonstrate an isointense or slight hyperintense rim on T1WI and isointense or hypointense rim on T2WI; the edema around the lesion is hyperintense on T2-weighted image. The necrosis is usually located in the central area of lesion and has restricted water diffusion on DWI. The lesion shows diffuse or nodular enhancement at first, then progressing to thick ringlike enhancement, according to the evolution of the central necrosis (Fig. 8.5).

When the capsule formation is complete, the capsule manifests as a hyperattenuated round or ovoid area; the central necrosis and peripheral edema also are found on precontrast CT images (Fig. 8.6). The sharp border of capsule is hypointense on T2WI, hyperintensity on T1WI, and hypointensity on gradient-echo images, probably due to collagen or paramagnetic material within macrophages. The restriction to water diffusion persists on DWI. The post-contrast images display obvious and smooth rim-like enhancement of the capsule with edema reduction (Fig. 8.7). Daughter abscess appears in this phase. In the later abscess phase, the central necrotic area of lesion decreases in size, and the capsule becomes iso- or hyperintense on T2-weighted images. The enhancement of abscess capsule may persist or disappear eventually.

During the process of brain pyogenic infection, extra fluid may collect in the subdural and epidural spaces. Subdural empyema is usually caused by retrograde thrombophlebitis via the skull emissary veins from an infected area nearby. It is necessary to differentiate subdural effusion from subdural empyema because the latter may cause complications such as thrombophlebitis and encephalitis. The empyema is slightly denser than cerebrospinal fluid on CT images, and it presents higher signal than cerebrospinal fluid on T1-weighted and FLAIR images because of higher concentrations of proteins. On enhanced T1-weighted images, the verge of empyema also enhanced (Figs. 8.8 and 8.9). Of course recently the differentiation has been easily done because of the use of DWI; the empyema shows higher signal and low ADC values like in abscess.

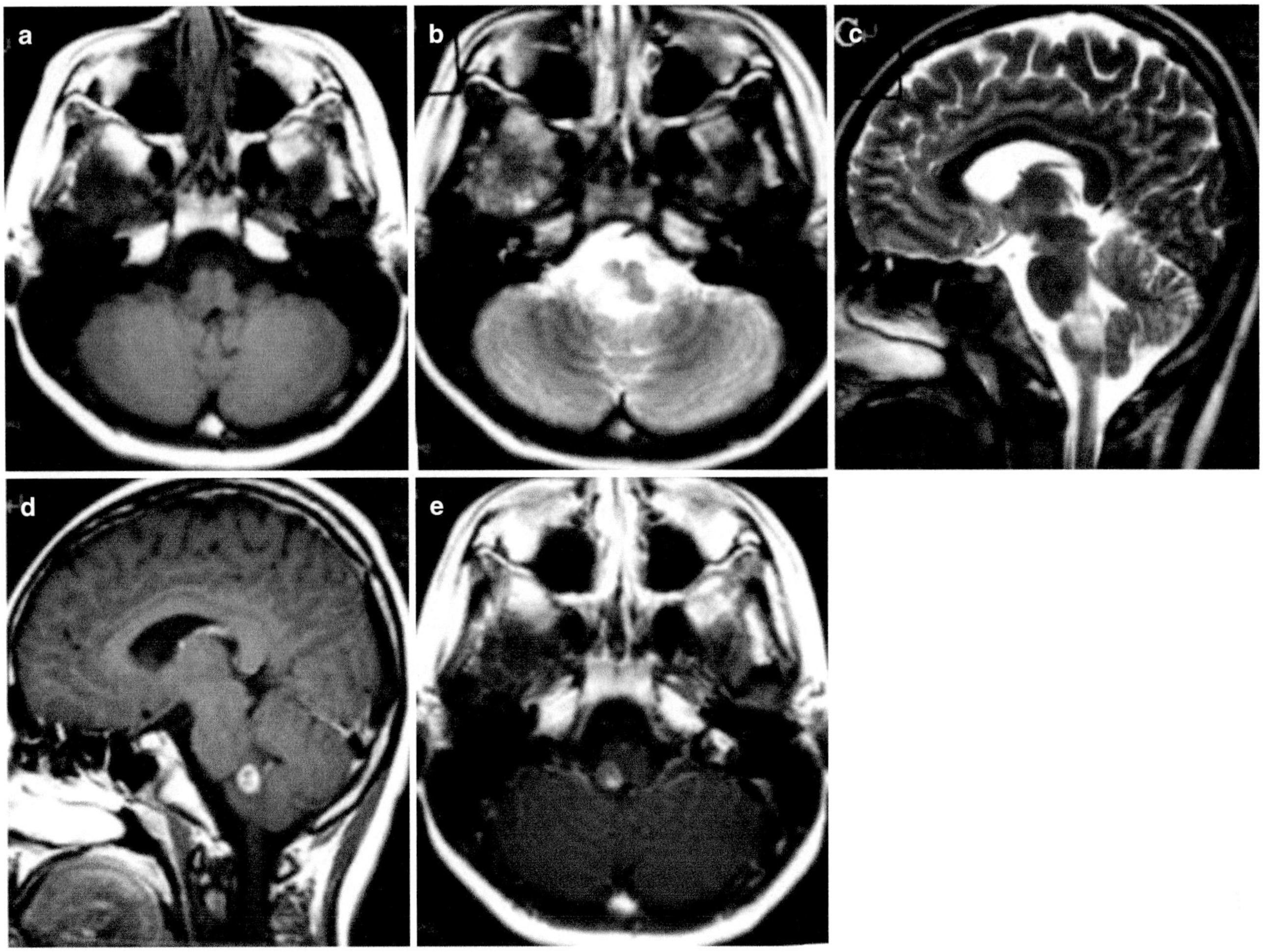

Fig. 8.4 Cerebritis. (**a**, **b**) The lesion is located in the right inferior cerebellar peduncle, which is hypointense signal on axial T1WI (**a**) and hyperintense signal on axial (**b**) and sagittal (**c**) T2WI; the lesion is indistinguishable from around edema. (**c**) Diffusion-weighted sequence demonstrates central hyperintense signal. (**d**) On sagittal (**d**) and axial (**e**) post-contrast T1-weighted MR imaging, the lesion demonstrates mild rim enhancement

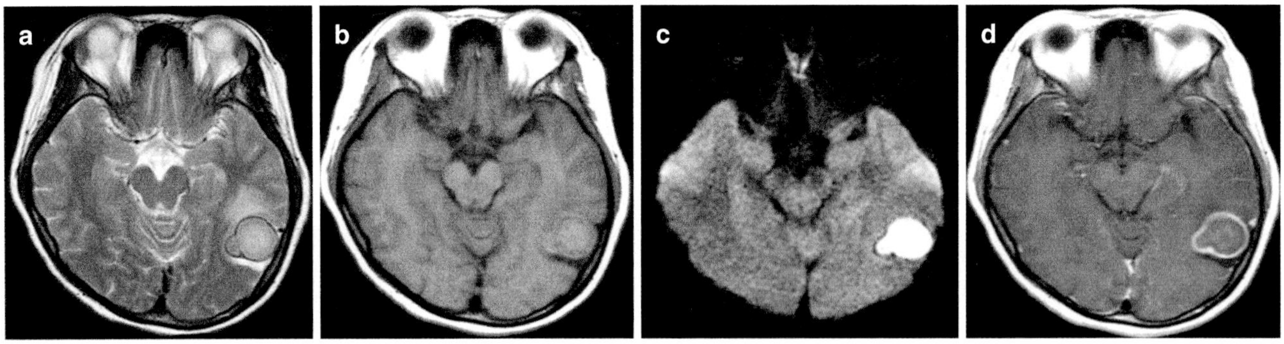

Fig. 8.5 Brain abscess. The lesion is located in the left temporal lobe, which margin is hypointensity on T2WI (**a**) and isointensity on T1WI (**b**). (**c**) Diffusion-weighted sequence demonstrates central hyperintense signal. (**d**) On axial post-contrast T1-weighted MR imaging, the lesion demonstrates rim enhancement

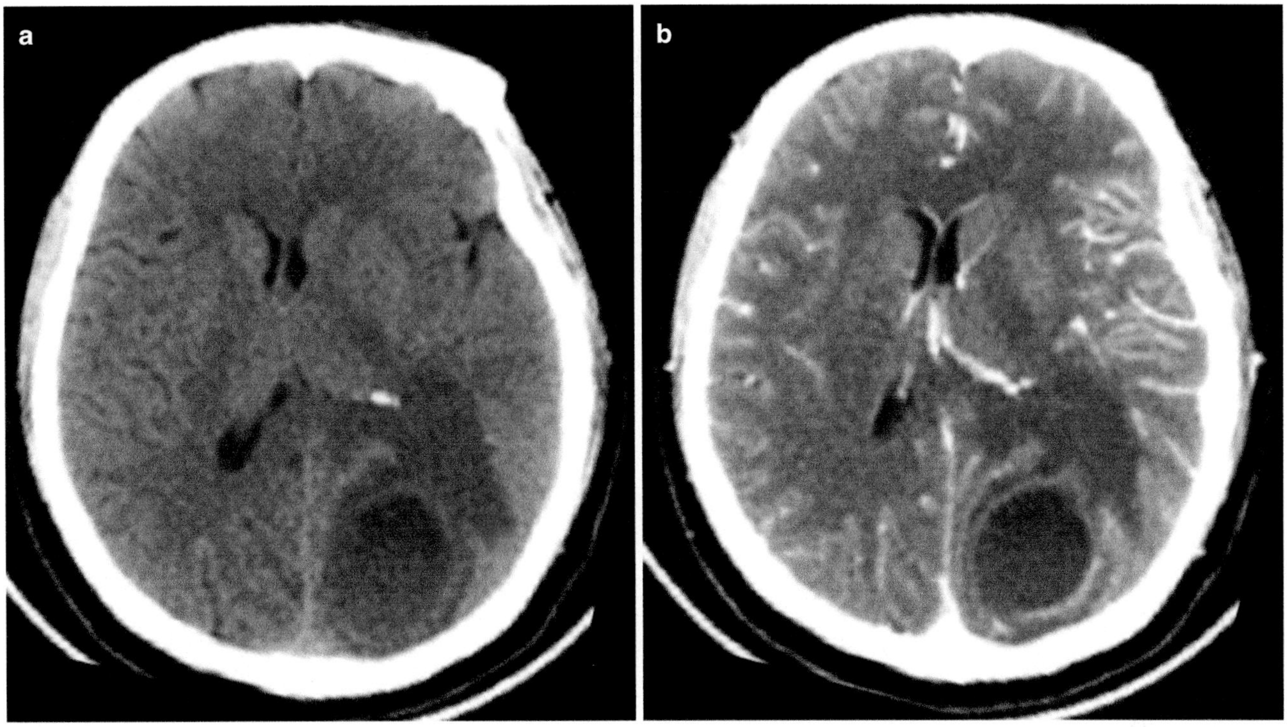

Fig. 8.6 Left occipital lobe abscess. (**a**) A hyperattenuated round area is demonstrated on pre-contrast CT image. (**b**) Post-contrast CT image reveals a well-defined ringlike enhancement corresponding to abscess, with central necrosis and peripheral edema

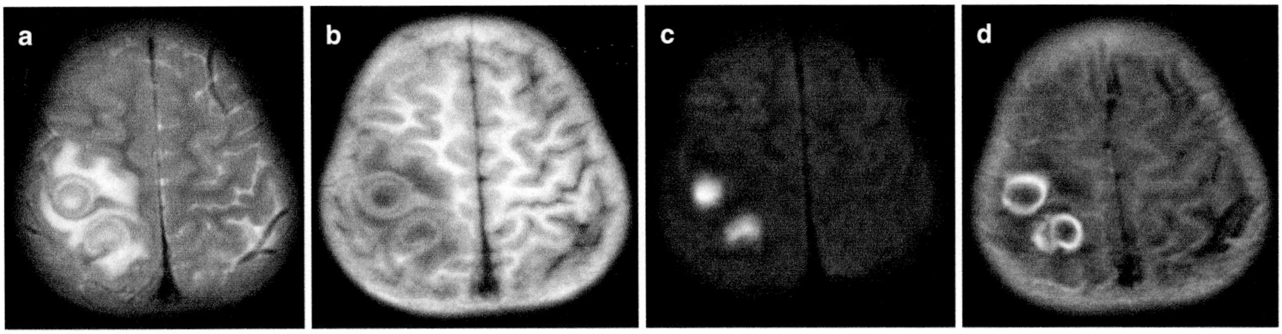

Fig. 8.7 Right parietal lobe abscess. The wall of abscess is hyperintense and is divided into three layers, and the pus cavity is hypointense on T2WI (**a**, **b**). Corresponding DWI sequence confirms restricted diffusion within the abscess cavity (**c**). Axial T1 post-contrast sequence demonstrates typical smooth ring enhancement of abscess (**d**)

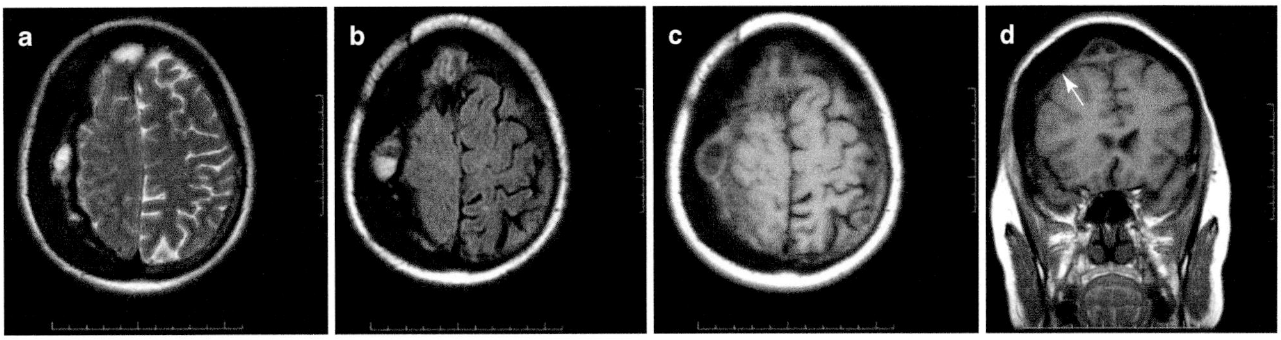

Fig. 8.8 Epidural empyema. (**a**, **b**) Axial MR image shows an extra-axial crescentic mass along the ventral frontal margin with hyperintense signal on T2WI and hypointense signal on T1WI. (**c**) Axial DWI shows hyperintensity in the mass. (**d**) Coronal T1WI shows the epidural empyema crossing the midline, superficial to the superior sagittal sinus (arrow), a finding that confirms an epidural location

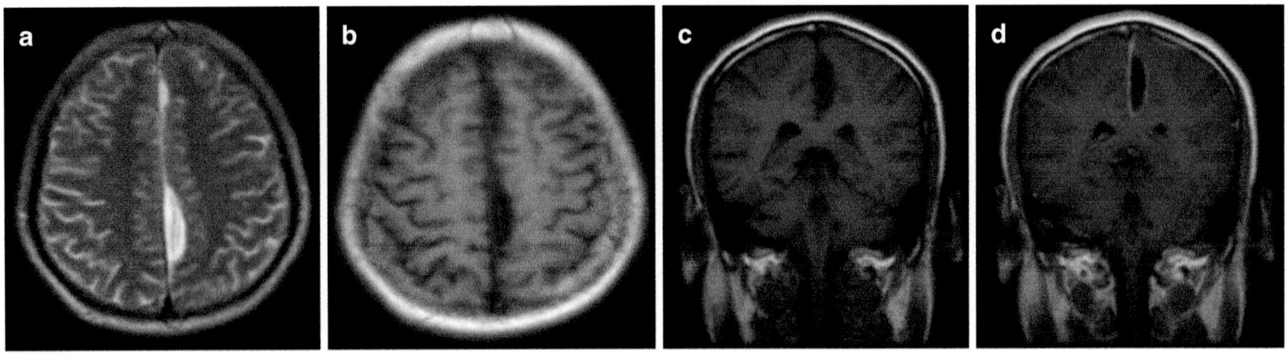

Fig. 8.9 Epidural empyema. (**a**, **b**) Axial MR image shows an extra-axial crescentic mass next to the cerebral falx with hyperintense signal on T2WI and hypointense signal on T1WI. (**c**, **d**) Coronal T1WI pre-contrast and post-contrast sequences demonstrate an epidural empyema

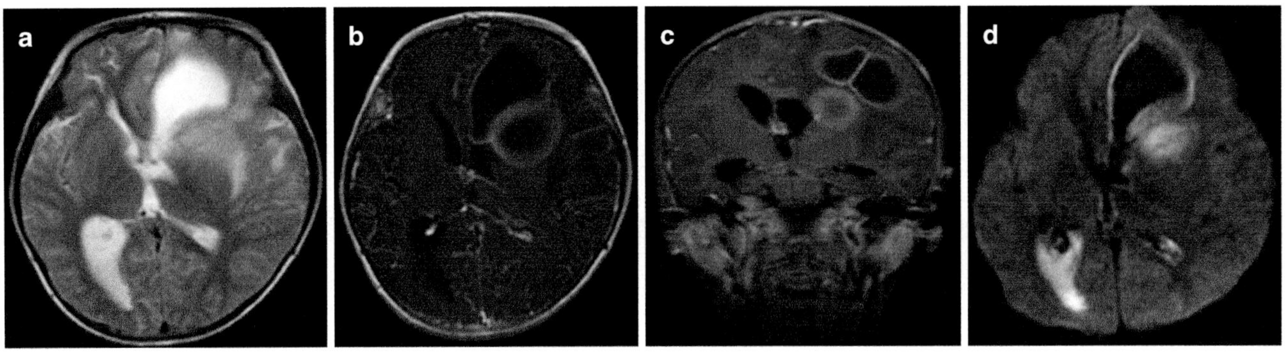

Fig. 8.10 Intraventricular rupture of abscess and ventriculitis. Axial T2WI and coronal T1 post-contrast images demonstrate multiple bilateral abscesses communicated with the ventricular system (**a**–**c**). (**d**) DWI sequence confirms intraventricular rupture and ventriculitis, with debris layering dependently in the ventricular system

The symptom and process of epidural abscess are insidious and benign, due to the empyema being localized outside the dura mater. The CT and MR image features are the same as subdural empyemas, except the shape of convex.

Ventriculitis

Ventriculitis is a common complication of meningitis or caused by the rupture of brain abscess into adjacent ventricular system. FLAIR and DWI are sensitive for demonstrating increased signal of pus in the ventricular system. After contrast agent injected intravenously, both CT and MR images show line-like enhancement of ependyma (Figs. 8.10 and 8.11).

As mentioned before, DWI is helpful in distinguishing pyogenic abscess from other ring-enhancing lesions such as primary neoplasm, metastasis, and hematoma. The central non-enhancing portion of brain abscess usually demonstrates restricted diffusion, while other ring-enhancing lesions demonstrate facilitated diffusion, which is a characteristic but not pathognomonic feature of brain abscess. In the meanwhile, the apparent diffusion coefficient (ADC) values on the ADC map are reduced. ^{1}H-MR spectroscopy may complement DWI and conventional MR imaging. The necrotic fluid of bacterial abscess in late stage lacks normal brain metabolites such as N-acetylaspartate (NAA), choline, and creatine. Meanwhile, the increased peak values of cytosolic amino acids (0.9 ppm) and lactate (1.3 ppm) are the characteristics of untreated pyogenic abscess, accompanied with or without acetate (1.9 ppm) and succinate (2.4 ppm) [5]. When cytosolic amino acids (valine, leucine, and isoleucine) are present, it is an important feature of pyogenic abscess [6]. Neuroimaging is most useful for excluding herniation and detecting complications, such as hydrocephalus, pyocephalus (Fig. 8.10), venous thrombosis, or parenchymal or subdural infection.

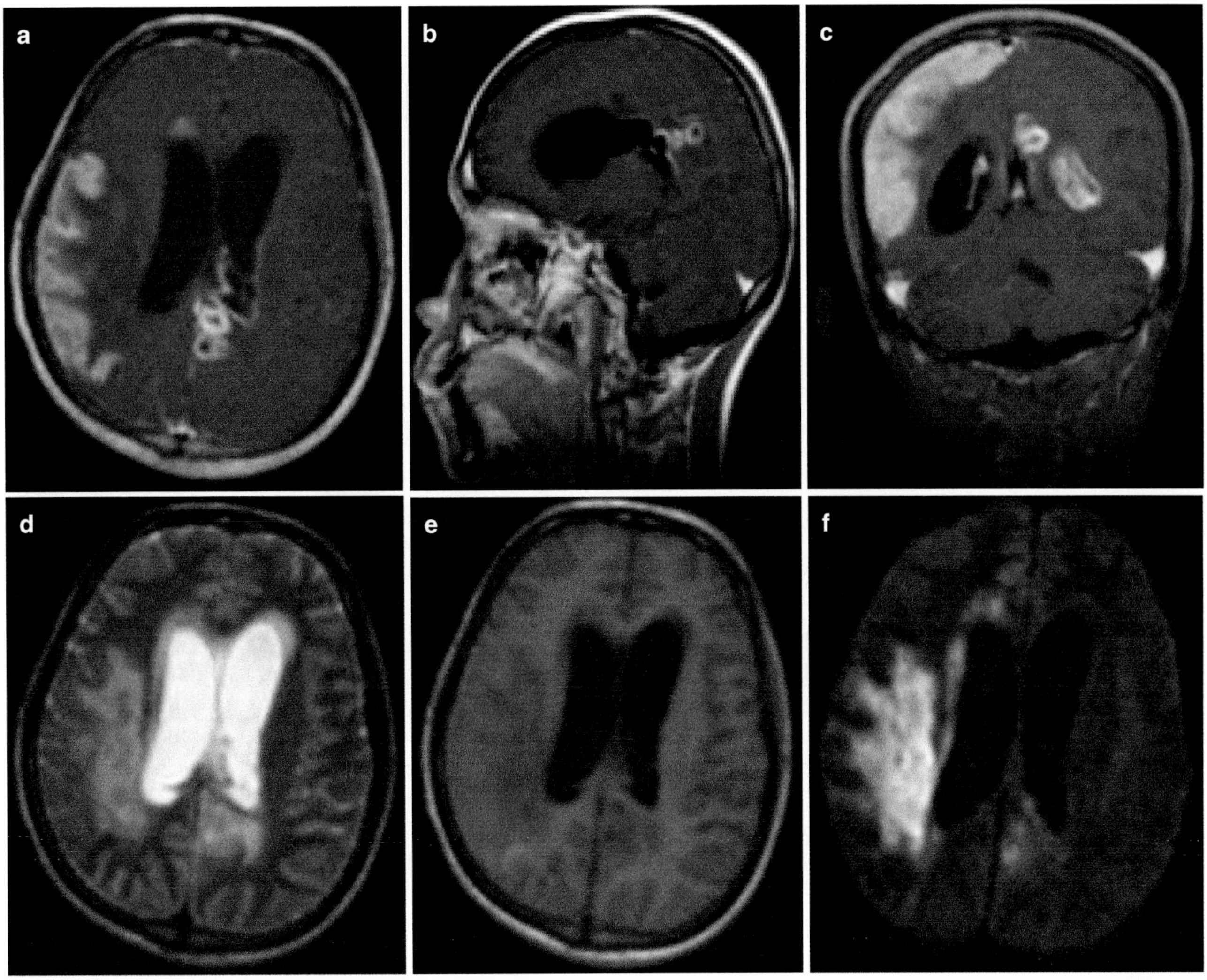

Fig. 8.11 Intraventricular rupture of abscess, ventriculitis, and vasculitis. Axial T2WI, T1WI, and DWI show multiple bilateral abscesses next to the lateral ventricle (**a**–**c**). T1W post-contrast images confirm the ventriculitis with the ventricular enhancement of left ventricle and the vasculitis with the gyriform enhancement of right temporal lobe (**d**–**f**)

8.2 Central Nervous System Tuberculosis

8.2.1 Introduction

Central nervous system disease due to *Mycobacterium tuberculosis* is highly disastrous, although its incidence seems to have decreased recently. According to the World Health Organization (WHO) report, 1.3 million deaths were caused by TB in 2008. Among all other forms of TB, CNS TB accounts for about 1% and has the highest mortality [7]. Although diagnostic assessment includes various biochemical investigations, molecular and microbiological pathologic imaging modalities have an important diagnostic value. Imaging helps in early diagnosis as well as in preventing morbidity and mortality. Imaging is essential in showing complications besides diagnosis of CNS TB.

8.2.2 Pathophysiology

Mycobacterium tuberculosis is the most common organism causing tuberculous infection of CNS. It usually recruits mononuclear phagocytes (monocytes) instead of lacking suppuration, which mature into organized collections of macrophages (granulomas) in chronic disease process. Granulomas with caseating necrosis are typical of tuberculosis, which is probably the prototypical atypical bacterial infection. During the initial pulmonary infection, tuberculous bacteria may enter the systemic circulation and subsequently reach the oxygen-rich CNS, establishing a focus called the Rich focus. This kind of focus may be located in the subpial, meninges, or subependymal region of the spinal cord or brain. Later, this may rupture into the ventricular system or subarachnoid space leading to meningitis. The probability of the organism reaching the brain depends on the immune response of the host and the extent of bacteremia. Meninges may be secondarily involved because of rupture of miliary tubercles in miliary TB or rupture of a tuberculoma into a vessel in the subarachnoid space. There can be adjacent spread of infection from the contiguous bone, but this is uncommon. Cell-mediated immunity is responsible for the formation of gelatinous, dense, inflammatory exudate along the basal surface of the cerebrum. Severe cases may display leptomeningeal involvement over the cerebral convexities and extension into the ventricular system, which can cause ependymitis and choroid plexitis. Parenchymal tuberculous focus can develop into brain abscess or tuberculoma in the presence of a sizable tuberculous focus or in the absence of adequate immunity.

8.2.3 Clinical Features

Adults with tuberculous meningitis (TBM) can often present with the classic meningitis symptoms of fever, stiff neck, and headache along with behavioral changes, alterations in consciousness, and focal neurological deficits. Children with TBM often present with fever, seizures, stiff neck, and abdominal symptoms such as vomiting and nausea. Depending on the stage of presentation, neurological symptoms range from agitation and lethargy to coma. Cranial nerve palsies occur in 20–30% of patients and may be the presenting clinical manifestation of TBM. The sixth cranial nerve is most commonly involved [8]. Vision loss resulted from optic nerve involvement may occasionally be a dominant presenting illness. Third ventricular compression of optic chiasma (if hydrocephalus develops), optic nerve granuloma, and optochiasmatic arachnoiditis are possible factors for vision loss in these patients.

8.2.4 Imaging Features

Imaging of CNS TB can be divided into tuberculous meningitis (TBM) and parenchymal TB (including tuberculous abscess, tuberculomas, tuberculous encephalopathy, tuberculous cerebritis).

TBM

The most specific CT feature for TBM is hyperdensity in the basal cisterns on plain scan (Fig. 8.12). The most sensitive feature of TBM is basal enhancement (Fig. 8.13). Presence of infarction on the non-contrast and hydrocephalus is as specific as pre-contrast hyperdensity in the basal cisterns but has a lower sensitivity [7, 8].

Non-contrast MR imaging displays little or no evidence of meningitis in the early stages. Mild shortening of T1 and T2 relaxation times of cerebrospinal fluid occurs as the disease progresses. Compared with contrast-enhanced CT and non-contrast MR imaging, contrast-enhanced MR imaging has the extra advantage of showing meningitis and its associated complications. Abnormal meningeal enhancement is seen in the Sylvian fissures and basal cisterns (Fig. 8.14); late-stage

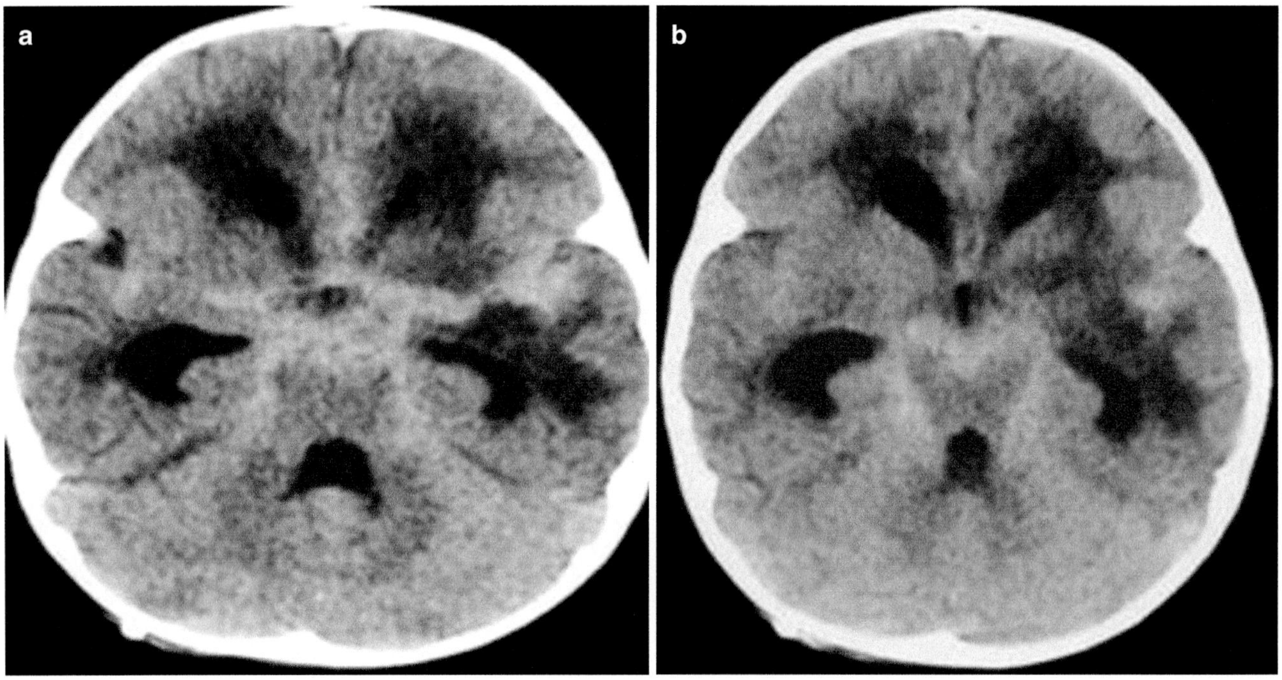

Fig. 8.12 Hyperdense exudates on non-contrast CT. (**a**) Non-contrast CT scans show hyperdense material occupying the suprasellar and middle cerebral artery cisterns. (**b**) The ambient and Sylvian cisterns are also involved. There is associated hydrocephalus with periventricular lucency

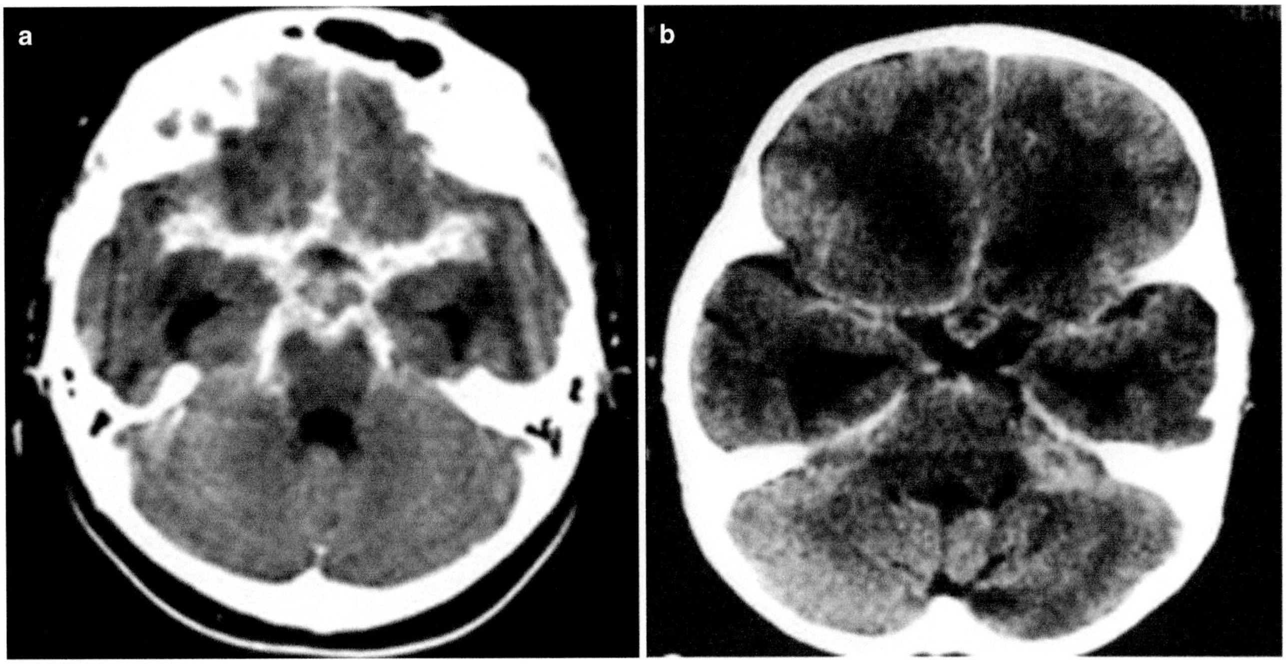

Fig. 8.13 Objective criteria for determining the presence of basal enhancement. (**a**) Contrast medium filling the cisterns with obliteration of CSF that surrounds normal vascular enhancement. (**b**) Enhancement of the posterior aspect of the infundibular recess of the third ventricle in the suprasellar cistern. There is no known vessel that lies here that can be confused with meningeal enhancement

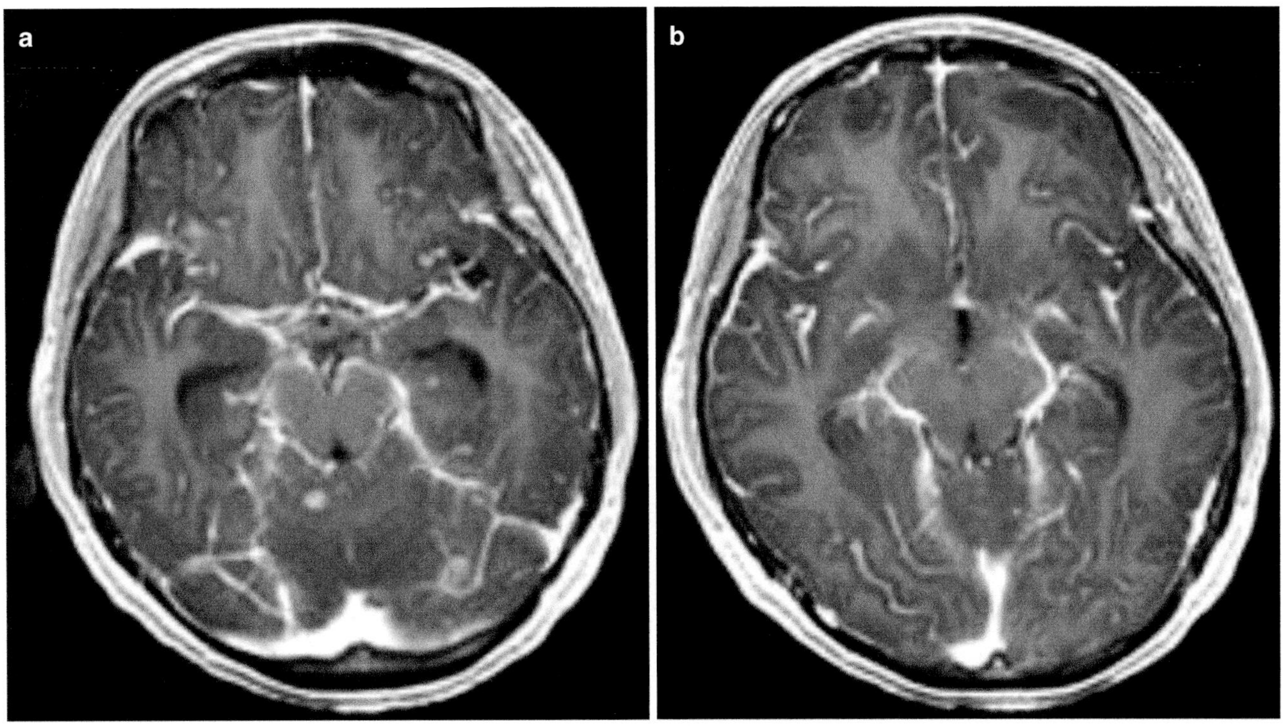

Fig. 8.14 Tuberculous meningitis. Fat-saturated post-contrast T1-weighted (T1W) images (**a**, **b**) show abnormal meningeal enhancement along the basal cisterns and interpeduncular cistern

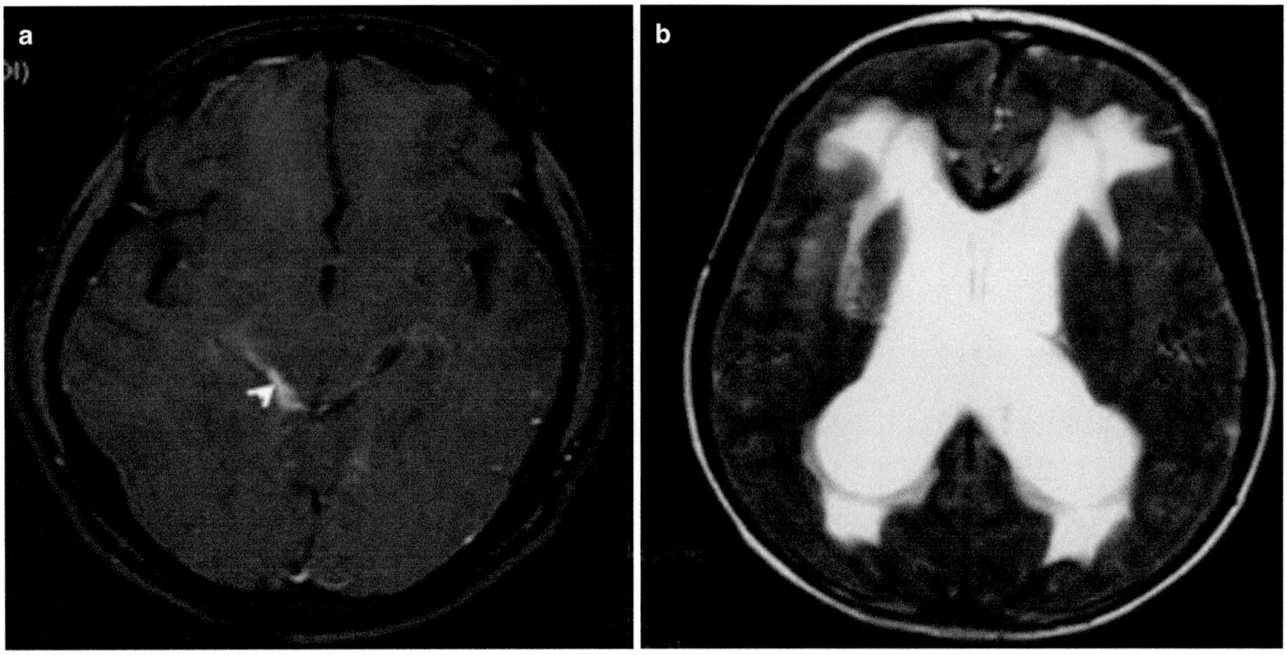

Fig. 8.15 Border zone encephalitis. (**a**) Post-contrast T1W image shows abnormal enhancement along the right perimesencephalic cistern (arrowhead) CNS tuberculoma (single or multiple). (**b**) T2WI shows moderate communicating hydrocephalus with periventricular hyperintensity

and severe TBM can show enhancement over the convexities. Tentorial and cerebellar meningeal involvement is less common [9]. The brain parenchyma immediately adjacent to the inflammatory exudate shows edema, a microglial reaction, and perivascular infiltration, known as border zone reaction (Fig. 8.15a). Hydrocephalus can be communicating, noncommunicating, or complex in patients with TBM [10–12]. It occurs because of obstruction to cerebrospinal fluid flow in the basal cisterns by inflammatory exudate (Fig. 8.15b). Vasculitis with cranial nerve involvement and infarct in TBM are seen in some of patients.

Tuberculomas

Tuberculomas are among the most common manifestations of parenchymal TB and the most common intracranial TB mass lesions. Imaging findings depend on the stage of tuberculoma, whether it is caseating or noncaseating with liquid or solid center. Solid noncaseating granuloma is slightly hypodense or isodense to the surrounding brain parenchyma on CT. A central calcification on pre-contrast images or nidus surrounded by ring enhancement on post-contrast images is considered pathognomonic of tuberculoma. Miliary tuberculomas are usually associated with meningitis, and most of these patients inevitably have primary pulmonary infection. On MR imaging, solid noncaseating granuloma shows hypointense on both T1WI and T2WI and homogeneous enhancement on post-contrast scans (Fig. 8.16). A caseating granuloma usually shows isointense to hypointense on both T1WI and T2WI and isointense to hyperintense rim on T2WI. It shows rim enhancement on post-contrast images (Fig. 8.17). Miliary tuberculomas may not be seen on conventional spin-echo images or usually seen as tiny hyperintense foci on T2W images. They show homogeneous enhancement on post-contrast images. Liquid caseating lesions show restricted diffusion, whereas solid caseating lesions do not reveal restriction of diffusion on DWI. MR spectroscopy is specific for the diagnosis of tuberculoma [13, 14]. In vivo spectroscopy shows only a lipid peak in lesions with a T2 hypointense center, whereas those with heterogeneous appearance reveal a choline peak at 3.22 ppm in addition to lipid.

Tuberculous Cerebritis and Tuberculous Encephalopathy

Tuberculous cerebritis is not a usual clinicoradiological pattern scene in patients without AIDS. Marked focal gyral enhancement with associated edema can be seen on maps. Tuberculous protein causes a delayed type IV hypersensitivity reaction with an immunologic mechanism, which prompts tuberculous encephalopathy to occur. Significant brain edema, which sometimes seriously affects cerebral hemisphere, can be showed on images [15].

Tuberculous Abscess

Imaging findings are often nonspecific. Large, usually multiloculated, ring-enhancing lesions, which accompany with perilesion edema and mass effect, are apparent. Central liquid caseation of tuberculous abscess is similar to granuloma. The diameter of abscesses, with thin walls, is usually >3 cm on imaging, which are often multiloculated and solitary.

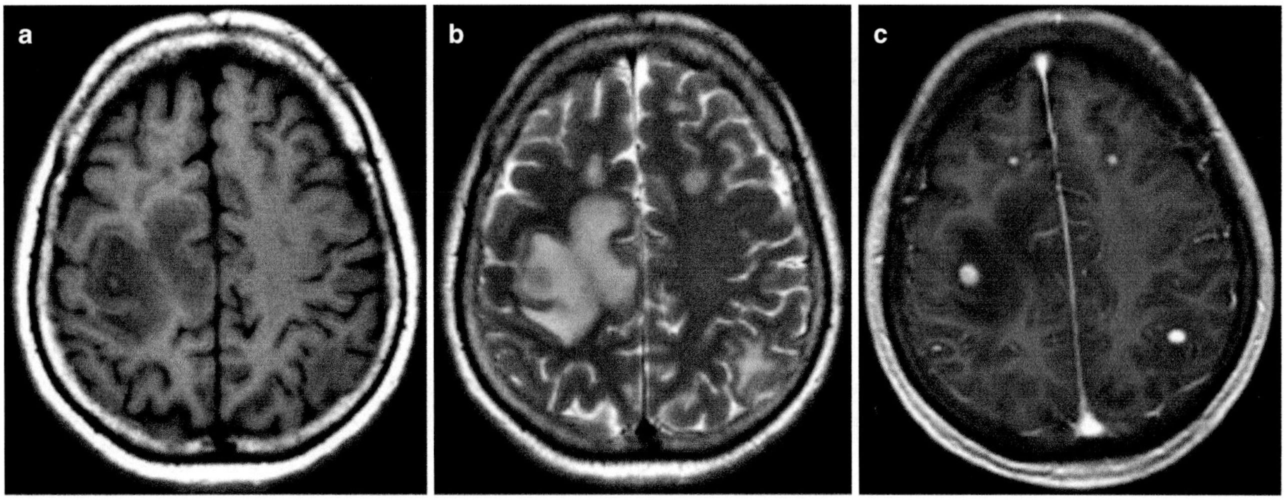

Fig. 8.16 Noncaseating disc-enhancing tuberculoma. Axial T1W (**a**) and T2W (**b**) images show an oval isointense lesion in the right frontal lobe that shows solid disc enhancement on post-contrast axial T1W image (**c**)

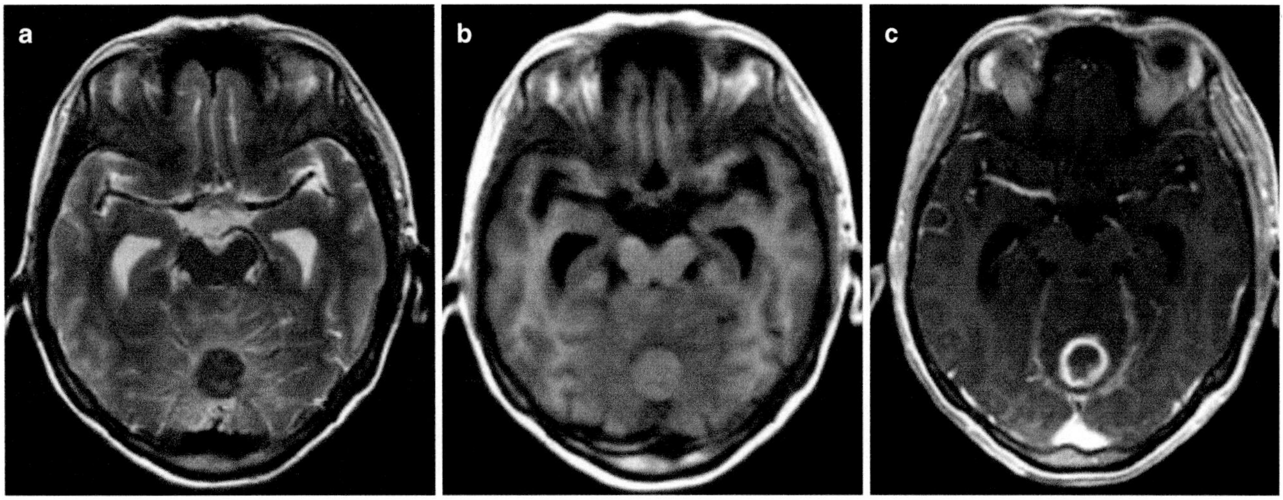

Fig. 8.17 Ring-enhancing typical tuberculoma. Axial T2W (**a**) and T1W (**b**) images show an oval hypointense lesion in the vermis cerebelli region. It shows ring enhancement on post-contrast axial (**c**)

It restricts water diffusion on DWI, accompanying low apparent diffusion coefficient (ADC) values. MR spectroscopy is useful to detection of tuberculous abscess and those of pyogenic and fungal causes. In contrast with pyogenic abscess, MR spectroscopy reveals lipid, lactate, and phosphoserine without evidence of cytosolic amino acids [16, 17].

8.3 Spirochete

8.3.1 Introduction

Spirochetes are long, thin, spiral-shaped mononuclear extracellular microorganisms, with a spiral motion caused by their flagella. Three genera of human pathogens are *Treponema*, *Borrelia*, and *Leptospira*. Syphilis and Lyme disease are the most commonly encountered diseases caused by *Treponema pallidum* and *Borrelia burgdorferi*, respectively. *Treponema pallidum* is sexually transmitted by direct inoculation at cutaneous or membranous sites, but it can also be transmitted transplacentally or by blood transfusion. The treatment of penicillin is sensitive to this disease; clinical recovery can be achieved in early syphilis. Despite this, the incidence continues to rise. This is a result of increased travel, the sex industry, and human immunodeficiency syndrome (HIV).

Lyme borreliosis is a multisystemic infectious disease caused by the spirochete *Borrelia burgdorferi*. First described in 1977 by Steere and colleagues, Lyme disease has been increasingly recognized in the Eastern United States as well as certain areas of the Pacific Northwest and Midwest. This disease is transmitted to human by the bite of infected ticks, characterized by skin rash and neurologic and arthritic findings. Most of the Lyme diseases are exposed in May to July when the nymphal stage of the ticks is most active.

8.3.2 Pathophysiology

Pathologically, syphilis infection in CNS mainly presents leptomeningeal and perivascular inflammation with predominant lymphocyte infiltration. Vascular neurosyphilis occurred as two types of vascular involvement: Heubner endarteritis and Nissl-Alzheimer endarteritis. The mechanism of Heubner endarteritis is fibroblastic proliferation of intima, thinning of the tunica media, and adventitial inflammatory changes. This endarteritis affects large- and medium-sized arteries, resulting in an irregular luminal narrowing and ectasia. Nissl-Alzheimer type of arteritis is characterized by thickening of the adventitia more than the endothelium, typically affecting small vessels. The pathological change of gummas mainly revealed mononuclear epithelial and fibroblastic cells with occasional giant cells and perivasculitis, generally appeared as circumscribed mass of granulation tissue. In tabetic neurosyphilis, the inflammation is mostly in the middle posterior and dorsal roots with interstitial neuritis. In paretic neurosyphilis, the inflammation varies from mild to severe, which is severer in the frontal and temporal lobes, milder in subcortical white matter and the dorsal hemispheres, and absent in the occipital lobe. Chronic inflammation can result in tissue injury, fibrosis, and thickening of meninges and blood vessels. Fibrosis is severer around the optic nerve and chiasm.

Borrelia burgdorferi has a predisposition for hematogenous dissemination and may cause lymphocytic arthritis and meningitis. The underlying neuropathophysiology is still unclear. For CNS injury, several mechanisms including direct cytotoxicity, secretion of neurotoxic mediators, or triggered autoimmune reactions are proposed. Migration of the spirochetes along the peripheral nerves is an alternative route. Localized LNB-associated inflammation usually occurs in the dorsal root ganglia, nerve roots, or leptomeninges with the infiltration of T-lymphocytes and plasma cells, not in the brain parenchyma.

8.3.3 Clinical Features

As a chronic infection, syphilis usually occurs through three well-characterized stages. The first stage is presented with a painless hard chancre at the point of inoculation and painless regional lymphadenopathy. If left untreated, a maculopapular rash can present on the palms of the hand and soles of the feet by hematological dissemination in a secondary stage. This rash is usually seen in 2–8 weeks after the chancre appears. About one-third of patients with secondary syphilis progress to tertiary syphilis. The tertiary stage usually occurs after a latent period of at least 5 years and mainly presents with cardiovascular syphilis, neurosyphilis, or syphilitic gummas. Neurosyphilis occurs at tertiary stage more commonly than any other stage of systemic infection. Approximately one-third of tertiary syphilis can develop to neurosyphilis, and about one-third of neurosyphilis cases can be asymptomatic. Meningovascular neurosyphilis and paretic and tabetic neurosyphilis are symptomatic syphilis. Meningeal neurosyphilis usually occurs within the first 2 years after infection and may present headache, meningeal signs, and cranial nerve palsies. The seventh and eighth cranial nerves are most frequently involved; facial paralysis, sensorineural hearing loss, and vertigo mainly are presented. Syphilitic gummas are another manifestation of meningovascular neurosyphilis. Vascular neurosyphilis usually occurs around 5–10 years after infection and presents headache, vertigo, and commonly ischemic syndrome in a young adult. Paretic neurosyphilis usually occurs in 10–20 years after the initial infection. The parenchymal damage may lead to modification of personality, delusions, hallucinations, loss of memory, and judgment. Tabetic neurosyphilis usually presents with dysuria, ataxia, areflexia, and loss of proprioception, with a latent period of 15–20 years.

Similar to syphilis, Lyme disease develops with three main stages clinically: early localized disease, early disseminated disease, and persisting late disease. During the early stage, spirochetes multiply in the dermis at the site of the tick bite and later spread centrifugally. Migrant erythema as characteristic skin lesion and accompanied flu-like symptoms and lymphadenopathy will present in this stage; it usually disappears in 4–12 weeks. In the second stage, lymphocytic meningitis, cranial neuropathy, and arthralgia can occur due to spirochete spread throughout the body. Cardiac disease with conduction defects and myopericarditis can present in some patients. If left untreated, chronic arthritis of large joints, polyneuropathy, and encephalitis can be present in a late disseminated stage generally after 2 or 3 years [18].

8.3.4 Imaging Features

Syphilis

On meningeal neurosyphilis, meningeal and cranial nerve enhancement can be present, most frequently involving the seventh and eighth nerve in basilar meningitis.

Neurovasculitis usually presents with focal areas of hyperintensity on T2WI and FLAIR, caused by parenchymal edema and gliosis or related to meningeal inflammation in small vessels and increased permeability of the blood-brain barrier. It can be observed at subcortical white matter, deep white matter or gray matter, but most frequently occurs in the area such as mesiotemporal and limbic system (hippocampus, thalamus, basal ganglia). Bilateral or asymmetrical mesiotemporal

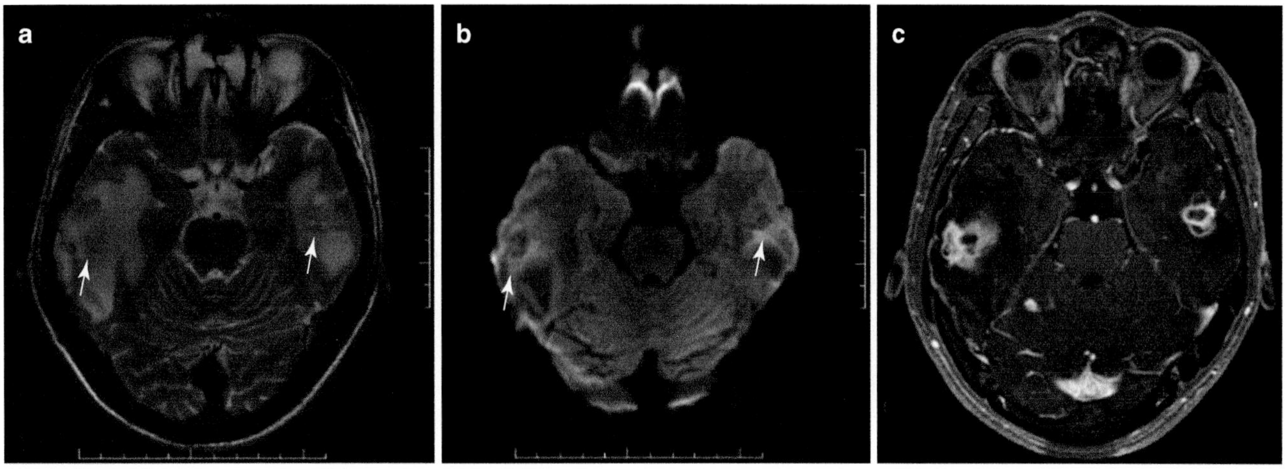

Fig. 8.18 Syphilitic gumma. (**a**) Axial T2-weighted image shows hypointense nodules with significant edema in bilateral temporal lobes (white arrows). (**b**) Diffusion-weighted image reveals restricted diffusion at the edge of the lesions (white arrow). (**c**) Enhanced T1-weighted image shows irregular lesions with irregular enhancing margin in bilateral temporal lobes

hyperintensity on T2WI and FLAIR is difficult to differentiate from the viral limbic encephalitis. Neurosyphilis typically presents with atrophy of the mesiotemporal lobes, differentiated from the global atrophy in viral encephalitis. Multiple areas of infarction in different vascular regions are suggestive of cerebral vasculitis. MR perfusion demonstrates the cerebral perfusion deficits and ischemic lesions. DWI is sensitive to show the ischemic changes. Direct imaging signs of cerebral vasculitis are vessel wall thickening with contrast enhancement, particularly involving the middle cerebral artery and branches of the basilar artery [19, 20].

Gummas usually present as circumscribed solitary or multiple mass lesions with nodular or ring enhancement, usually located on the cerebral convexities of the frontal, temporal, and parietal lobes. Sometimes, associated dural tail sign can be seen (Fig. 8.18). It is difficult to differentiate from other intracranial mass lesions, especially brain neoplasms and tubercular meningitis.

The MRI findings of tabes dorsalis are similar to those seen in subacute combined degeneration, which is characterized by intramedullary hyperintensities in the dorsal roots and posterior spinal columns with no enhancement and cord atrophy.

MRI Findings on Lyme Disease

Many cases of Lyme disease have no obvious neuroimaging findings, even in patients with neurologic symptoms. Similar to syphilis, smooth abnormal leptomeningeal enhancement with cranial or spinal nerve root involvement may be seen, especially the third, fifth, and seventh cranial nerve enhanced. Perivascular extension of the lymphocytic inflammation may lead to foci of T2 prolongation in periventricular, callososeptal, and infratentorial white matter, which is similar to the multiple sclerosis. Basal ganglia and the brain stem may also be involved. Other manifestations like subarachnoid hemorrhage, intracerebral hemorrhage, and rare vasculitis may also be present in some cases. Prominent Virchow-Robin spaces can be seen in pediatric cases.

8.4 Central Nervous System Rickettsiosis

8.4.1 Introduction

Rickettsia is named for Howard Taylor Ricketts, who studied Rocky Mountain spotted fever and then died of another rickettsial illnesses (typhus) while investigating a disease outbreak in Mexico City in 1910 [21]. This disease occurs in a minority of patients for now, although it is often rapid in onset and can be fatal, specially rickettsiosis in the central nervous system (CNS). So some characteristic imaging findings play an important role in the early determination of CNS rickettsiosis.

8.4.2 Pathophysiology

Rickettsia is a third kingdom of atypical bacteria, which is a genus of obligate intracellular pathogens that phylogenetically occupy a position between bacteria and viruses. *Rickettsia* causes diseases in humans and animals, to which it is transmitted by arthropod vectors such as fleas, lice, mites, or ticks [22]. Hematogenous dissemination of the organism and subsequent invasion of the endothelium of the arterioles and capillaries are participated in the pathophysiological mechanism of rickettsial infection of the CNS. *Rickettsia* causes meningitis with diffuse systemic small-vessel thrombovasculitis.

8.4.3 Clinical Features

An abrupt onset of high-grade fever, rash, and unremitting headache are the classic clinical triad. The neurological manifestations including lethargy, altered consciousness, confusion, disorientation, headache, ataxia, aphasia, paralysis, seizure, stupor, and coma are altered [23].

8.4.4 Imaging Features

CT Findings
The head CT without contrast agent is interpreted as normal. Contrast-enhanced CT images show diffuse leptomeningeal enhancement.

MRI Findings
Abnormal multiple punctate high signal intensity foci in the subcortical and deep white matter scatter bilaterally, particularly in a perivascular distribution, which can be found on T2WI and FLAIR images can occur, but this finding is nonspecific. The largest number of the nidus is high signal intensity on DWI, resembling a scene of a "starry sky" [24]. Contrast-enhanced T1-weighted MR images show diffuse leptomeningeal enhancement. MR imaging is sensitive for detection of meningeal enhancement, different degrees of cerebral edema, and/or focal regions of periventricular and subcortical infarction secondary to concomitant vasculitis.

Rickettsial infection shares common imaging findings with many other infections, so additional laboratory examination, specifically CSF analysis, is required to initiate confirmation of the rickettsial disease [24].

References

1. Britt RH, Enzmann DR. Clinical stages of human brain abscesses on serial CT scans after contrast infusion. Computerized tomographic, neuropathological, and clinical correlations. J Neurosurg. 1983;59(6):972–89.
2. Mathisen GE, Johnson JP. Brain abscess. Clin Infect Dis. 1997;25(4):763–79. quiz 80-1.
3. Bartt R. Acute bacterial and viral meningitis. Continuum (Minneap Minn). 2012;18(6 Infectious Disease):1255–70.
4. Singer MB, Atlas SW, Drayer BP. Subarachnoid space disease: diagnosis with fluid-attenuated inversion-recovery MR imaging and comparison with gadolinium-enhanced spin-echo MR imaging--blinded reader study. Radiology. 1998;208(2):417–22.
5. Pal D, Bhattacharyya A, Husain M, et al. In vivo proton MR spectroscopy evaluation of pyogenic brain abscesses: a report of 194 cases. AJNR Am J Neuroradiol. 2010;31(2):360–6.
6. Grand S, Passaro G, Ziegler A, et al. Necrotic tumor versus brain abscess: importance of amino acids detected at 1H MR spectroscopy--initial results. Radiology. 1999;213(3):785–93.
7. Moodley M, Bamber S. The operculum syndrome: an unusual complication of tuberculous meningitis. Dev Med Child Neurol. 1990;32(10):919–22.
8. Hosoglu S, Ayaz C, Geyik MF, et al. Tuberculous meningitis in adults: an eleven-year review. Int J Tuberc Lung Dis. 1998;2(7):553–7.
9. Kioumehr F, Dadsetan MR, Rooholamini SA, et al. Central nervous system tuberculosis: MRI. Neuroradiology. 1994;36(2):93–6.
10. Lamprecht D, Schoeman J, Donald P, et al. Ventriculoperitoneal shunting in childhood tuberculous meningitis. Br J Neurosurg. 2001;15(2):119–25.
11. Saremi F, Helmy M, Farzin S, et al. MRI of cranial nerve enhancement. AJR Am J Roentgenol. 2005;185(6):1487–97.
12. Shah GV. Central nervous system tuberculosis: imaging manifestations. Neuroimaging Clin N Am. 2000;10(2):355–74.
13. Harisinghani MG, McLoud TC, Shepard JA, et al. Tuberculosis from head to toe. Radiographics. 2000;20(2):449–70. quiz 528-9, 32.
14. Nogami K, Nomura S, Kashiwagi S, et al. Fluid-attenuated inversion-recovery imaging of cerebral infarction associated with tuberculous meningitis. Comput Med Imaging Graph. 2000;24(5):333–7.
15. Gupta RK, Haris M, Husain N, et al. Relative cerebral blood volume is a measure of angiogenesis in brain tuberculoma. J Comput Assist Tomogr. 2007;31(3):335–41.
16. Kumar R, Pandey CK, Bose N, et al. Tuberculous brain abscess: clinical presentation, pathophysiology and treatment (in children). Childs Nerv Syst. 2002;18(3-4):118–23.
17. Saxena S, Prakash M, Kumar S, et al. Comparative evaluation of magnetization transfer contrast and fluid attenuated inversion recovery sequences in brain tuberculoma. Clin Radiol. 2005;60(7):787–93.
18. Akgoz A, Mukundan S, Lee TC. Imaging of rickettsial, spirochetal, and parasitic infections. Neuroimaging Clin N Am. 2012;22(4):633–57.
19. Saunderson RB, Chan RC. Mesiotemporal changes on magnetic resonance imaging in neurosyphilis. Intern Med J. 2012;42(9):1057–63.
20. Czarnowska-Cubala M, Wiglusz MS, Cubala WJ, et al. MR findings in neurosyphilis--a literature review with a focus on a practical approach to neuroimaging. Psychiatr Danub. 2013;25(Suppl 2):S153–7.
21. Shih RY, Koeller KK. Bacterial, Fungal, and parasitic infections of the central nervous system: radiologic-pathologic correlation and historical perspectives. Radiographics. 2015;35(4):1141–69.
22. Novakova M, Costa FB, Krause F, et al. Rickettsia vini n. sp. (Rickettsiaceae) infecting the tick Ixodes arboricola (Acari: Ixodidae). Parasit Vectors. 2016;9:469.
23. Crapp S, Harrar D, Strother M, et al. Rocky Mountain spotted fever: 'starry sky' appearance with diffusion-weighted imaging in a child. Pediatr Radiol. 2012;42(4):499–502.
24. Lim CC, Sitoh YY, Hui F, et al. Nipah viral encephalitis or Japanese encephalitis? MR findings in a new zoonotic disease. AJNR Am J Neuroradiol. 2000;21(3):455–61.

Parasitic Infections

9

Tijiang Zhang, Xiaoxi Chen, Yanan Wang, and Zhen Zeng

9.1 Neurocysticercosis

9.1.1 Etiology and Epidemiology

Cysticercosis is a common parasitic infection of the central nervous system (CNS) caused by the larval form of the pork tapeworm *Taenia solium*. This parasite is widely distributed around the world, particularly in South American and Far Eastern areas. It is prevalent in the northeastern, northern, northwestern, and southwestern regions of China. Humans are the only definitive host for this tapeworm. The adult worm attaches itself in the gastrointestinal tract of humans.

9.1.2 Pathology and Pathogenesis

Tapeworm infection is usually asymptomatic. Tapeworm eggs passed in the feces are ingested by pigs, wild boars, or other intermediate hosts where the development of the cysticerci is completed. If the infected pork is eaten by a human, the cysticerci remain in the intestinal tract and grow to adulthood. However, when humans directly ingest the eggs, they become the intermediate host in the life cycle of this tapeworm, and the eggs will develop into cysticerci inside the human body. Cysticerci can be disseminated to various parts of the body through the bloodstream, especially to the brain, muscle, and subcutaneous tissue [1–3]. Cysticerci that lodge in the brain cause neurocysticercosis.

The cysticercus is oval in shape and filled with transparent fluid. The diameter of the cyst is 4–5 mm, and the thickness of the capsule is 0.05–0.1 mm. It has an eccentric scolex, which may reach a length of 2–3 mm. Larvae can lodge in the brain parenchyma, ventricles, and meninges. When the larva is alive, it has no toxic effects on brain tissue and does not cause edema. However, once the larva degenerates or decomposes, tissue edema, inflammatory reaction, glial cell proliferation, and vasculitis develop around the dying parasite. Further degeneration and death of larvae lead to the formation of granuloma or abscesses with diffuse brain edema. When multiple cysticerci lodge in the ventricle (usually the fourth ventricle) with a diameter of up to 3–4 cm, they can easily block the cerebrospinal fluid passage. They also release toxins that stimulate the choroid plexus to secrete more cerebrospinal fluid (CSF), thereby causing hydrocephalus.

Cysticerci in the meninges, usually involving the pia mater and subarachnoid space, are often scattered throughout the basal cistern and sylvian fissure cistern where they induce adhesions and influence CSF circulation. Parenchymal cysticercus evolution can be divided into four stages:

1 Vesicular stage: the larva is alive.
2 Colloidal vesicular stage: the larva degenerates or decomposes, has a thickened capsule, and releases certain metabolites that cause a severe inflammatory reaction and brain edema. Patients may display onset of seizure or local neurologic signs.
3 Granular nodular stage: the necrotic larva continues to shrink and has a thickened capsule and calcified scolex. Brain edema around the parasite decreases or even disappears.
4 Nodular calcified stage: active inflammation and cerebral edema disappear with the formation of necrosis, organization, and calcification of the larva.

9.1.3 Clinical Manifestations

Neurocysticercosis can be seen in patients of any ages; however, it is particularly seen in young adults. Headache and seizures are the most common symptoms . Usually, seizures are the primary or only symptom. Some patients with increased intracranial pressure may have severe headache, nausea, vomiting, blurred vision, or impaired vision.

T. Zhang (✉) · X. Chen · Y. Wang · Z. Zeng
Department of Radiology, Affiliated Hospital of Zunyi Medical University, Zunyi, China

B. Gao et al. (eds.), *Imaging of CNS Infections and Neuroimmunology*, https://doi.org/10.1007/978-981-13-6904-9_9

9.1.4 Imaging

Imaging manifestations depend on the location and number of cysts and the course of disease. Neurocysticercosis is classified into four types according to its location: (1) parenchymal type, (2) ventricular type, (3) meningeal type, and (4) mixed type.

Parenchymal Type

CT and MRI can reflect the pathological changes of the cysticercus at different stages.

Early Stage In the acute stage, the cysticercus is round or oval and pea-sized. Often, there are multiple cysts located in the brain parenchyma, and more cysts are found in the cerebrum than in the cerebellum. The occurrence of these cysts is more common in the cerebral cortex and white matter and less common in the basal ganglia. A large number of cysticerci entering the brain and inducing an inflammatory reaction are referred to as "encephalitis cysticercosis" [4]. CT findings are as follows: if the inflammation is mild and focal, the scan may appear normal. A severe inflammatory reaction can manifest as reduced cerebral hemisphere density, flattened or absent sulci, and narrowed cisterns and ventricles. There is no advantage to using contrast-enhanced CT scans. MRI is more sensitive than CT in detecting cerebral edema caused by mild focal inflammation. The patchy lesion is hypointense on T_1WI and markedly hyperintense on T_2WI and FLAIR. A more severe inflammatory reaction can appear as a considerably low signal on T_1WI and a high signal on T_2WI and FLAIR in the hemispheres with narrowed ventricles and disappeared sulci and cisterns. There is no enhancement or only patchy enhancement.

Middle Stage Three to twelve months after infection, the cysticerci mature, and the cysts are filled with liquid and manifest as a liquid-containing cystic lesion on imaging. CT shows either a single or multiple, small, round or oval cystic low-density areas with a diameter of 0.5–1 cm in the brain parenchyma, with no enhancement. Sometimes, there are varying degrees of peripheral edema and narrowed ventricles without midline shift. Large cystic lesions can present as round, oval, or lobulated cystic low-density areas with mass effect. The CT value is close to that of CSF and, generally, cannot be enhanced. MRI reveals multiple cystic lesions with a diameter of 0.5–1 cm. These lesions are usually located at the gray matter or gray-white matter junction areas and have a signal similar to that of CSF (hypointense on T_1WI and hyperintense on T_2WI, no enhancement). If the larva is alive, there is no edema around the lesion. Sometimes, a visible, small, dot-like protrusion, 1–2 mm in size, can be seen; this is the scolex. Its signal is consistent with that of the brain parenchyma. MRI is superior to CT in observing scolex and polycystic lesions in the cerebral convexity and posterior fossa.

Degeneration or Death Stage In this stage, there is significant inflammation and edema around the larva. CT findings are as follows: The lesion (granuloma or cystic small abscess) manifests as a low-density patch on the edge of the cerebral convexity with nodular or small ring-like enhancements. If the larva is completely degenerated and calcified, and peripheral edema completely disappears, CT will reveal either single or multiple spot-like calcifications in the brain parenchyma. MRI findings are as follows: The patchy lesion is hypointense on T_1WI, hyperintense on T_2WI, and hypointense on FLAIR, with hyperintense edema surrounding it. Sometimes, a slightly hyperintense scolex is visible. The MRI enhancement pattern is similar to that of CT [5]. As the thickened cyst wall alongside protein aggregation can shorten T_1 relaxation time, cyst fluid has higher signal intensity than the CSF on T_1WI and proton density-weighted imaging (PDWI), and the fluid cannot be distinguished from edema on T_2WI MRI. But the cyst wall and scolex have lower signals than edema (Fig. 9.1).

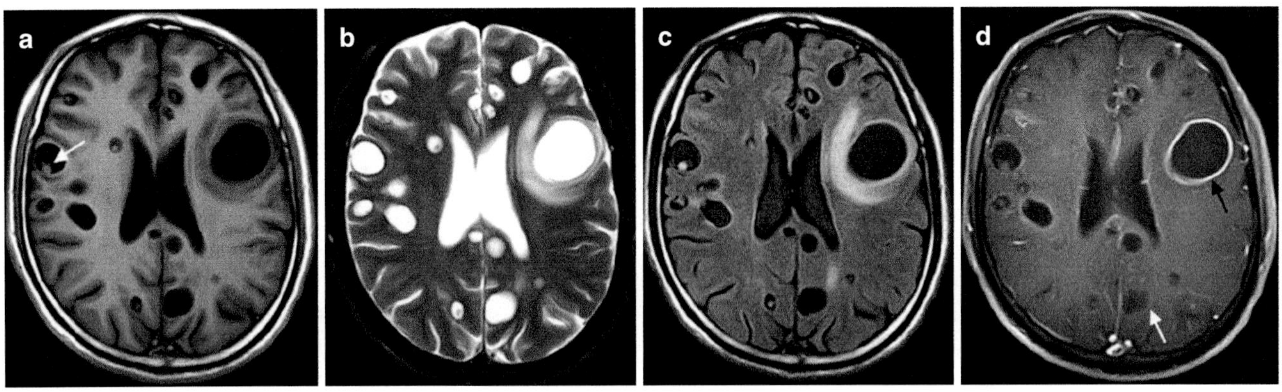

Fig. 9.1 Neurocysticercosis at different stages. MR imaging shows multiple, different-sized, round or oval cystic hypointense on T_1WI and hyperintense on T_2WI in bilateral hemisphere. An eccentric scolex can be seen in some lesions which manifested as mural nodule (**a** white arrow). The lesion located in the left frontal lobe is surrounded by vasogenic edema (**b**, **c**). Axial contrast-enhanced T_1WI shows that lesion in the left frontal lobe is ring-shaped enhancement (**d** black arrow) and some lesions are without enhancements (**d** white arrow)

Ventricular Type

Approximately 15% of larvae are located in the ventricles, especially the fourth ventricle [6]. CT findings are as follows: As the cyst wall is thin and the density of the fluid within it is close to that of CSF, the cyst wall shows no enhancement. Thus, it can sometimes be difficult to identify an intraventricular cyst. Therefore, CT-based diagnosis of intraventricular cysticercosis mainly relies on indirect signs such as local asymmetric enlargement of the ventricle, compression of the choroid plexus, or obstructive hydrocephalus. In rare cases, spherical enhancement or calcification can be seen. MRI is more sensitive than CT at identifying intraventricular cysts, which manifest as round or oval cystic signals similar to that of CSF. Usually, the cyst wall and scolex are visible and the diagnosis is easy. However, it can be difficult to identify a cyst on T_2WI because the signal intensity of fluid within it is similar to that of CSF. Cine MRI can show the flow of CSF around the cyst. The cyst wall can be enhanced after secondary infection [7].

Meningeal Type

Meningeal-type cysticercosis mainly affects the subarachnoid space and adjacent meninges, especially at the base of the brain. Often the cysts are located in the cerebellopontine angle cistern or suprasellar cistern. Unlike the parenchymal type, the cysts of the meningeal type can be large, lobulated, blister-like (single cyst), or grape-like (multiple cysts). This type can cause chronic arachnoiditis and adhesions, leading to hydrocephalus. The scolex can be difficult to identify. CT findings are as follows: low-density cyst or enlargement of the cisterns with slight mass effect. Blockade of CSF circulation caused by arachnoid adhesions can result in hydrocephalus and symmetrical enlargement of the ventricles. Using contrast-enhanced CT, the meninges can be enhanced, and, occasionally, the contour of a cyst is visible after mild enhancement of the cyst wall. MRI findings are as follows: single cyst or grape-like polycystic lesions in the cerebellopontine angle area or suprasellar cistern. The signal intensity within the cyst is similar to that of CSF. Sometimes, the enlarged cisterns and asymmetrical subarachnoid space are the only manifestations, with the cyst wall and scolex not being obvious. Secondary chronic meningitis can lead to blockage of CSF circulation and hydrocephalus. Vasculitis may result in cerebral infarction. Pia mater at the base of the brain can be enhanced.

Mixed Type

Namely, two or more types of cysticercosis coexist. MRI is superior to CT in diagnosing meningeal and ventricular mixed type. In addition, when MRI cannot identify the scolex because of the ovoid cystic low signal intensity inside and the homogeneous cyst wall, cine MRI can detect the bypassing of CSF around the cyst, providing high tissue contrast and precise scolex and cyst wall localization.

9.1.5 Diagnosis and Differential Diagnosis

The most common clinical manifestation of neurocysticercosis is the onset of seizure. It is easy to diagnose this disease according to typical CT and MRI findings combined with epidemiological history. However, for the single large cystic, meningeal, and ventricular types, other brain parasitic diseases and arachnoid cysts should be considered as differential diagnoses. The scolex in the cyst is a typical manifestation seen in neurocysticercosis, and MRI is the best imaging tool available to detect this. Cysticercosis granuloma and small abscesses in the degenerative stage should not be confused with tuberculosis granuloma, bacterial brain abscesses, and metastases. Tuberculosis granuloma and abscesses can aggregate together and become polycyclic. Bacterial abscesses are usually large and hyperintense in DWI. Cysticercosis abscesses are generally less than 2 cm in size. Metastases often develop in elderly patients with a clinical history of primary malignant tumor, presenting as irregular enhancement and obvious edema. MRS is useful for diagnosing and distinguishing brain cysticercosis and metastases when patients do not present with a history of primary malignant tumors.

9.1.6 Treatment and Prognosis

Symptomatic treatment mainly includes administration of anti-epileptic drugs, intracranial pressure reduction, and surgery. The prognosis of neurocysticercosis depends on the number and location of cysts, length of treatment, and initiation of therapy. Most patients can be cured by using effective anti-parasitic and symptomatic treatments [8]. A number of patients who do not receive timely treatment can be left with serious parenchymal damage and varying degrees of neurological disorder.

9.2 Hydatid Disease

9.2.1 Etiology and Epidemiology

Hydatid disease, also known as echinococcosis, is a disease caused by the larvae of *Echinococcus* tapeworm parasitizing the brain. It is a zoonotic disease that occurs naturally in pastoral areas. This disease occurs sporadically in pastoral areas worldwide. It is prevalent in Xinjiang, Inner Mongolia, Gansu, Qinghai, Tibet, and other pastoral regions of China.

9.2.2 Pathology and Pathogenesis

The genus *Echinococcus* contains many species, and human infection is mainly caused by *E. granulosus*. The adult worms lodge in the small intestines of dogs or wild animals such as wolves and foxes, and their eggs are excreted in the feces. If a human accidentally ingests the eggs, they will hatch into oncospheres in the duodenum, penetrate the intestinal wall, enter the liver through the portal vein, and usually produce hydatid cysts in the hepatic sinus [9]. A few oncospheres can reach the brain or other distant organs via the blood circulation, resulting in cerebral hydatid disease. In addition, ruptured primary hydatid cysts can enter the brain via the blood. Hydatid disease is a systemic disease most commonly involving the liver, followed by the lungs. Cerebral hydatid disease is rare, accounting for 2% of all hydatid diseases.

E. granulosus in the brain presents as cysts of different sizes filled with transparent fluid. Its wall is differentiated into outer and inner layers. The inner layer (germinal layer) is hydatid own cyst and is a colorless transparent envelope. Brood capsules can develop into daughter cysts away from the germinal layer. The outer layer is a thick fibrous membrane consisting of the hosts' own reactive tissue. Hydatid cysts are mainly located in the area of the middle cerebral artery, especially the frontal and parietal lobes. In rare cases the cerebellum, ventricles, base of the brain, and epidural space can be involved. The lesion is generally solitary; however, it may progress if the primary cyst ruptures. When combined with infection, its manifestation is similar to that of a brain abscess.

9.2.3 Clinical Manifestations

Cerebral hydatid disease is commonly seen in not only children and young adults but also the elderly. Its occurrence is higher in men than in women. Most patients have a history of pastoral life or close contact with dogs and sheep. Some patients also suffer from visceral hydatid diseases. This disease is mainly characterized by signs and symptoms such as increased intracranial pressure, for instance, headache, vomiting, papilledema, and decreased visual acuity [10]. Focal neurologic signs including epilepsy and hemi-paralysis are also observed. Large cysts can lead to brain herniation.

9.2.4 Laboratory

Routine blood examinations show an elevated eosinophil count. Gasoni intracutaneous test and complement fixation tests have specific diagnostic value in hydatid diseases [11]. However, the positive rate of these tests for cerebral hydatid disease is usually less than 50%, which is significantly lower than that in visceral hydatid disease. Combining more than two types of laboratory methods can improve the sensitivity and positive rate of diagnosis.

9.2.5 Imaging

Radiography
The diagnostic value of X-ray is limited. A localized bulge and thinning of the skull adjacent to the cyst are observed along with widened cranial sutures. The eggshell or curved calcification of the cyst wall with spot-like and striped calcification inside can be seen.

CT

Type I (Simple Type) This type is a simple cystic lesion without daughter cyst and cyst wall calcification. The noncontrast CT scan shows a large, spherical-shaped, cystic lesion with a density similar to that of CSF and obvious mass effect [10, 12]. However, edema is absent around the lesion. Normally there is either no enhancement or slight enhancement. Hemorrhage in a cyst can be easily shown on CT (Fig. 9.2).

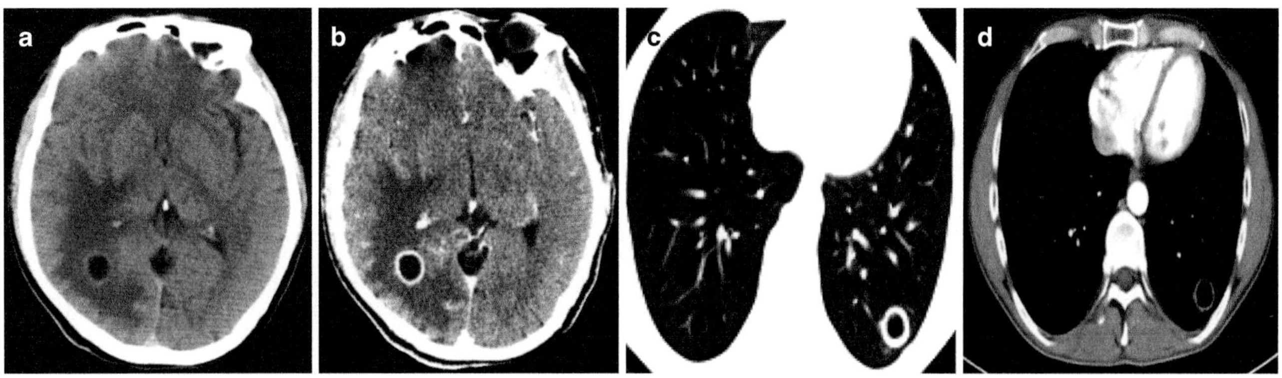

Fig. 9.2 Hydatid disease. CT imaging shows a simple cystic lesion surrounded by prominent vasogenic edema in the right temporal lobe (**a**). Contrast-enhanced CT shows ring-shaped enhancement (**b**). Lung CT of the same patient shows cystic hypodense in the inferior lobe of the left lung (**c**, **d**)

Type II (Multiple Daughter Cysts Type) The presence of multiple daughter cysts within the mother cyst is a typical feature of cerebral hydatid disease. The number and size of daughter cysts differ. A small number of daughter cysts form a wheel-shaped assembly in the periphery, while other daughter cysts fill the mother cyst in a honeycomb-like pattern. The density of a daughter cyst is lower than that of a mother cyst, and the density of a new daughter cyst near the periphery is slightly lower than that of an old one near the center. There is no edema around the cysts and sometimes the calcification of the cyst wall is visible. The cyst wall can be slightly enhanced [10, 12].

Rupture and infection are the most common complications of cerebral hydatid disease, presenting as increased density of cystic fluid, a thickened cyst wall, peripheral edema, and the formation of multiple hydatid cysts on CT. Hydrocephalic changes, such as dilated ventricles, can be observed when CSF circulation is obstructed by hydatids.

MRI

MRI manifestations: round or oval cystic lesion, no peripheral edema, hypodense on T_1WI, and hyperdense on T_2WI [10, 12–14]. The cyst wall has continuously low signal intensity. Daughter cysts within a mother cyst are the typical manifestation in this disease. The signal of a mother cyst is higher than that of daughter cysts. Separated cyst walls can be observed. Calcified cystic walls mostly present as low signal intensity. When infection occurs concurrently, edema is observed around the cystic lesion with obvious enhancement of the cyst wall.

9.2.6 Diagnosis and Differential Diagnosis

According to typical imaging findings and epidemiological history, it is easy to diagnose cerebral hydatid disease. Simple hydatid cysts should not be confused with arachnoid cysts, and large hydatid cysts should be differentiated from supratentorial ependymoma. Concurrent infection should be distinguished from brain abscesses. A brain abscess has a thicker wall, stronger enhancement, and more obvious edema surrounding it. Calcified hydatid disease can be distinguished from brain tumors with calcification, such as oligodendroglioma and craniopharyngioma, of which the location, shape of calcification, and internal density differ from that in hydatid disease.

9.2.7 Treatment and Prognosis

Surgical resection is the first line of treatment for this disease. Albendazole and mebendazole have certain therapeutic effects against cerebral hydatids, the former being superior to the latter [9, 15].

When the lesion is large, drugs often have limited therapeutic effects, and surgery can lead to the development of central nervous system sequelae in many patients; thus the disease prognosis is dismal [15].

9.3 Cerebral Schistosomiasis

9.3.1 Etiology and Epidemiology

Brain schistosomiasis is a parasitic brain disease caused by the deposition of schistosome eggs in the brain via the blood circulation, manifesting as schistosomal granuloma. Statistics suggest that the incidence rate of brain schistosomiasis is 1.5–4.3% among patients with schistosomiasis. Schistosoma is also known as blood fluke due to the lodgement of adult worms in blood vessels. The causative agents for human schistosomiasis include *S. japonicum*, *S. mansoni*, *S. haematobium*, *S. mekong*, and *S. intercalatum*, among others [16]. This disease is prevalent in Asia, Africa, South America, and the Middle East. Epidemic areas include Japan, the Philippines, Indonesia, and China [17]. Schistosomiasis in China is mainly caused by *S. japonicum*, which is found at epidemic proportions in the Yangtze River basin and the southern rural and mountainous areas.

9.3.2 Pathology and Pathogenesis

Schistosomiasis is a disease caused by the schistosome parasitizing the human venous system. When schistosome eggs escape from the portal system and lodge in the brain, brain schistosomiasis develops. Eosinophilic granuloma and pseudotuberculosis nodules can form in the superficial layers of gray and white matter, under the pia mater [18]. Acute cerebral schistosomiasis may be an immune reaction caused by eggs located in the brain parenchyma.

Schistosomal granuloma is a chronic pseudotuberculosis nodule, which mainly presents as nodule under the cerebral cortex with swelling of brain tissue and shallow or absent sulci. Under the microscope the nodular center contains eosinophilic necrosis and ruptured eggs, while around the nodule, new granulomatous tissue can be found.

9.3.3 Clinical Manifestations

This disease is mainly seen in young adult men. Clinically, this disease can be divided into three types: (1) encephalitis, (2) epilepsy, and (3) stroke. Grand mal seizures and paresis are the most common symptoms. Symptoms associated with increased intracranial pressure such as headache, vomiting, and papilledema are also observed [19]. Encephalitis type often features high fever, mental disorders, disturbance of consciousness, and positive pyramidal signs.

9.3.4 Imaging

CT

Lesions are usually located in unilateral cerebral hemisphere; sometimes, they can be found in the cerebellum. In terms of pathological changes, CT results are divided into four types: (1) encephalitis, (2) infarction, (3) granuloma, and (4) atrophy.

Encephalitis Type Allergic and toxic encephalitis caused by the secretion of metabolites from the eggs manifests as patchy and ill-defined hypodensity in one or more lobes of the brain with mass effect. The lesion may have heterogeneous patchy enhancement.

Infarction Type Brain tissue ischemic necrosis induced by egg-obstructed cerebral arteries manifests as triangle- or wedge-shaped hypodensity conforming to the arterial territory with its base facing the brain surface. Small ovoid hypodensity can also be seen.

Granuloma Type This is the most common type of cerebral schistosomiasis. Deposition of eggs can induce granuloma and brain edema, manifesting as a variable number of isodensity nodules of different sizes in the "fingerstall-like" brain edema area [20]. The nodules, which are mainly located in the cortical and subcortical area, have irregular margins and can fuse together. Based on nodule size and pathological findings, granuloma type can be subdivided as follows:

1. Multiple small nodules type: nodules with a diameter of 0.2–0.9 cm have scattered or plexiform distribution and do not fuse together. Enhanced scan shows "starry sky" sign.
2. Single large nodule type: nodules with a diameter >1.5 cm manifest as isodensity or slight hyperdensity near cerebral convolutions and heterogeneous enhancement.
3. Mixed nodules type: this type demonstrates enhanced large nodules with a diameter of 1–3 cm and multiple small peripheral nodules with a diameter of 0.2–0.9 cm.
4. Ring-enhanced nodule type: this type is most common in children. Owing to the fact that schistosome eggs can deposit in children's brain and trigger local allergies, which are stronger than that in adults, acute egg nodules featuring eosinophilic necrosis can develop. These nodules with a diameter of 1 cm can be ring-enhanced.

Atrophy Type This type shows fibrous tissue proliferation and scar formation, manifesting as well-defined, irregular, and non-enhanced low-density areas on CT with an enlarged ipsilateral ventricle, widened and deepened cisterns, and cortical sulci.

MRI

The cerebral schistosomal granuloma nodule is hypointense on T_1WI and isointense on T_2WI. "Fingerstall-like" or "Buddha's-hand-like" edema with low signal intensity on T_1WI and high signal intensity on T_2WI is found around the lesions [16, 19, 21]. MRI enhancement pattern is similar to that of CT; however, MRI is more sensitive in displaying enhanced small nodules than CT (Fig. 9.3).

9.3.5 Diagnosis and Differential Diagnosis

Cerebral schistosomiasis should be considered when the patient has a history of contact with infected water and the imaging indicates granuloma. However, it is insufficient to

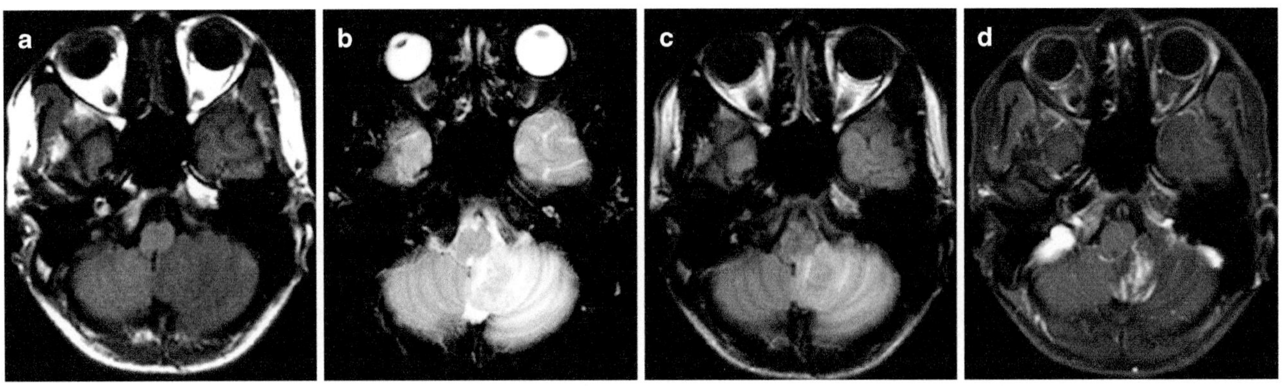

Fig. 9.3 Granuloma-type brain schistosomiasis. MR imaging shows multiple small nodular isointense on T_1WI and T_2WI surrounded by prominently vasogenic edema in the left cerebellum (**a**–**c**). Contrast-enhanced T_1WI showed nodular and patchy enhancement (**d**)

diagnose cerebral schistosomiasis based purely on imaging findings. Diagnosis of this disease should also consider clinical signs as follows:

1 Schistosome infection evidence: positive stool examination, positive biopsy of the rectal mucous membrane, and positive serology (cercarien hullen reaction, circumoval precipitin test).
2 Brain symptoms appear after infection and the treatment for cerebral schistosomiasis is effective.

Encephalitic type should not be confused with acute cerebral infarction. Granulomatous type should mainly be differentiated from glioma, metastatic tumors, and brain tuberculoma, among other conditions.

9.3.6 Treatment and Prognosis

Praziquantel has excellent therapeutic effect in the treatment of cerebral schistosomiasis [22]. Its short-term efficacy is as high as 100% and long-term efficacy can attain 90%. Chinese scholars believe that anti-schistosomiasis treatment can be performed even when the diagnosis of brain lesions is unknown. If the lesions shrink or disappear, the disease is confirmed.

9.4 Cerebral Paragonimiasis

9.4.1 Etiology and Epidemiology

Cerebral paragonimiasis is a severe complication caused by intracephalic heterotrophic parasitism of lung flukes, with an incidence rate of 2~27%. *P. westermani* and *P. miyazaki* are the most common lung flukes. Lung flukes can be found throughout Southeast Asia, Western Africa, Latin America, and Northeast, Northern, Eastern, and South Central China.

9.4.2 Pathology and Pathogenesis

Paragonimiasis is a parasitic disease caused by lung flukes. When humans ingest undercooked freshwater crabs and crayfish, metacercariae will first hatch into larvae in the intestinal canal, and then larvae migrate into the abdominal cavity through the intestinal wall, enter the thoracic cavity through the diaphragmatic muscle, and finally grow and develop into adult worm in the lung where they ovulate. The adult worms in pleural cavity and peritoneal cavity migrate along the loose tissues around the carotid artery, through the carotid canal or foramen lacerum into the brain. Allergic, toxic, and xenobiotic reaction of brain tissues can be caused by the migration, oviposition, and secretion of metabolites.

Its pathology is divided into three stages:

1 The tissue necrosis stage: the adult worms migrate into the brain and form tunnels. Metabolites produced by adult worms can cause vasculitis, resulting in inflammatory exudation, infarction, hemorrhage, and hollow necrosis in brain tissues.
2 Cyst formation stage: granulomatous cyst walls are formed owing to hemorrhage, liquefactive necrosis, and infiltration of eosinophils and monocytes in the necrosis periphery. Lung fluke eggs can disperse in the inner layer of cyst wall and cystic fluid. Cysts are often multiple, different in size and number, with granulomatous nodules in some lesions.
3 Fibrous scar stage: lesions will organize and calcify with different degrees of encephalatrophy when adult worms die or leave.

9.4.3 Clinical Manifestation

Clinical symptoms mainly include headache, vomiting, epilepsy, hemiplegia, aphasia, blurred vision, and meningeal irritation sign [23]. Laboratory tests show that eosinophils, serum immunoglobulins, and eosinophils and protein level in cerebrospinal fluid (CSF) are increased. Intracutaneous, sputum, and CSF tests for lung fluke eggs are positive, and serum- or CSF-specific IgG levels are increased, i.e., the enzyme-linked immunosorbent assay (ELISA) test for cerebral paragonimiasis, which shows high sensitivity, is positive.

9.4.4 Imaging

CT

On the basis of the results of pathological tests and CT scans, this disease can be divided into four types. Hemorrhagic type is frequently encountered in children [23].

Encephalitic Type This is the tissue necrosis phase of this disease. Non-enhanced CT (NECT) indicates multiple ill-defined patchy and irregular heterogeneous low-density areas. Contrast-enhanced CT (CECT) demonstrates no enhancement or mild enhancement, with mild mass effect.

Cystic Type NECT shows multiple unequally sized isodense rings in low-density areas. CECT indicates smooth and ring-like enhancement. The typical manifestation of the cystic type is three to five conglomerate ring-shaped enhancements (i.e., grape cluster form). Both cerebral edema and mass effect are obvious.

Calcification Type This is the end stage of cerebral paragonimiasis. NECT indicates patchy, nodular, or annular calcification. The typical manifestation of the calcification type is clustered and annular calcification. The low-density areas around the calcification indicate adhesive arachnoid cysts or cerebromalacia. Dilated ventricles along with widened sulci and fissures can also be seen.

Hemorrhagic Type This type is mostly seen in children. As children have thinner blood vessel walls and fragile tissues, lung flukes migrating in the brain can cause mechanical injury, local congestion, and vasculitis. Increased vascular permeability and ruptured blood capillaries result in hemorrhage. CT indicates single or multiple, punctate, striped, and patchy and irregular high density in the junctional zone between the cortex and medulla.

MRI

Manifestation of encephalitic type demonstrates punctate, multiple patchy long T_1 and long T_2 signals without enhancement or slightly heterogeneous enhancement. Imaging of cystic type shows a large irregular area with long T_1-weighted and long T_2-weighted signals; enhanced scan presents as multiple ring-enhanced lesions with different sizes gathering

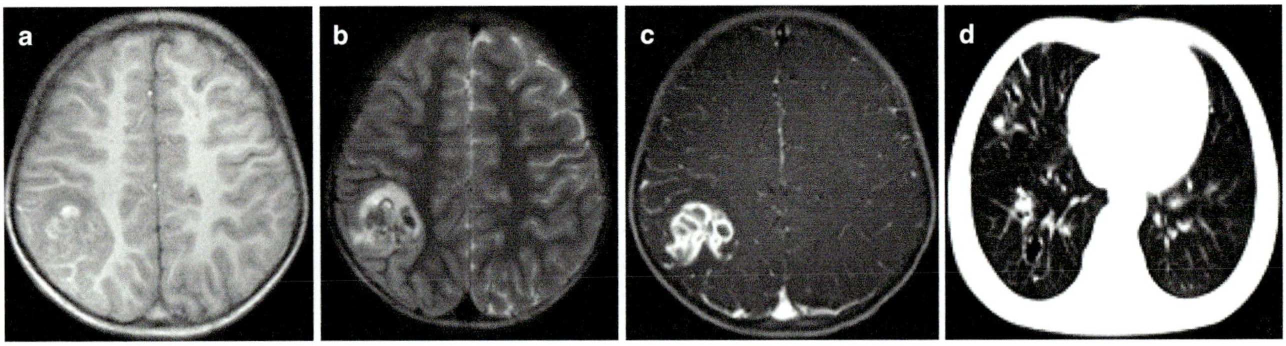

Fig. 9.4 A 7-year-old boy presented with general convulsive seizures and paroxysmal limb spasticity. MR imaging showed multiple ring-like hyperintense on T_1WI and T_2WI in the right parietal lobe (**a**, **b**). Axial contrast-enhanced T_1WI showed conglomerate, multiple, ring-shaped enhancements (**c**). Lung CT showed multiple cystic hypodense in the middle and inferior lobe of the right lung (**d**)

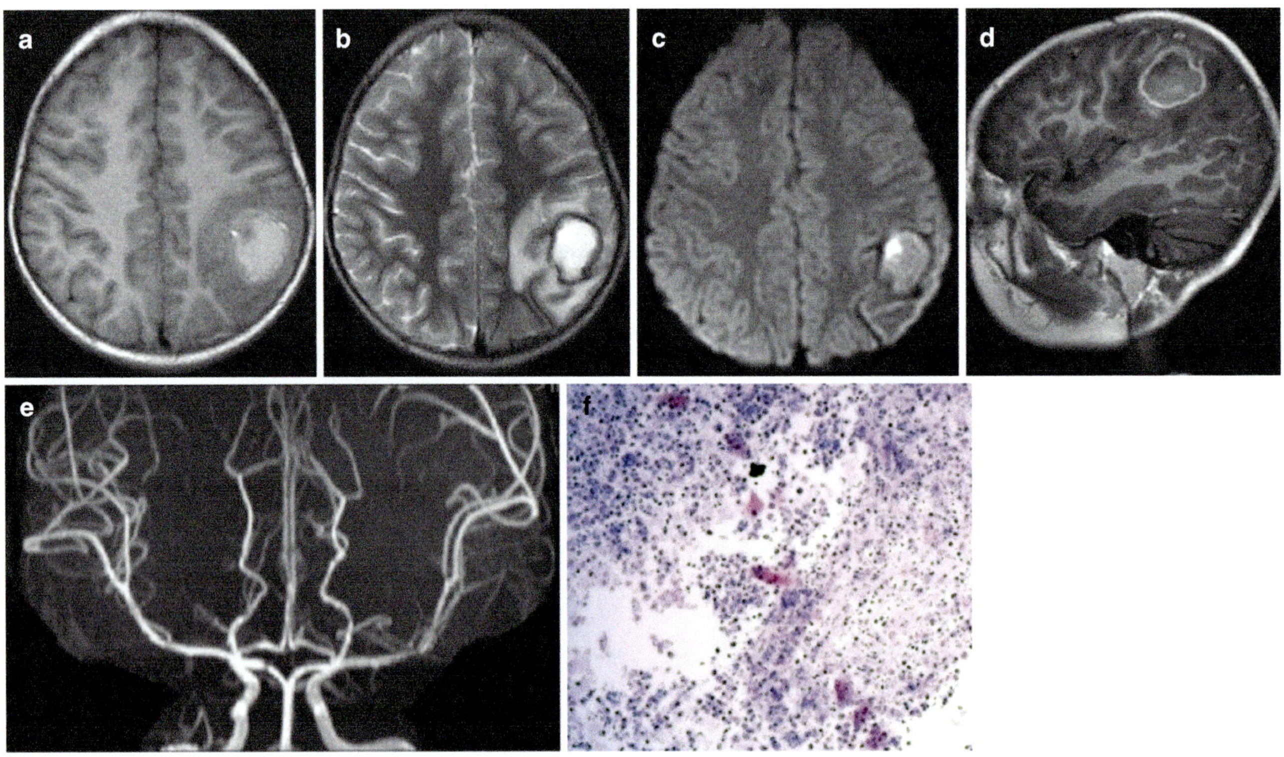

Fig. 9.5 A 6-year-old girl presented with paroxysmal headache associated with simultaneous vomiting. MR imaging showed oval hyperintense on T_1WI and T_2WI surrounded by prominently vasogenic edema (**a**–**c**). Sagittal contrast-enhanced T_1WI showed ring-like enhancement, the lesion located in the subcortical areas of left occipital lobe (**d**). MRA was normal (**e**). Hematoxylin-eosin staining (×100) revealed a large quantity of eosinophils, accompanied with scattering hemorrhage (**f**)

like grape cluster. In some cases, tunnel signs also appear [24]. Manifestation of intraparenchymal hemorrhagic type shows single or multiple punctate, sheetlike, cordlike, or oval short T_1 and long T_2 signals (Figs. 9.4 and 9.5).

9.4.5 Diagnosis and Differential Diagnosis

The diagnosis of cerebral paragonimiasis should be performed on the basis of clinical history (living in epidemic areas, consuming uncooked crabs, suffering from lung fluke diseases), neurological signs and symptoms, laboratory tests, imaging results, observations during treatment, and postoperative pathological results. This disease must also be distinguished from viral encephalitis, tuberculosis, and fungal infection. Herpes simplex virus infections are mostly seen in the temporal lobe, without clustered and annular enhancement. Tuberculosis or fungal infection may present as single or multiple ring-like foci in the brain but seldom with hemorrhage. Hemorrhagic cerebral paragonimiasis should be distinguished from vascular malformation and tumors, among other conditions. Digital subtraction angiography (DSA) or magnetic resonance angiography (MRA) can help identify vascular malformations. Contrast-enhanced scans can show enhanced tumor parenchyma. The manifestations of cerebral paragonimiasis in magnetic resonance spectroscopy (MRS) are normal choline (Cho), normal choline/creatine (Cho/Cr), and slightly decreased or normal N-acetylaspartate (NAA) levels, which indicate nonneoplastic lesions.

9.4.6 Treatment and Prognosis

Neurological symptoms in cerebral paragonimiasis are caused not only by egg granuloma but also by vasospasm and vasculitis. Operation is invasive and fails to solve these problems. Praziquantel, however, has the advantages of excellent therapeutic effect, short duration of action, and few side effects. The therapeutic effect of chronic cerebral paragonimiasis is poor, and intracranial hypertension crises may develop during conventional treatment, which may require surgical intervention.

9.5 Cerebral Toxoplasmosis

9.5.1 Etiology and Epidemiology

Toxoplasma gondii is one of the key pathogens that cause zoonotic parasitic disease. The acquired infection of cerebral toxoplasmosis in humans is caused by consumption of oocysts from contaminated food or water. Congenital cerebral toxoplasmosis occurs by placenta transmission of tachyzoites from the mother to the fetus after a primary infection during pregnancy. Cerebral toxoplasmosis is found worldwide with the infection rate ranging from 0.1% to 30% in humans. Humans are generally easily infected, especially where patients are immunocompromised due to posttransplantation therapy, HIV infection, or following bone marrow transplantation. Cerebral toxoplasmosis is more likely to occur in females.

9.5.2 Pathology and Pathogenesis

There are three developmental stages of *Toxoplasma gondii* in human tissues: oocysts, bradyzoites, and tachyzoites, all of which can cause toxoplasmosis in humans. During the acute infection period, oocysts rupture to deliver sporozoites that divide and develop into tachyzoites, which in turn eventually infect neurocytes. These cells simultaneously produce a variety of inflammatory factors that can cause damage to the nervous system while countering *T. gondii* infections [25]. When the immune response is tolerable, tachyzoites breed and aggregate in tissue cysts and form bradyzoites, which are characteristic of the chronic stage of infection. Bradyzoites can persist for months, years, or even the lifetime of an individual.

The lesions of cerebral toxoplasmosis can be divided into the following three zones. The central zone is a nonvascular area without microorganisms, which shows nonvascular coagulative necrosis. The middle zone is the congestive vascular area, where the inflammatory reaction is the most intense, and shows swelling of endothelial cells, lymphocytes, plasma cells, and macrophages around the small peripheral vein with a large number of free tachyzoites appearing in or out of capillaries. There are considerable numbers of bradyzoites and a small number of tachyzoites in the peripheral zone that show decreased tissue necrosis and do not show vascular abnormalities. Congenital toxoplasmosis of the CNS manifests as brain tissue necrosis, inflammatory cell infiltration, and scattered calcification, mainly in the periventricular zone. Acquired cerebral toxoplasmosis is mainly located in the basal ganglia and corticomedullary zone.

9.5.3 Clinical Manifestations

Human toxoplasmosis falls under two categories: congenital and acquired infections. Congenital infection is far more severe than acquired infection. Congenital cerebral toxoplasmosis occurs because of maternal sporadic placental transmission to the fetus. *T. gondii* infection in early pregnancy can cause miscarriage or stillbirth, while infection in late pregnancy can result in premature births and/or neurologic deficits shortly after birth. Early symptoms of infection of the central nervous system include neurological deficits, convulsions, rigidity, and retinochoroiditis. The most common consequences of infection are mental retardation, hydrocephalus, microcephaly, nystagmus, and optic atrophy. Approximately 80% of patients with cerebral toxoplasmosis presented without symptoms at birth, although patients could present with neurological symptoms and a decompensated stage within a few months to years or even in adulthood. Acquired toxoplasma infection is typically an asymptomatic recessive infection and can heal itself in immunocompetent hosts. Patients can acquire lifelong immunity after an infection. However, *T. gondii* in HIV-positive individuals can cause severe multi-organ damage involving the brain, eye, heart, lungs, and other organs. Central nervous system symptoms manifest as headache, fever, a change in mental status, confusion, epilepsy, and focal neurological deficits.

9.5.4 Imaging

CT

Due to the different pathological changes of cerebral toxoplasmosis in early and late stages, the imaging results are different. Early acute infection manifests as massive cerebral necrosis associated with perivascular lymphocytic infiltration, which is mainly caused by blood embolism. Manifestations of early acute infection include encephalitis and meningitis, which show multiple irregular, asymmetric low-density areas located in the corticomedullary junction and the basal ganglia of bilateral cerebral hemispheres. Contrast-enhanced scans show linear and nodular enhancement. In the final stage of infection, calcification is present in the cerebral necrosis center. Brain CT not only shows calcification in the subependymal region, basal ganglia, and cortex, which manifests as multiple nodular or curvilineal form high densities, but also simultaneously exhibits brain deformities caused by congenital *Toxoplasma* infection such as microcephaly, neuronal migrational disorder, and atelencephalia. The earlier a fetus is infected, the more severe the brain malformations that occur. Hydrocephalus is commonly image in patients with congenital infection. Hydrocephalus occurs due to aqueductus mesencephali obstruction caused by debris from necrotic brain tissue and cerebrospinal fluid circulation obstruction caused by the lesions of the aqueductus wall itself.

MRI

Cerebral toxoplasmosis is one of the most common opportunistic infections in patients with acquired immunodeficiency disorder (AIDS). The corticomedullary junction and basal ganglia are most frequently involved. The infectious lesions in early stages present as bilateral, multiple, irregular, and asymmetric hypointensity on T_1WI and hyperintensity on T_2WI. The isointensity or hypointensity on T_2WI represents coagulative necrosis. Hemorrhage is often observed in the lesion. Granuloma of *T. gondii* infection manifests as an intraparenchymal nodular mass with extensive perifocal edema and significant mass effect. The lesions show nodular or curvilinear enhancement [26, 27]. Some authors suggest that the "eccentric target sign" is a characteristic feature of toxoplasmosis on contrast-enhanced images which demonstrate an eccentric innermost enhancing core surrounded by an intermediate hypointense region and a peripheral enhancing rim (Fig. 9.6) [28]. However, this indication is seen in <30% of cases. The infectious lesions involve the subependymal area and appear hyperintense on T_2WI which represent necrotic lesions, with periventricular ependymal curvilinear enhancement after contrast administration in the early stage. The calcifications are hypointense on MRI. The concomitant congenital malformation in patients with cerebral toxoplasmosis is better demonstrated on MRI.

9.5.5 Diagnosis and Differential Diagnosis

Diagnostic evidence relies on the isolation of pathogens. Diagnosis of congenital toxoplasmosis relies on serological evaluation. Toxoplasma-specific IgM in infected patients is positive after 7–14 days; the concentration will peak in 6–8 weeks and can persist for several years.

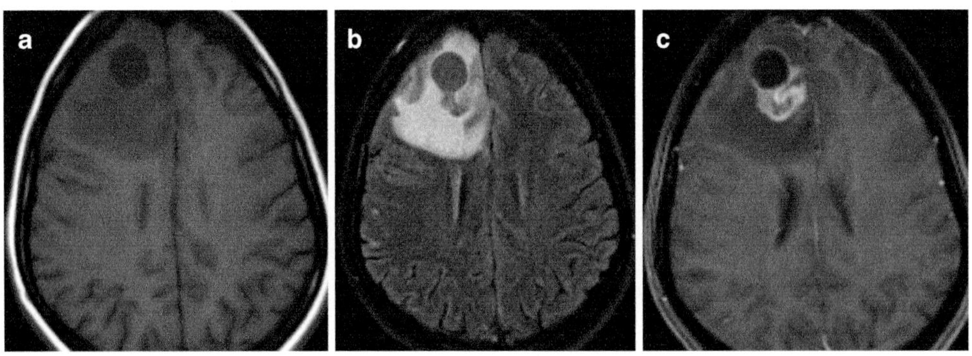

Fig. 9.6 A 23-year-old female HIV patient presented with altered mental status. MRI showed oval hypointense on T_1WI and FLAIR surrounded by prominently vasogenic edema in the subcortical areas of right frontal lobe (**a**, **b**). Post-contrast T_1WI showed ring-like, patchy enhancement (**c**)

The neuroradiological manifestations of cerebral toxoplasmosis are not pathognomonic; it should be differentiated from primary central nervous system lymphoma (PCNSL), fungal infection, tuberculosis, cytomegalovirus infection, etc. Magnetic resonance spectroscopy (MRS) is helpful in distinguishing between cerebral toxoplasmosis and lymphoma. The contractible scope of the disease and reduced degree of perifocal edema after effective anti-toxoplasmosis therapy provide clinical diagnostic evidence.

9.5.6 Treatment and Prognosis

Cerebral toxoplasmosis is treated with drugs such as sulfadiazine, pyrimethamine, and clindamycin. The clinical symptoms of cerebral toxoplasmosis can improve significantly after treatment.

References

1. Galan-Puchades MT, Fuentes MV. Updating Taenia asiatica in humans and pigs. Parasitol Res. 2016;115(11):4423–5.
2. Udare A, Juvekar S, Medhi S, et al. Disseminated cysticercosis: role of whole body magnetic resonance imaging. Ann Parasitol. 2016;62(2):149–51.
3. Vaidya A, Singhal S, Dhall S, et al. Asymptomatic disseminated cysticercosis. J Clin Diagn Res. 2013;7(8):1761–3.
4. Xiao A, Zeng H, Xiao J, et al. Imaging features of neurocysticercosis: analysis of 57 consecutive patients. Turk Neurosurg. 2017;27(3):386–94.
5. Cangalaya C, Bustos JA, Calcina J, et al. Perilesional inflammation in neurocysticercosis - relationship between contrast-enhanced magnetic resonance imaging, evans blue staining and histopathology in the pig model. PLoS Negl Trop Dis. 2016;10(7):e0004869.
6. Jensen TO, Post JJ. Intraventricular neurocysticercosis: Presentation, diagnosis and management. Asian Pac J Trop Med. 2016;9(8):815–8.
7. Mahale RR, Mehta A, Rangasetty S. Extraparenchymal (Racemose) neurocysticercosis and its multitude manifestations: a comprehensive review. J Clin Neurol. 2015;11(3):203–11.
8. Garcia HH, Lescano AG, Gonzales I, et al. Cysticidal efficacy of combined treatment with praziquantel and albendazole for parenchymal brain cysticercosis. Clin Infect Dis. 2016;62(11):1375–9.
9. Mcmanus DP, Zhang W, Li J, et al. Echinococcosis. Lancet. 2003;362(9392):1295.
10. Bükte Y, Kemaloglu S, Nazaroglu H, et al. Cerebral hydatid disease: CT and MR imaging findings. Swiss Med Wkly. 2004;134(31-32):459–67.
11. Sarkari B, Rezaei Z. Immunodiagnosis of human hydatid disease: where do we stand? World J Methodol. 2015;5(4):185–95.
12. Teke M, Göçmez C, Hamidi C, et al. Imaging features of cerebral and spinal cystic echinococcosis. La Radiologia Medica. 2015;120(5):458–65.
13. Guzel A, Tatli M, Maciaczyk J, et al. Primary cerebral intraventricular hydatid cyst: a case report and review of the literature. J Child Neurol. 2008;23(5):585–8.
14. Pandey S, Pandey D, Shende N, et al. Cerebral intraventricular echinococcosis in an adult. Surg Neurol Int. 2015;6:138.
15. Turgut M. Intracranial hydatidosis in Turkey: its clinical presentation, diagnostic studies, surgical management, and outcome. A review of 276 cases. Neurosurg Rev. 2001;24(4):200–8.
16. Olveda DU, Olveda RM, Lam AK, et al. Utility of diagnostic imaging in the diagnosis and management of schistosomiasis. Clin Microbiol. 2014;3(2):142.
17. Weerakoon KG, Gobert GN, Cai P, et al. Advances in the diagnosis of human schistosomiasis. Clin Microbiol Rev. 2015;28(4):939–67.
18. Kristensson K, Masocha W, Bentivoglio M. Mechanisms of CNS invasion and damage by parasites. Handb Clin Neurol. 2013;114:11–22.
19. Ross AG, Mcmanus DP, Farrar J, et al. Neuroschistosomiasis. J Neurol. 2012;259(1):22–32.
20. Wu L, Wu M, Tian D, et al. Clinical and imaging characteristics of cerebral schistosomiasis. Cell Biochem Biophys. 2012;62(2):289–95.
21. Abdel Razek AA, Watcharakorn A, Castillo M. Parasitic diseases of the central nervous system. Neuroimaging Clin N Am. 2011;21(4):815–21.
22. Barda B, Coulibaly JT, Puchkov M, et al. Efficacy and safety of moxidectin, synriam, synriam-praziquantel versus praziquantel against schistosoma haematobium and s. mansoni infections: a randomized, exploratory phase 2 trial. PLoS Negl Trop Dis. 2016;10(9):e0005008.
23. Chen J, Chen Z, Lin J, et al. Cerebral paragonimiasis: a retrospective analysis of 89 cases. Clin Neurol Neurosurg. 2013;115(5):546–51.
24. Xia Y, Chen J, Yan J, et al. Characteristic CT and MR imaging findings of cerebral paragonimiasis. J Neuroradiol. 2016;43(3):200–6.
25. Parlog A, Schlüter D, Dunay IR. Toxoplasma gondii-induced neuronal alterations. Parasite Immunol. 2015;37(3):159–70.
26. Mahadevan A, Ramalingaiah AH, Parthasarathy S, et al. Neuropathological correlate of the "concentric target sign" in MRI of HIV-associated cerebral toxoplasmosis. J Magn Reson Imaging. 2013;38(2):488–95.
27. Maschke M, Kastrup O, Forsting M, et al. Update on neuroimaging in infectious central nervous system disease. Curr Opin Neurol. 2004;17(4):475–80.
28. Correia CDC, Lacerda HR, Costa VMDA, et al. Cerebral toxoplasmosis: unusual MRI findings. Clin Imaging. 2012;36(5):462–5.

Opportunistic Infections

10

Guiquan Shen, Mu-xi Wu, and Bo Gao

10.1 Introduction

Over 60% AIDS patients have neurologic manifestations, which is the first symptom in 10–20% patients before highly active antiretroviral therapy (HAART) [1, 2]. HIV crosses the intact blood–brain barrier, infects the monocyte–macrophage lineages, and results in CNS injury [3]. Neurologic complications may arise from HIV infection itself, or from secondary opportunistic infections or neoplasms, or is drug therapy related complications [4]. Impaired cellular immunity contributes to the host susceptible to such opportunistic CNS infections as toxoplasmosis, cryptococcosis, progressive multifocal leukoencephalopathy, and cytomegalovirus (CMV) encephalitis. Additionally, CNS tuberculosis (TB) and neurosyphilis may also occur with a relatively higher frequency compared to immunocompetent patients [1, 4]. The imaging findings seen in AIDS-related diseases of the CNS are often varied and challenging.

10.2 HIV Encephalopathy

HIV encephalopathy is the result of the direct involving of HIV virus via blood–brain barrier (BBB) in the early course, then precipitating the inflammatory response process and ultimately resulting in white matter demyelination or gliosis. Progressive subcortical dementia also known as AIDS dementia complex (ADC) is usually manifested in such patients in clinical practice. Generalized atrophy out of proportion to age is the most sensitive imaging finding in patients with ADC, especially in patients with advanced immunosuppression (Fig. 10.1). Symmetric signal abnormalities on MRI or hypo-attenuation on CT in periventricular and deep white matter can also be noted sometimes [5]. HIV encephalopathy does not result in mass effect or enhancement after contrast enhancements (Fig. 10.2).

10.3 Toxoplasmic Encephalitis

Toxoplasmic encephalitis (TE) is a necrotizing inflammation caused by protozoa Toxoplasma gondii. Clinically, patients present either acutely or insidiously with variable symptoms. The lesions on T2WI are quite variable of signal abnormalities and the presence of extensive vasogenic edema is usually classical. Hemorrhage may be seen occasionally but is characteristic to differentiate toxoplasmosis from lymphoma. Multiple nodular or ring-enhancing lesions can be seen on postcontrast T1WI (Fig. 10.3). Multi-modalities MR may aid in differentiating between TE and lymphoma [6].

10.4 Cytomegalovirus Infection

Cytomegalovirus is latent in majority of the population but may reactivate under the condition of impaired cellular immunity. It has two frequently overlapping forms recognized in CMV encephalitis: microglial nodular encephalitis and ventriculoencephalitis. Its characteristic focal neurologic signs include nystagmus, ataxia, and cranial nerve palsies. Demyelination can result in diffuse white matter abnormalities appearing hypo-attenuation on CT or hyperintensity on T2WI. In CMV meningoencephalitis or ventriculitis, low attenuation may be seen in the white matter, and ependymal enhancement may be seen in contrast-enhanced CT images. MRI demonstrates increased T2 hyperintensity in white matter, as well as ependymal, subependymal, and periventricular [7].

G. Shen · M.-x. Wu · B. Gao (✉)
Department of Radiology, Affiliated Hospital of Guizhou Medical University, Guiyang, Guizhou, China

B. Gao et al. (eds.), *Imaging of CNS Infections and Neuroimmunology*, https://doi.org/10.1007/978-981-13-6904-9_10

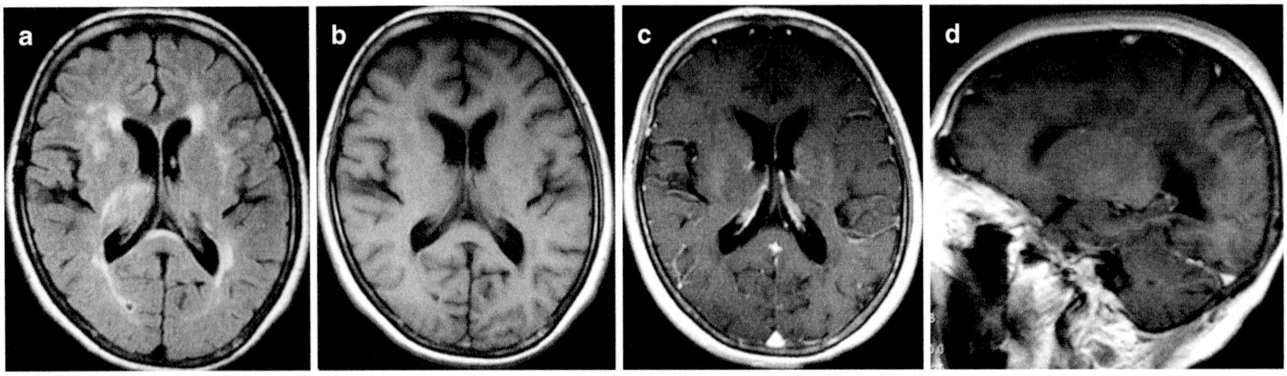

Fig. 10.1 AIDS dementia complex in a 37-year-old man with progressive dementia and ataxia. (**a**, **b**) Axial FLAIR shows diffuse atrophy and symmetric periventricular hyperintensity corresponding sightly hypointensity on T1WI; (**c**, **d**) Postcontrast axial and sagittal T1WI shows no enhancement in the regions of abnormalities (courtesy of Hongjun Li MD, Department of Radiology, You'an Hospital, Capital Medical University, China)

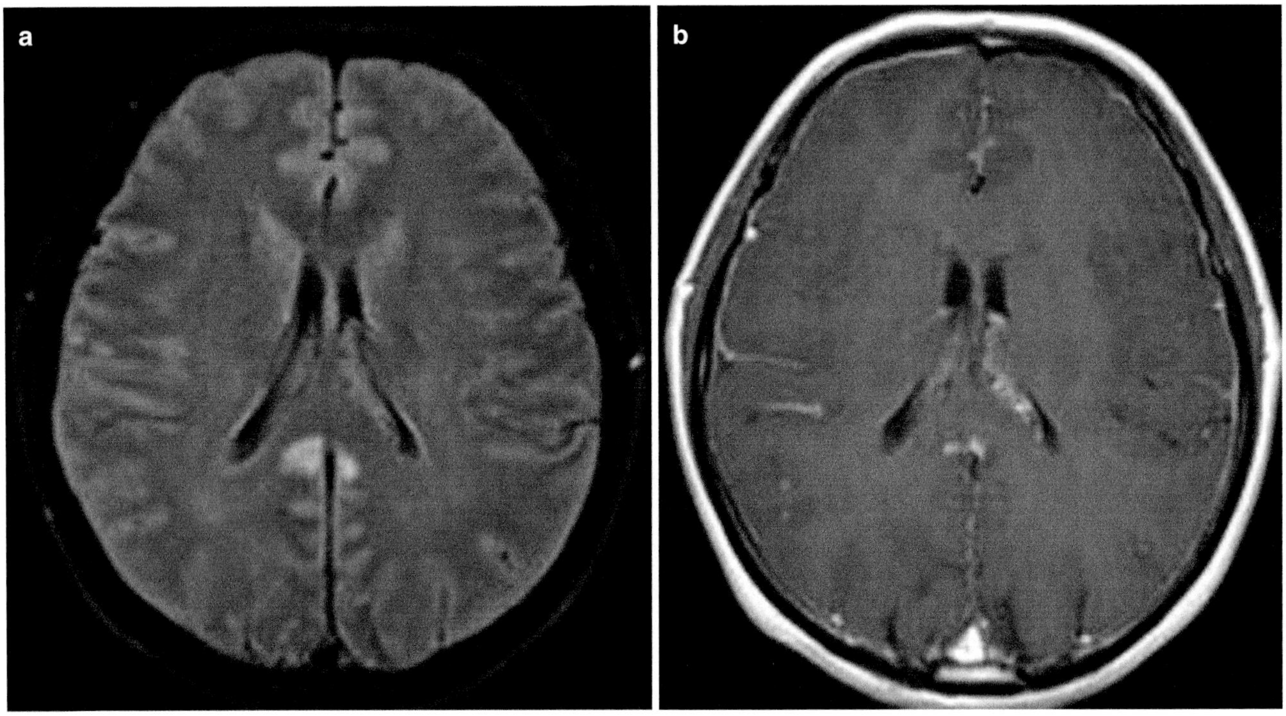

Fig. 10.2 HIV encephalopathy in a 53-year-old man with progressive consciousness and fevers. (**a**) Axial FLAIR image demonstrates focal hyperintensity in posterior cingulate and diffuse minor hyperintensity in bilateral hemispheres; (**b**) Postcontrast T1-weighted image shows dot-like enhancement (courtesy of Su Lyu MD, Department of Radiology, Huaxi Hospital, Sichuan University, China)

10.5 Progressive Multifocal Leukoencephalopathy

Progressive multifocal leukoencephalopathy (PML) is an opportunistic infection caused by the reactivation of JC virus in immunocompromised patients. Typically, it results in a progressive neurologic decline, cognitive impairment, altered mental status, and personality changes [8]. In a minority of individuals, the recovery of immune function with HAART therapy can precipitate immune reconstitution inflammatory syndrome (PML-IRIS). CT reveals asymmetric focal hypoattenuation involving periventricular and subcortical white matter. MRI shows single or multifocal asymmetric signal abnormalities and may be confluent with disease progression.

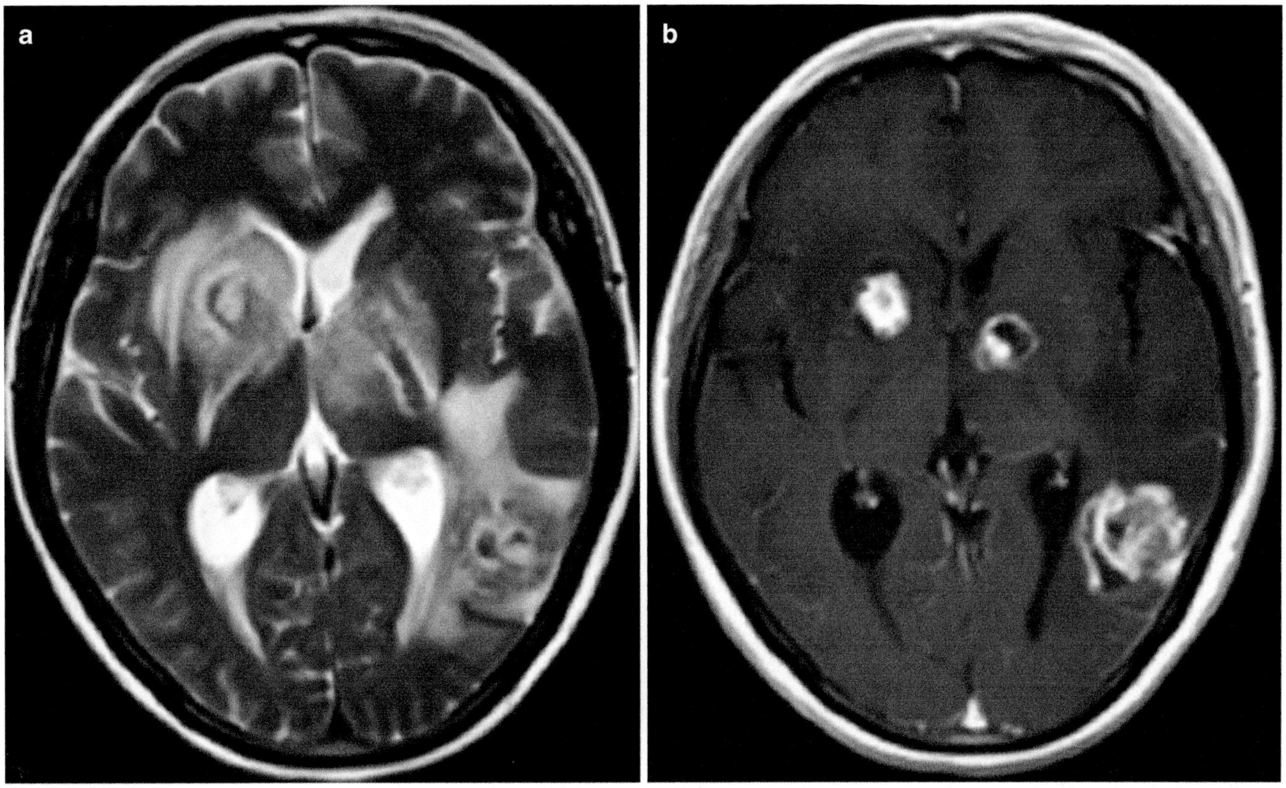

Fig. 10.3 A HIV patient accompanied with toxoplasma infection. (**a**) T2WI showed multiple lesions in bilateral basal ganglia and left posterior temporal region with surrounding edema; (**b**) postcontrast T1WI showed significant ring-like enhancement with mural nodules (courtesy of Hongjun Li MD, Department of Radiology, You'an Hospital, Capital Medical University)

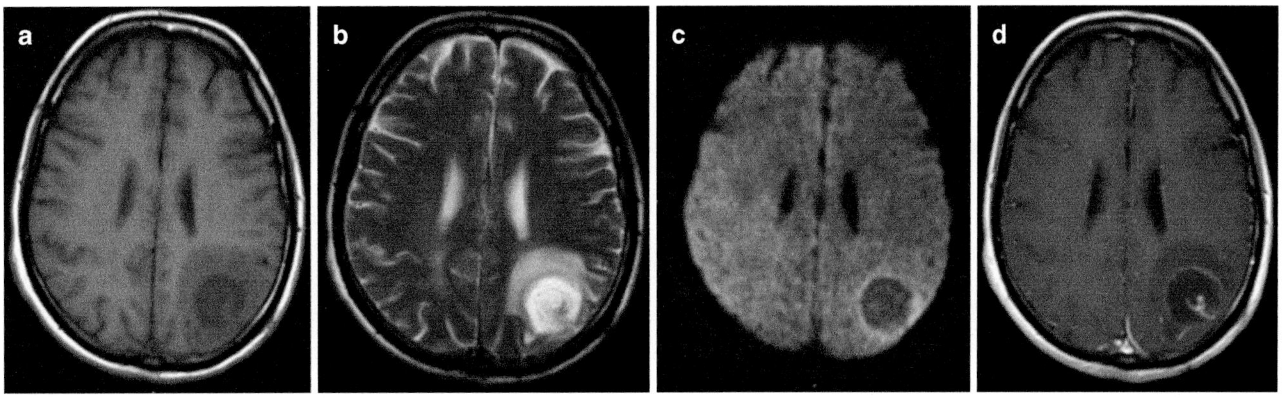

Fig. 10.4 HIV patient accompanied with cryptococcus infection. (**a**, **b**) The lesion was located in subcortical white matter of the left parietal lobe along with moderate edema, and hypointensity on T1WI and hyperintensity on T2WI; (**c**) DWI showed hyperintensity at the edge of the lesion with hypointensity in center; (**d**) after injection of contrast medium the lesion was ring-like enhanced with mural nodule in posterior lateral wall (courtesy of Li Li MD, Department of Radiology, Youan Hospital, Capital University, China)

10.6 Cryptococcosis

Cryptococcus neoformans is an encapsulated, ubiquitous yeast-like fungus contaminated by bird excreta. Patients may present with nonspecific symptoms and signs of meningitis or meningoencephalitis [9]. The radiologic findings of CNS cryptococcal infection are highly variable and sometimes minimal [10]. The classic neuroimaging features include dilated VR spaces, gelatinous pseudocysts, meningitis, hydrocephalus, and intraparenchymal cystic masses (Fig. 10.4). MRI is superior to CT in detecting the presence and extent of cryptococcal lesions [11] (Fig. 10.5).

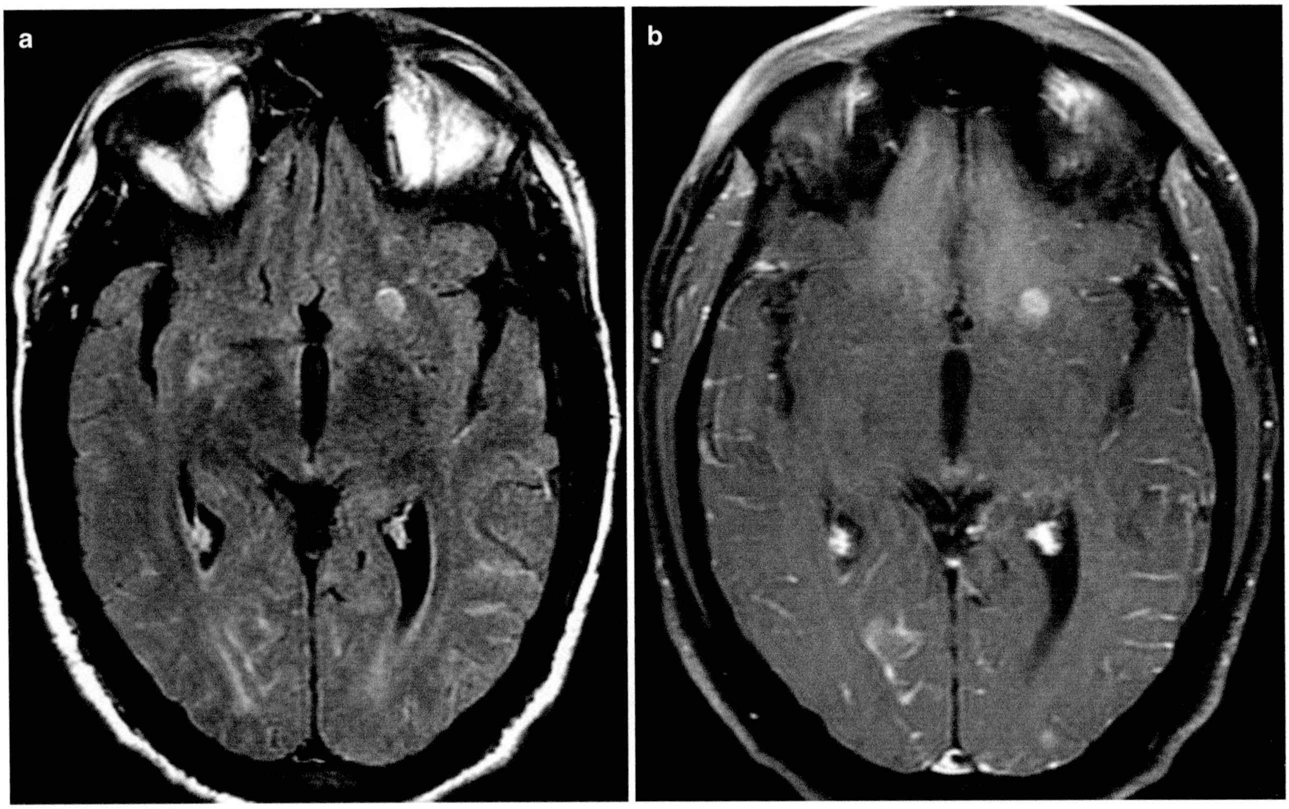

Fig. 10.5 Cryptococcal meningoencephalitis in HIV patient. Axial FLAIR (**a**) basilar regions focal parenchymal hyperintense lesions, subarachnoid space-leptomeningeal hyperintensity, and on axial T1 + C (**b**) parenchymal and leptomeningeal enhancement bilaterally (courtesy of Fanny Morón MD, Department of Radiology, Baylor College of Medicine, USA)

10.7 Aspergillosis

Cerebral involvement by aspergillus is the result of hematogenous spread from a pulmonary focus, or directly invasion the brain via the sinus [12]. Involvement of the skull base and orbit from aspergillus would result in visual disturbance, cranial nerve palsies. Cerebral aspergillosis generally demonstrates multiple of low attenuation on CT images in cortical and subcortical regions. T2 hyperintensity on MRI with ring-enhancing pattern and dural thickening adjacent to lesions of the paranasal sinuses or calvaria could also be noted [13].

10.8 Tuberculosis

AIDS patients may go on to develop TB from early hematogenous spread or from "rich" foci seeding into subarachnoid space. Tuberculous meningitis usually has an insidious prodrome characterized by fluctuating fever, behavioral changes, and weight loss with mental status changes. Around half of patients may present meningeal and cranial nerves symptoms [2]. Tuberculous meningitis usually manifests as meningeal enhancement in the basal cisterns and sylvian fissures on imaging studies. DWI may help to differentiate infarction or cerebritis from tuberculosis [14]. Tuberculomas are granulomas resulting either from hematogenous spread or from CSF seeding via cortical veins or small penetrating arteries. Tuberculomas generally locate supratentorially and may be solitary or multiple (Fig. 10.6) [6].

10.9 Neurosyphilis

Neurosyphilis is a sexually transmitted disease resulting from spirochete Treponema pallidum. Its clinical manifestations usually are protean and variable, from asymptomatic to headaches, confusion, focal neurologic deficits, and dementia [15]. Mild to moderate atrophy, white matter lesions, infarctions, gummas, leptomeningeal enhancement, and arteritis have all been reported [6]. Infarcts may be medium to large and represent a vascular territory, like MCA, or they may alternatively occur in the basal ganglia or brainstem resulting from perforating vessel disease (Fig. 10.7).

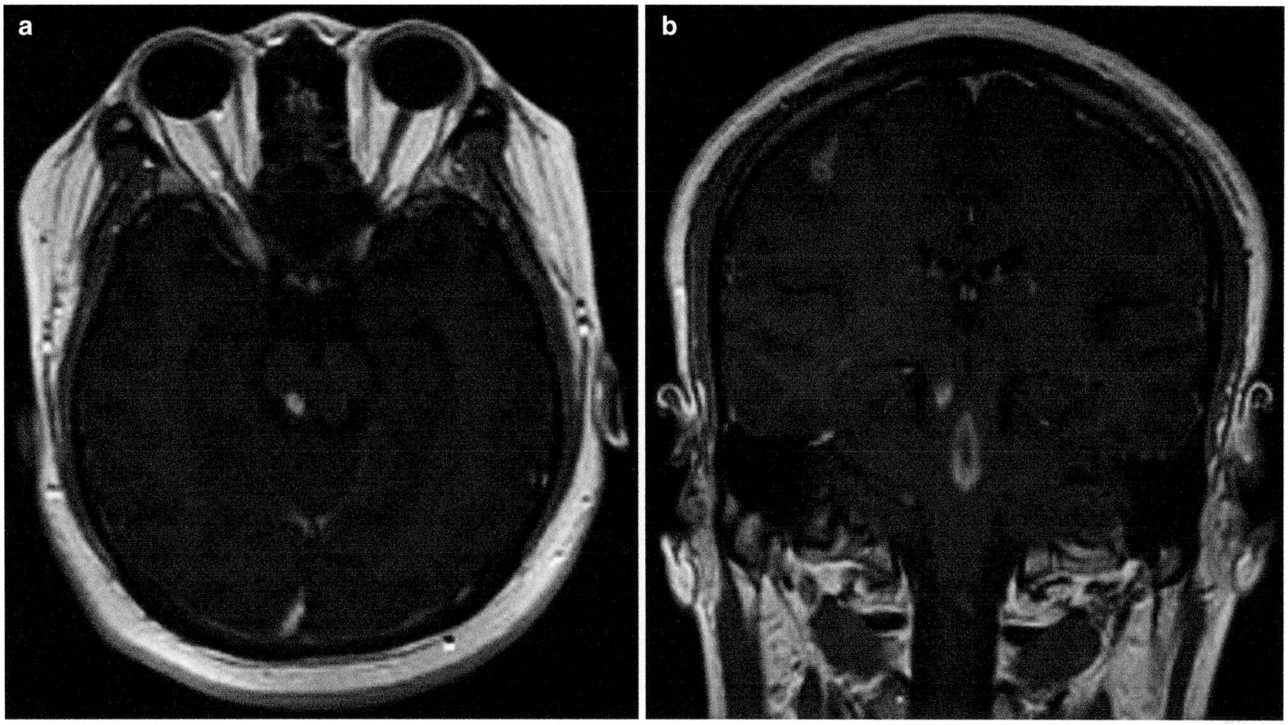

Fig. 10.6 A HIV patient accompanied with tuberculosis infection. Contrast-enhanced T1WI (**a**, **b**) showed significant nodular or circular enhancement lesions in the brainstem and hemispheres (courtesy of Li Li MD, Department of Radiology, Youan Hospital, Capital Medical University, China)

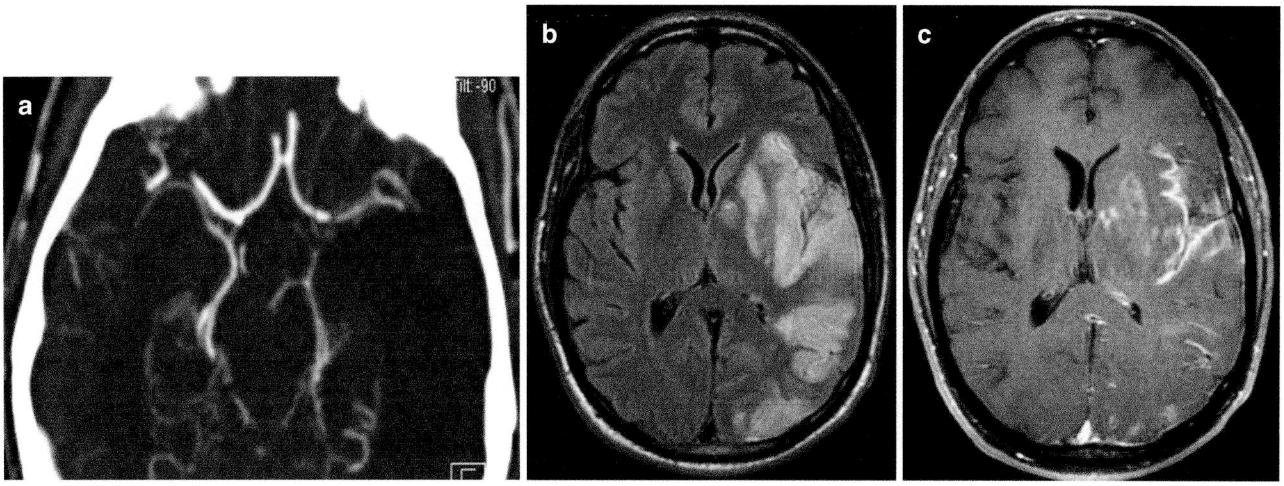

Fig. 10.7 Neurosyphilis on HIV patient with acute left MCA stroke (24 h) due to infective vasculitis. Axial CTA (**a**) images show diffuse narrowing of the left MCA and paucity of the distal branches. Axial FLAIR (**b**) showed intense hyperintensity in the left putamen, insula, and temporoparietal/occipital lobes, corresponding to the axial FLAIR. Axial T1 + C (**c**) shows diffuse leptomeningeal and gyriform enhancement in the affected areas, in part due to the infarction and to meningoencephalitis in this acute stage infarct (courtesy of Fanny Morón MD, Department of Radiology, Baylor College of Medicine, USA)

10.10 Immune Reconstitution Inflammatory Syndrome

HAART succeeds in suppressing HIV replication and improving cellular immunity, in this way protecting HIV-infected patients from opportunistic infections. However, partial restoration of specific immunity may worsen a preexisting disease with the resulting condition of immune reconstitution inflammatory syndrome (IRIS). Patients with IRIS demonstrate paradoxic deterioration for their rise of CD4 counts and viral replication is under control. IRIS occurs in the initial months

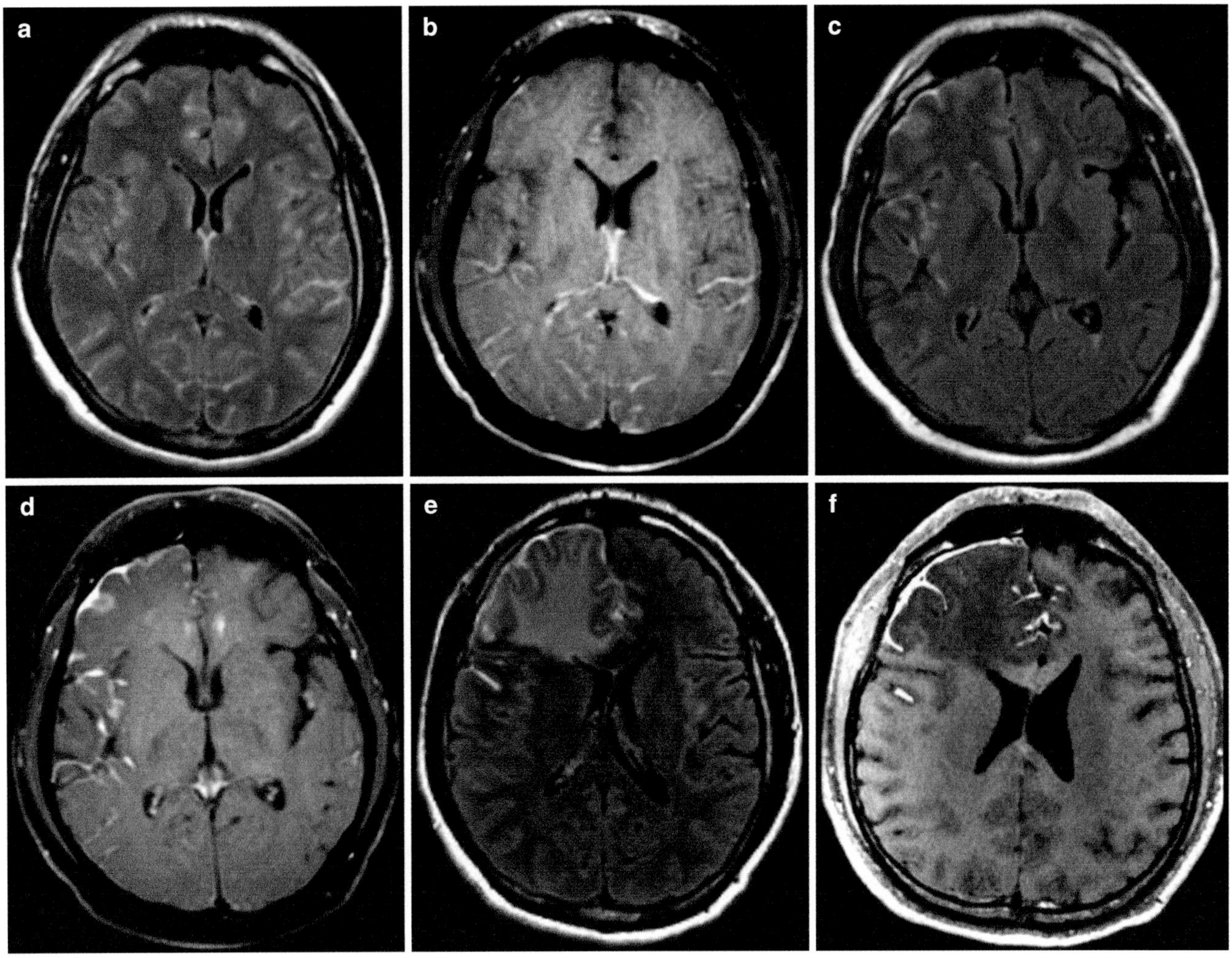

Fig. 10.8 HIV patient with cryptococcal meningitis was placed on HAART and antifungal medication. Subarachnoid FLAIR hyperintensity (**a**) and T1 leptomeningeal enhancement (**b**), on follow-up MRI improved subarachnoid FLIAR hyperintensity and enhancement (**c**, **d**) but developed new focal right frontal opercular FLAIR hyperintensities and gyriform enhancement (**e**, **f**), was thought to represent infarction; however, it evolved with worsening mass effect and enhancement, consistent with cryptococcal immune reconstitution inflammatory syndrome (IRIS) on pathology (courtesy of Fanny Morón MD, Department of Radiology, Baylor College of Medicine, USA)

after the onset of HAART. The neuroimaging findings may be atypical and depending on the underlying pathologic conditions, such as prominent, progressive enhancement, and mass effect seen in PML (Fig. 10.8) [16–18].

References

1. Albarillo F, O'Keefe P. Opportunistic neurologic infections in patients with acquired immunodeficiency syndrome (AIDS). Curr Neurol Neurosci Rep. 2016;16(1):10.
2. Bowen LN, Smith B, Reich D, et al. CNS infections: pathophysiology, diagnosis and treatment. Nat Rev Neurol. 2016;12(11):662–74.
3. Smith AB, Smirniotopoulos JG, Rushing EJ. From the archives of the AFIP: central nervous system infections associated with human immunodeficiency virus infection: radiologic-pathologic correlation. Radiographics. 2008;28(7):2033–58.
4. Tan IL, Smith BR, von Geldern G, et al. HIV-associated opportunistic infections of the CNS. Lancet Neurol. 2012;11(7):605–17.
5. Sarbu N, Shih RY, Jones RV, et al. White matter diseases with radiologic-pathologic correlation. Radiographics. 2016;36(5):1426–47.
6. Gottumukkala RV, Romero JM, Riascos RF, et al. Imaging of the brain in patients with human immunodeficiency virus infection. Top Magn Reson Imaging. 2014;23(5):275–91.
7. Renard T, Daumas-Duport B, Auffray-Calvier E, et al. Cytomegalovirus encephalitis: undescribed diffusion-weighted imaging characteristics. Original aspects of cases extracted from a retrospective study, and from literature review. J Neuroradiol. 2016;43(6):371–7.
8. Berger JR, Aksamit AJ, Clifford DB, et al. PML diagnostic criteria: consensus statement from the AAN neuroinfectious disease section. Neurology. 2013;80(15):1430–8.
9. Loyse A, Moodley A, Rich P, et al. Neurological, visual, and MRI brain scan findings in 87 south African patients with HIV-associated cryptococcal meningoencephalitis. J Infect. 2015;70(6):668–75.
10. Tan ZR, Long XY, Li GL, et al. Spectrum of neuroimaging findings in cryptococcal meningitis in immunocompetent patients in China—a series of 18 cases. J Neurol Sci. 2016;368:132–7.
11. Sarkis RA, Mays M, Isada C, et al. MRI findings in cryptococcal meningitis of the non-HIV population. Neurologist. 2015;19(2):40–5.

12. Siddiqui AA, Bashir SH, Ali Shah A, et al. Diagnostic MR imaging features of craniocerebral Aspergillosis of sino-nasal origin in immunocompetent patients. Acta Neurochir. 2006;148(2):155–66; discussion 166.
13. Guermazi A, Gluckman E, Tabti B, et al. Invasive central nervous system aspergillosis in bone marrow transplantation recipients: an overview. Eur Radiol. 2003;13(2):377–88.
14. Patkar D, Narang J, Yanamandala R, et al. Central nervous system tuberculosis: pathophysiology and imaging findings. Neuroimaging Clin N Am. 2012;22(4):677–705.
15. Akgoz A, Mukundan S, Lee TC. Imaging of rickettsial, spirochetal, and parasitic infections. Neuroimaging Clin N Am. 2012;22(4):633–57.
16. Post MJ, Thurnher MM, Clifford DB, et al. CNS-immune reconstitution inflammatory syndrome in the setting of HIV infection, part 1: overview and discussion of progressive multifocal leukoencephalopathy-immune reconstitution inflammatory syndrome and cryptococcal-immune reconstitution inflammatory syndrome. AJNR Am J Neuroradiol. 2013;34(7):1297–307.
17. Post MJ, Thurnher MM, Clifford DB, et al. CNS-immune reconstitution inflammatory syndrome in the setting of HIV infection, part 2: discussion of neuro-immune reconstitution inflammatory syndrome with and without other pathogens. AJNR Am J Neuroradiol. 2013;34(7):1308–18.
18. Guevara-Silva EA, Ramírez-Crescencio MA, Soto-Hernández JL, et al. Central nervous system immune reconstitution inflammatory syndrome in AIDS: experience of a Mexican neurological centre. Clin Neurol Neurosurg. 2012;114(7):852–61.

11 Cerebrovascular Complications of CNS Infections

Fanny Morón and Orlando Diaz

11.1 Infectious Intracranial Aneurysm

11.1.1 Epidemiology

Infectious intracranial aneurysm (IIA), also known as mycotic aneurysms, is rare and accounts for 0.7–6.5% of all intracranial aneurysms in the general population and up to 15% in children [1–3]. They are the result of a complicated systemic infective processes; a comprehensive review by Ducruet et al. found that 65% of patients with IIA had underlying endocarditis [1]. In contrast, only 10% of patients with endocarditis have been reported to demonstrate neurological signs attributed to IIA [4, 5]. IIA can also present as a complication of central nervous system (CNS) infections such as meningitis, dural venous sinus thrombophlebitis, and abscesses. Other infections associated with IIA include local head and neck infective foci such as orbital cellulitis and paranasal sinusitis.

The population at risk includes intravenous drug abusers, those with poor dental hygiene, immunocompromised patients with diabetes, chronic illness, malignancies, and HIV, and patients on chemotherapy or immunosuppressive medications. There is an increased risk associated to invasive procedures, such as lumbar punctures and spinal anesthesia. There is no reported significant gender predominance. The median age for patients with IIA is 35.1 years [1].

11.1.2 Presentation and Natural History

Infectious IA may be asymptomatic (silent in 10%) [6]. A major complication of IIA is subarachnoid hemorrhage secondary to rupture. This may be accompanied by parenchymal or intraventricular hemorrhage. Ruptured mycotic aneurysms have a high mortality of about 60–90% [7]. Other complications include septic cerebral infarction, focal neurologic deficits from ischemia, headache, fever, and seizures. Blood cultures are positive in only in 35% of the cases [1]; additional biomarkers of infection include leukocytosis, elevated erythrocyte sedimentation rate (ESR), and elevated C-reactive protein (CRP). The management of unruptured infectious IA is with broad-spectrum intravenous antibiotics. However, the risk of rupture on an infectious IA is not reduced during antibiotic therapy [3]. Thus, close monitoring with serial angiographic imaging starting in 1–2 weeks after initial diagnosis is recommended. If there is interval resolution or decreased in size of the aneurysm in the follow-up studies, the patient usually will not need an invasive treatment. In this setting antibiotic treatment for 4–6 weeks is required. If the aneurysm is unchanged in size or is larger in the follow-up study, or if there are new aneurysms, then further intervention is warranted.

There are no established treatment guidelines regarding surgery or endovascular intervention for IIA; however both techniques are safe and effective; treated patients with intervention have a higher survival compared to conservative management alone [8]. Endovascular treatment is favored in patients with high-risk aneurysm and with high surgical-risk patients. IIA is considered high risk if there is (1) circumferential vessel involvement and (2) proximal location and (3) the parent artery cannot be sacrificed due to significant neurologic deficit [9]. Patients are considered a high surgical risk if the patients are hemodynamically unstable, have severe comorbidities such as immunosuppression, or require acute cardiac valve repair due to delays with anticoagulation reversal.

Ruptured aneurysms carry a worse prognosis and require immediate intervention; the choice between endovascular treatment and open surgery should be made on a case-by-case bases (personalized) ([1, 4, 8, 11]). Various endovascular techniques exist: parent artery occlusion or direct embolization of the aneurysm. Parent artery occlusion can be achieved with different material (coils, liquid embolic agents such as Onyx, *N*-butyl 2-cyanoacrylate, NBCA, ethylene-vinyl alco-

F. Morón (✉)
Department of Radiology, Baylor College of Medicine, Houston, TX, USA
e-mail: fmoron@bcm.edu

O. Diaz
Neurovascular Center, Houston Methodist Hospital, Weill Cornell Medical College, Houston, TX, USA

B. Gao et al. (eds.), *Imaging of CNS Infections and Neuroimmunology*, https://doi.org/10.1007/978-981-13-6904-9_11

hol copolymer). Direct embolization can be achieved with coils, stent-assisted coiling, liquid embolic materials, and more recently flow diverter stents [9, 10]. Surgery is indicated in patients with ruptured infectious IA with associated large intraparenchymal hematoma and raised intracranial pressure. Surgical interventional techniques include trapping, clipping, bypassing, and wrapping the aneurysm; direct excision with parent vessel grafting can also be performed [4, 8, 11].

11.1.3 Pathophysiology

Infectious intracranial aneurysm is defined as a focal dilatation of the cerebral artery vessels due to microbacterial infection with associated inflammation of the arterial wall. The infection can reach the vessels through different routes: (1) septic embolization to the vessel wall through the vasa vasorum that then progresses to the adventitia and intima (because there is involvement of the muscular layer, IIA are pseudoaneurysms); (2) through the endothelium via the endoluminal vascular space; (3) direct extension from adjacent focus of infection, such as an abscess, dural sinus thrombophlebitis, and bacterial meningitis; (4) direct inoculation during trauma or surgery; and (5) hematogenous contamination of a preexisting aneurysm, injured wall, or atherosclerotic plaque. The inflammation of the vessel wall with polymorphic neutrophils, enzymes, and pro-inflammatory cytokines results in degradation of the layers of the vessel wall into a friable, often absent wall. The most common pathogens are bacterial: *Streptococcus* and *Staphylococcus* groups; far less common pathogens include fungal organism particularly *Aspergillus* and *Mucor* spp. (see additional information in the infectious vasculitis section), contrary to what the name suggest.

11.1.4 Imaging

Since more than 65% of patients with infectious IA have underlying infective endocarditis [1], it is recommended to perform cerebrovascular imaging in all patients with bacterial endocarditis that present with neurologic symptoms.

Initial imaging is a non-contrast head computed tomography (CT). This evaluates the presence of subarachnoid hemorrhage (SAH) and parenchymal, extra-axial, or intraventricular

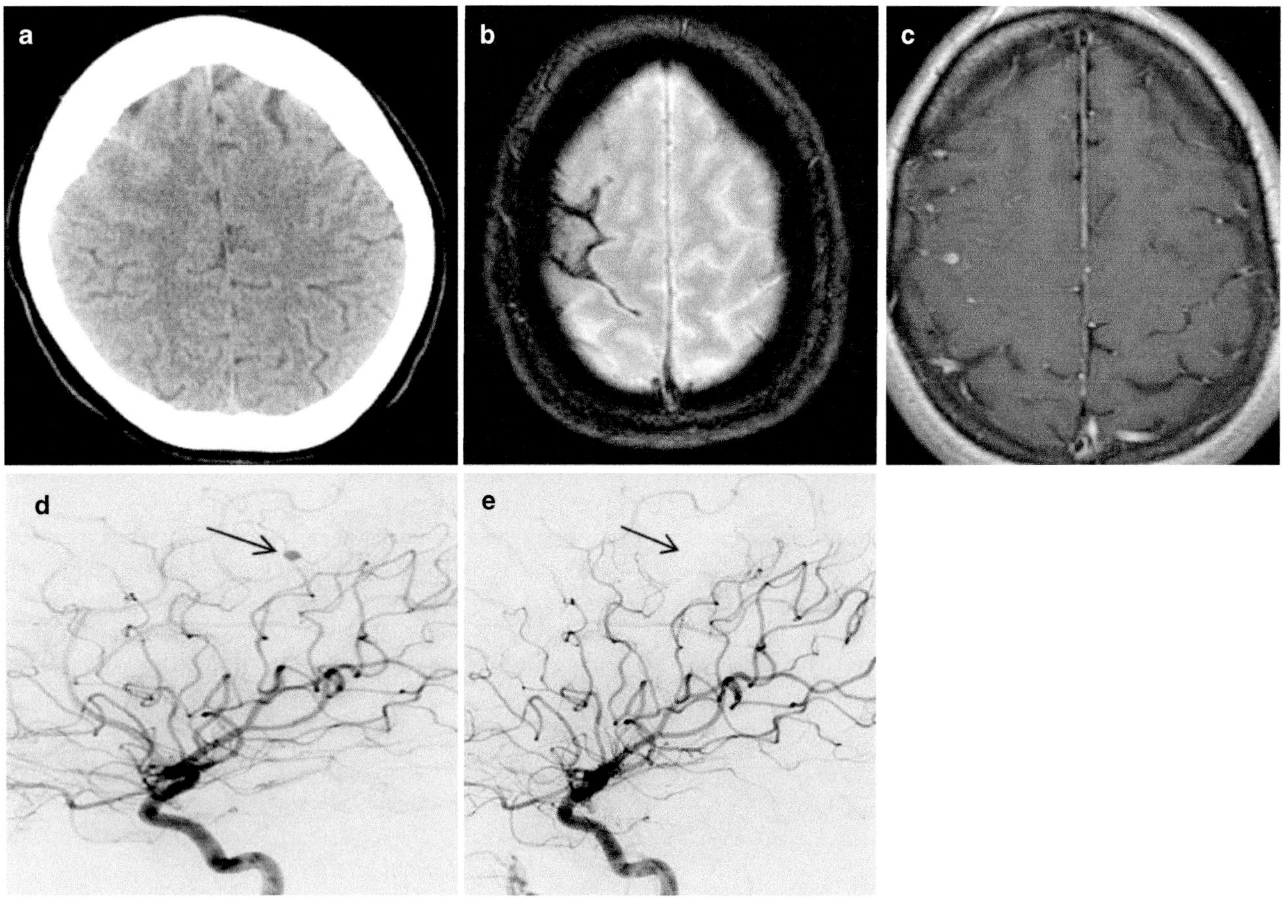

Fig. 11.1 Aspergillosis in leukemia patient with ruptured mycotic aneurysm. Axial non-contrast head CT (**a**) with right middle frontal sulcus hyperdensity, confirmed to represent hemorrhage on axial T2* (**b**). Post-contrast axial T1 (**c**) T1 shows mild leptomeningeal enhancement and small focus of pooling of contrast within the right middle frontal sulcus suggestive of aneurysm. Confirmed on DSA right ICA injection lateral projection (**d**) shows small peripheral right MCA (M4) infective aneurysm (black arrow). Post embolization using glue (nBCA) lateral projections (**e**) shows complete obliteration of the aneurysm (black arrow)

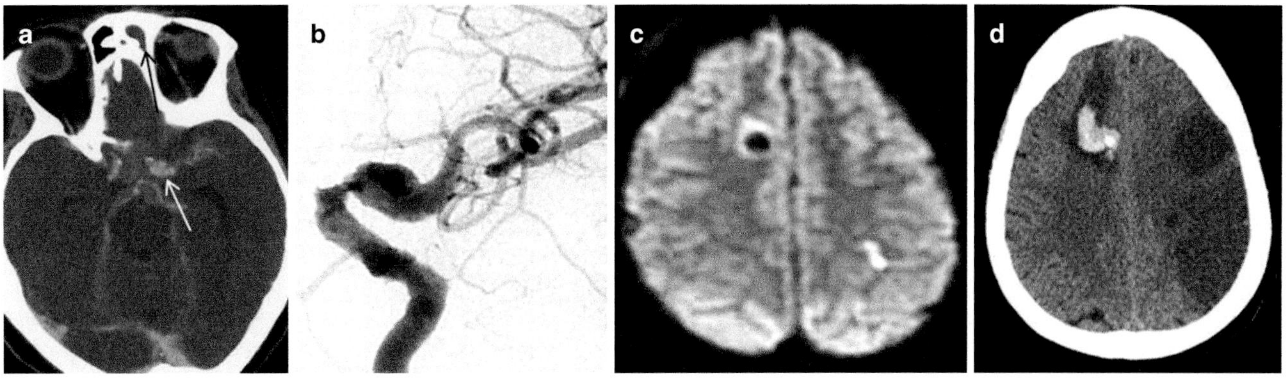

Fig. 11.2 Mucormycosis left frontoethmoidal sinusitis and orbit cellulitis with left ICA infective aneurysm. Axial CTA (**a**) shows left intraconal cellulitis and opacified left frontal and ethmoidal sinuses (black arrows) with dilatation and irregularity of the left supraclinoid ICA (white arrow). DSA left ICA injection. Magnified oblique projections (**b**) verified irregular fusiform aneurysmal dilatation of the ICA with large posterior communicating segment infective aneurysm. Axial DWI (**c**) with right frontal ventricular catheter and multiple small left parietal acute embolic lacunar infarcts, worsening symptoms with new large acute left MCA distribution. Acute ischemic infarct on CT (**d**) likely due to occlusion of the vessel

hemorrhage (Fig. 11.1). Contrast-enhanced CT angiography is the initial vascular imaging of choice for the detection of the aneurysm. There is high sensitivity (92.8–94%) and specificity (90.2–100%) for the detection of IIA. MR angiography (MRA) detects aneurysm with a high sensitivity (95–100%), comparable to CTA. Digital subtraction angiography (DSA) is comparable to CTA. However, the accuracy of DSA is reduced in smaller than 3 mm aneurysms (70.4–91.7%) [12, 13]. Magnetic resonance imaging (MRI) of the brain is recommended for the detection of early infection-related findings, for instance, leptomeningeal enhancement, brain edema, infarcts, and cerebritis.

The imaging characteristics of infectious IA are nonspecific, but the presence of multiple positive findings should favor the diagnosis. Infectious IA are usually located in the periphery (about 70%) and in the distal branches of the middle cerebral artery (segments M2 to M4) (Fig. 11.1). About 25% of mycotic aneurysms are multiple [14]. Usually they are fusiform (Fig. 11.2); up to 41% are saccular [1]. Associated neurovascular imaging findings to make the diagnosis include narrowed or stenotic vessels close to the aneurysm (often the parent vessel), wide or absent neck, multiplicity, rapid change in size or shape over time, or the appearance of a new aneurysm in follow-up angiogram (Figs. 11.1 and 11.2). Contrary to saccular aneurysm, the size of the IIA does not predict the risk of rupture [5].

Digital subtraction angiography (DSA) remains the gold standard and is recommended in the setting of a negative CTA or MRA if there is high clinical suspicion for IIA. Although DSA is an invasive technique, the risk of complications is less than 1% [1].

11.2 Infectious Vasculitis

11.2.1 Epidemiology

CNS infectious vasculitis is a feared complication that can result from infective endocarditis, central nervous system infections, or systemic bacteremia-sepsis.

In infective endocarditis (IE), neurological complications are the most severe extracardiac complications with up to 17% of patients with left-sided IE developing stroke symptoms [15]. Forty to 50 percent of the neurological complications of IE are acute cerebrovascular accidents. These are either embolic strokes or transient ischemic attacks (TIA) [16].

In bacterial meningitis, up to 25% of patients can present with cerebrovascular complications of infectious CNS vasculitis [17]. This carries a worse prognosis with often irreversible neurologic deficits. The most common presentation of infectious CNS vasculitis is an ischemic stroke and less commonly intracranial hemorrhage. This can be subarachnoid or parenchymal bleed (about 1–3% of patients) [18]. The most common bacteria are *Streptococcus pneumonia* and *Staphylococcus aureus* in 67% and 21% of patients, respectively [18].

In the setting of systemic infections, published data in large population studies suggest an association between ischemic strokes and systemic infections. Patients with systemic infections have been reported to have a higher risk of cardioembolic strokes [18, 19].

In addition, the risk of stroke can be transiently higher during the first 3 days after the diagnosis of a respiratory tract or a urinary tract infection [20]. Stimulation of the inflammatory response with vascular endothelial alteration and atherogenesis is thought to be the mechanism of action.

11.2.2 Presentation and Natural History

Left-sided IE-related atherothrombotic and cardioembolic ischemic insults to the CNS can be subclinical (silent areas of the brain), without neurological deficit in up to 48% of cases [21, 22]. A high clinical suspicion and imaging studies are required to make the diagnosis and establish appropriate clinical management to prevent this catastrophic complication.

Treatment of IE-related embolic ischemic insult to the CNS includes parental antibiotic. The use of steroids, anticoagulation, and a thrombolytic (alteplase) medication is controversial and should be tailored individually as no guidelines exist. The need of cardiac surgery should also be considered, particularly regarding the use of anticoagulation [18, 23]. Unfortunately, a stroke may present at any time, during or after completion of antibiotic treatment [24].

Patients with acute pyogenic meningitis may present with headache, fever, nuchal rigidity, altered mental status with confusion, and/or seizures (the absence of these symptoms does not rule out acute bacterial meningitis). Cerebral spinal fluid (SCF) shows elevated proteins, leukocytosis, and decreased glucose. At admission, focal neurologic deficits can be present in 46% of adult patients with bacterial meningitis. In 25% of patients with community-acquired bacterial meningitis (usually caused by *Streptococcus pneumonia* and *Neisseria meningitidis*), the neurological deficit is secondary to brain infarction [17]. The source for meningitis may be systemic with hematogenous dissemination or from contiguous spread from head and neck infections. The latter may be due to paranasal sinusitis, orbit-facial cellulitis, or otomastoiditis. Clinical features and poor prognostic factors of cerebral infarction in adults with community-acquired meningitis include older age, focal neurologic deficit on admission, low Glasgow Outcome Scale (GOS, <4), baseline chronic debilitating comorbidities, bacteremia, pneumonia, high erythrocyte sedimentation rates (ESR), and low CSF leukocyte count [17, 25, 26]. Elevation of the intracranial cerebral blood flow (CBF) measured with transcranial Doppler is associated with increased risk of stroke and unfavorable outcome in the setting of acute bacterial meningitis [25]. Prompt treatment of the bacterial meningitis with intravenous antibiotics and corticosteroids reduces the risk of CV complications [27].

In the setting of systemic infections, patients may present with signs and symptoms related to the primary site of infection such as dyspnea, dysuria, and hematuria. Clinical features associated with cerebrovascular complications of systemic infections are similar to other infections. These include focal neurologic deficits, altered level of consciousness, and seizures. Treatment and vaccine prevention when applicable of the systemic infection reduce the risk of CV complications [20].

11.2.3 Pathophysiology

Infections, regardless of the source, can cause cerebral infarction through two main routes. The first one is extracranial sources that disseminate hematogenously to the CNS, particularly cardioembolic strokes such as in the setting of patients with infective endocarditis. These emboli can affect large vessels with territorial infarcts and/or small vessels with lacunar mostly basal ganglia and peripheral and watershed distribution infarcts. These infarcts tend to be multiple and in different vascular territories. In addition, septic thrombi can deposit in the brain and these can also develop abscesses.

The second route of cerebrovascular involvement from central nervous system (CNS) infections is through infectious vasculitis and subsequent ischemia. In general, the affected vessels with infectious vasculitis have wall thickening from proliferative changes, which results in vessel lumen narrowing, and in turn will predispose to thrombosis, stenosis with insufficient cerebral perfusion, and infarcts [28, 29]. Vessels can be involved by different mechanisms in the setting of infection: (1) the vessel wall can narrow from sterile inflammation with reactive arteritis; (2) the vessels can directly be infected and degraded by microorganisms as the vessel traverses the infected spaces; usually vessels passing through basilar cistern exudate get infected and allow the infection to travel along the perivascular spaces which results in basal ganglia infarcts; (3) the vessel can narrow as the result of immune-mediated parainfectious process leading to vasospasm in which no vasculitic changes are seen in the vessel wall; and (4) due to hypercoagulable state, atherogenesis, atherosclerosis plaque rupture, and thrombosis due to inflammatory cascade and resultant ischemic strokes [18].

11.2.4 Imaging

Conventional imaging with CT and MRI as well as angiographic imaging with CT angiography (CTA), MR angiography (MRA), or digital subtraction angiography (DSA) of the cervical and intracranial vessels plays an important role in the diagnosis of cerebrovascular complications of infections. These techniques have also an impact on decision-making process regarding clinical management.

Non-contrast-enhanced initial CT is usually negative in infectious CNS vasculitis. The most common imaging finding is that of a stroke. Infarctions can be present in about 21% of patients with pneumococcal meningitis [29]. In the non-contrast CT examination, areas of ischemia correspond to regions of hypodensity with loss of the gray-white matter differentiation, variable mass effect, and sulci effacement. Infarcts are located in the deep gray nuclei, thalami, may be multifocal peripheral in the gray-white junction, or involve a major cortical vascular territory (Fig. 11.3). Less commonly seen on the non-contrast CT is the presence of subarachnoid or parenchymal hemorrhage (reported data varies from 1% to 9%) [26, 29]. The small foci of hemorrhage are better visualized on gradient recalled echo (GRE) scans and are even more conspicuous on susceptibility-weighted images (SWI) (Fig. 11.4). MRI is more accurate in detecting early

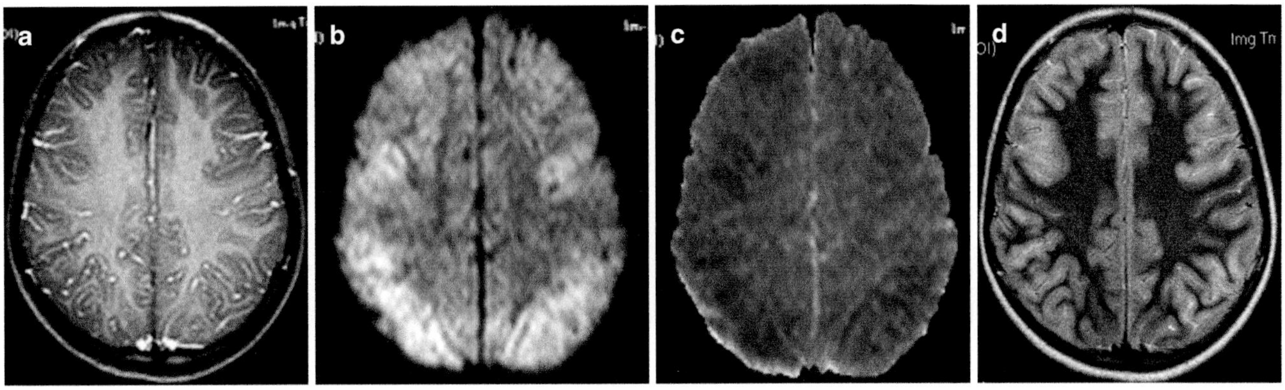

Fig. 11.3 Bacterial meningococcal meningoencephalitis with bilateral acute infarcts. Axial T1 with contrast enhancement (**a**) shows diffuse leptomeningeal enhancement. Axial DWI/ADC (**b**, **c**) with restricted discussion in a bilateral parieto-occipital watershed cortical distribution and corresponding FLAIR cortico-subcortical hyperintensity (**d**)

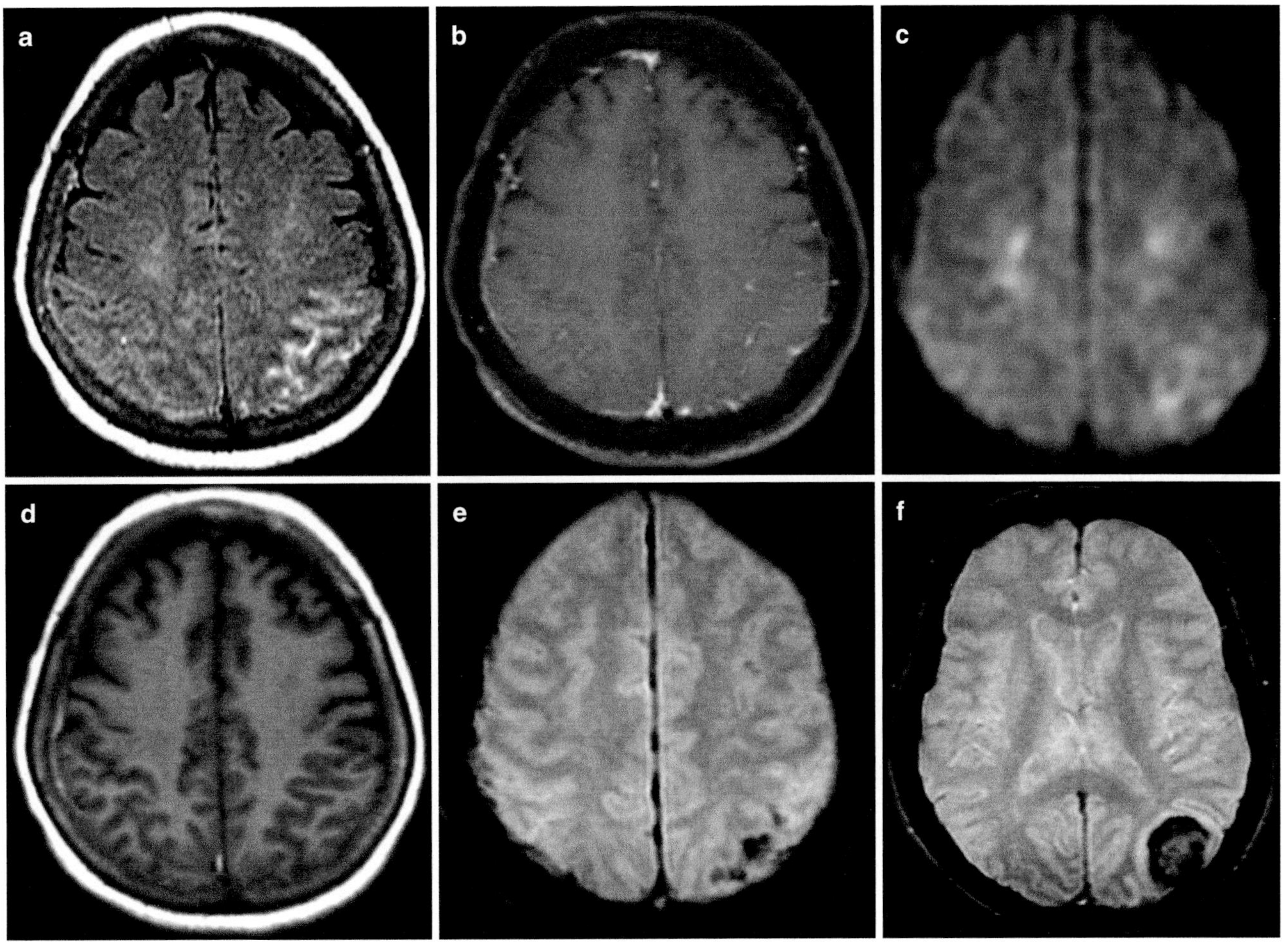

Fig. 11.4 *Streptococcus* meningitis with ischemic and hemorrhagic infarcts. At centrum semiovale level, left > right posterior FLAIR (**a**) subarachnoid hyperintensity and T1 (**b**) leptomeningeal enhancement (sparing of frontal lobes), DWI (**c**) with bilateral internal border zone centrum semiovale watershed infarcts. Axial T1 without contrast enhancement (**d**) shows parietal gyri swelling but fails to demonstrate small foci of left parietal cortico-subcortical hemorrhage, better depicted on T2* (**e**). Lateral ventricles level, T2*WI demonstrates left occipitoparietal juxta-subcortical focal hemorrhage with prominent blooming (**f**)

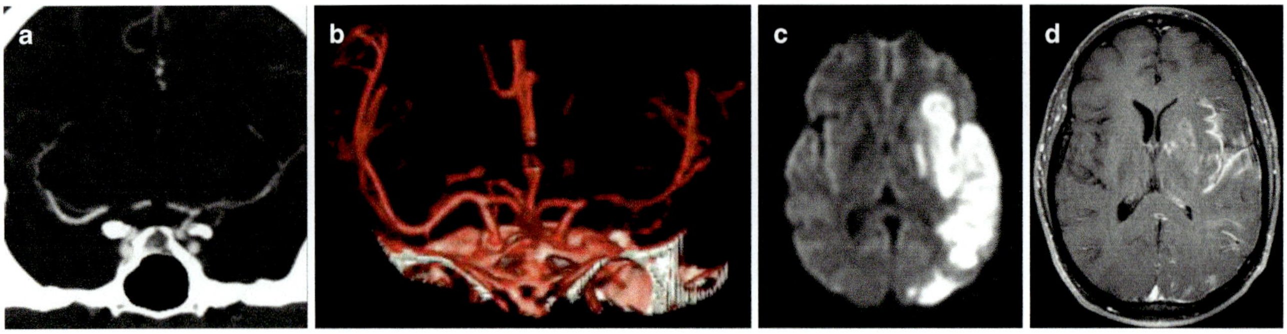

Fig. 11.5 Neurosyphilis on HIV patient with acute left MCA stroke (24 h) due to infective vasculitis. Axial and coronal CTA (**a**) images show diffuse narrowing of the left MCA and paucity of the distal branches. 3D reconstruction (**b**) confirms vessel stenosis. Axial DWI (**c**) showed intense restricted diffusion in the left putamen, insula, and temporoparietal/occipital lobes. Axial T1+C (**d**) shows diffuse leptomeningeal and gyriform enhancement in the affected areas, in part due to the infarction and to meningoencephalitis in this acute stage infarct that otherwise would not enhance

acute infarctions and small lacunar infarcts. These are seen as hyperintense on the diffusion-weighted images (DWI) with a corresponding decreased apparent diffusion coefficient values (ADC), indicative of restricted diffusion. These areas are low on T1W and high on T2W-FLAIR signal intensity with variable mass effect and sulci effacement. In the subacute phase of the infarcts, there is unrestricted diffusion on DWI and characteristic gyriform enhancement on post-contrast T1W images.

For CTA, MRA, and DSA, the angiographic vascular pattern of vasculitis with arterial narrowing and dilatations with "beaded appearance" (Fig. 11.5) is not specific of infectious vasculitis and is similar to noninfectious vasculopathy. DSA is considered the gold standard. In a small series of patients with the diagnosis of infectious vasculitis with stroke symptoms, 65% of patients demonstrated abnormalities with conversional digital subtraction angiography (DSA) [26, 30].

Vessel wall imaging can be performed with MRI. The vessels are seen with high-resolution black-blood contrast-enhanced T1-weighted MRI technique. This allows the evaluation of the arterial wall characteristics and not just the luminal evaluation that is obtained with conventional angiographic imaging modalities (CTA, MRA, and DSA). Vessel wall imaging findings of infectious vasculitis include smooth wall thickening of medium- and small-size arteries. The thickening is usually concentric but can also be eccentric, and wall enhancement is present during active inflammation [31–34].

11.3 Specific Pathogens

11.3.1 Bacterial

15–25% of patients with bacterial meningitis develop CNS vascular complications; of these 30% are associated with pneumococcal meningitis [17, 18, 25, 26, 29]. Vascular complications may be present in the acute phase of the meningovasculitis or appear days to weeks later after initiation of treatment and normalization of the cerebrospinal fluid (CSF). Patients are an overall higher risk for stroke within a year after the CNS infection [25, 30, 35]. Patients with CNS vascular complications present with focal neurologic deficit in up to 46% of cases [17]. One or more than one vascular territory can be affected.

MRI allows the early detection of acute territorial vascular infarcts. This may be seen along specific vascular territories or in a watershed distribution (either inner zone or cortical zone) as well as small perforating vessel lacunar infarcts in the basal ganglia, brain stem, and thalami (Fig. 11.6). There is T2/FLAIR/DWI hyperintensity with decreased ADC values consistent with restricted diffusion. Gyriform enhancement secondary to the breakdown of the blood-brain barrier (BBB) and from luxury perfusion is seen in the subacute phase. Nonspecific and non-territorial cortical foci of restricted diffusion on DWI and foci of GRE/SWI hypointensity related to micro-bleeds have also been described [36]. Blood products appear as hyperdensity on CT and hypointensity on GRE/SWI sequences on MRI. This may be seen in the subarachnoid space from spontaneous subarachnoid hemorrhage usually along the convexities. Intracerebral bleed associated to vasculitis can be present in up to 9.2% of patients with pneumococcal meningitis (Fig. 11.4) [26]. Angiographic imaging can demonstrate vasculopathic changes in up to 50% of patients with bacterial meningitis [30]. These are areas of vessel wall irregularity, segmental narrowing, and dilatations of the vessels, stenosis, and thrombosis involving the circle of Willis vessels at the basilar cistern level, as well as the supraclinoid segment of the ICA and occlusion of distal branches of the MCA. Large- and medium-size vessels are affected. Focal abnormal parenchymal blush has also been described in DSA [30, 36].

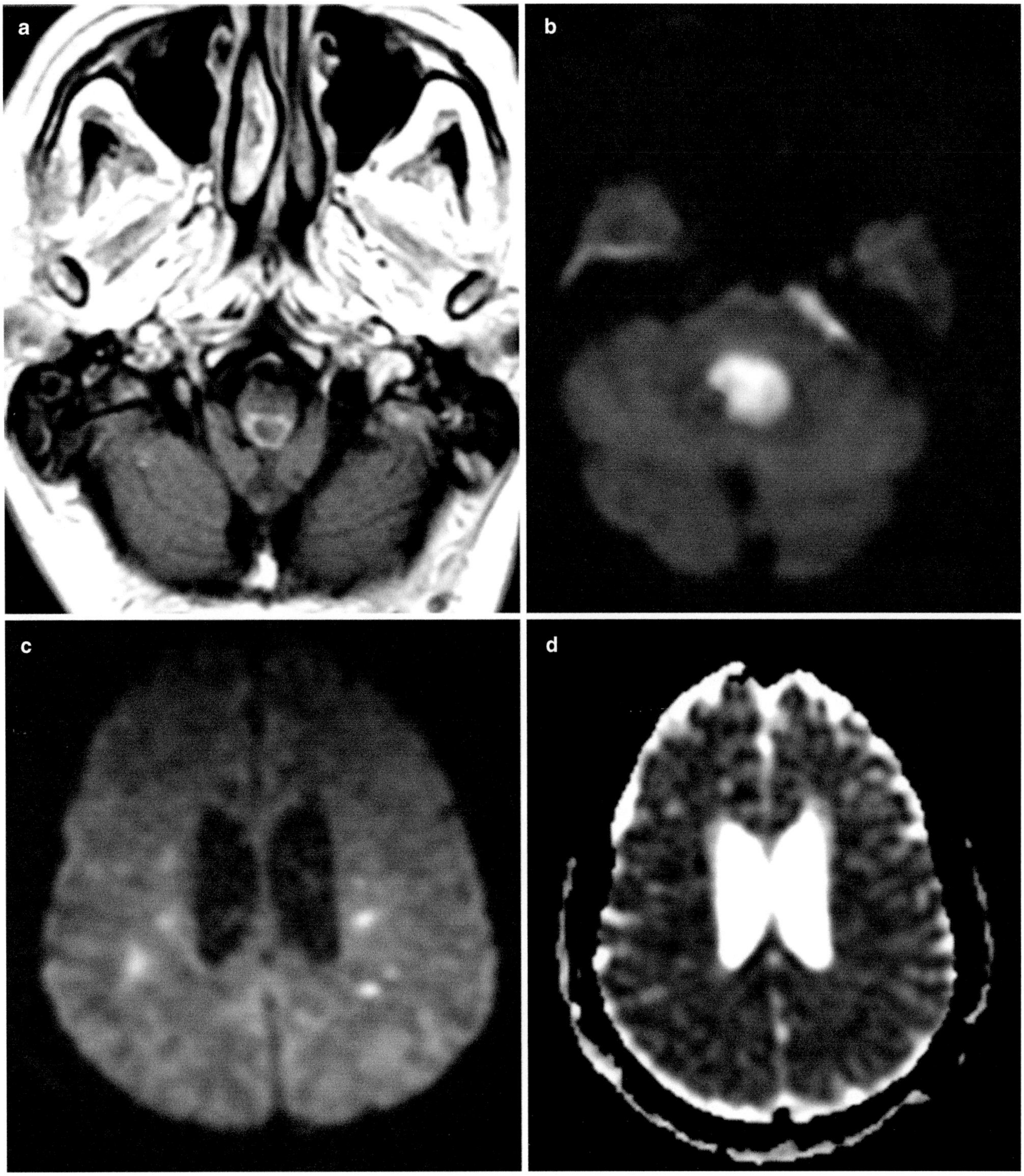

Fig. 11.6 MRSA Bulbo-medullary abscess and embolic infarcts; diabetic patient who presented with quadriplegia and ventilator dependent. Axial T1 post contrast (**a**) shows ring enhancing bulbo-medullary junction abscess. Evacuation of abscess with piocele within the 4th ventricle shows restricted diffusion on DWI (**b**) and bilateral corona radiata acute lacunar infarcts with restricted diffusion on DWI/ADC (**c**, **d**)

11.3.2 Syphilis

Approximately 5–10% of untreated syphilitic patients will develop neurosyphilis [37]. And meningovascular syphilitic infection is present in 15–23% of patients with neurosyphilis [29]. Most patients are asymptomatic or present with nonspecific symptoms. About 10–20% of these patients have brain infarctions, usually in young adults without cerebrovascular risk factors [18, 38]. About 30% of patients with neurosyphilis have negative imaging studies [38]. Syphilis was nearly eradicated with the use of penicillin; however the prevalence increased since the HIV-AIDS epidemic. Since syphilis is sexually transmitted, there is an increase coinfection of HIV and syphilis, both of which potentiate each other, putting patients at a higher risk for more aggressive and faster involvement of the CNS by both organisms [29, 39]. Patients with early form of neurosyphilis either meningitis or meningovasculitis (more commonly seen in the setting of HIV-AIDS) have symptoms of meningitis with altered mental status, cranial nerve palsies, and acute or subacute focal neurologic deficits from vasculitis and infarcts. Over the entire course of the disease, the most common neurologic manifestation is psychiatric symptomatology with personality changes and cognitive impairment. The spirochete (*Treponema pallidum*) enters the cerebrospinal fluid (CSF) early in the course of infection, but it could take decades before manifesting any neurological symptomatology; early form presents within 2–7 years after the infection, and late form which is almost never seen anymore takes more than two decades; however HIV patients have a more accelerated course of syphilitic infection [39]. The bacterium infects the vascular endothelial cells. There is thickening of the intima from proliferation of fibroblasts. There is thinning of the media and adventitial inflammation and fibrosis, which result in the so-called obliterative endarteritis or Heubner arteritis. Progression of vasculopathy with luminal narrowing and thrombosis will lead to strokes [18].

MRI findings in meningovascular neurosyphilis are not very specific, but MRI is very sensitive in the detection of periventricular and juxtacortical white matter T2-FLAIR hyperintense foci (due to small microvascular involvement), leptomeningeal enhancement, cranial nerve (CN) enhancement in cranial neuritis, and cortical- or dural-based gummas [38, 40]. Cerebrovascular imaging finding is usually related to infectious arteritis of medium- and large-size vessels (commonly the middle cerebral and basilar arteries). This results in territorial infarctions (Fig. 11.7). Lacunar infarcts in the basal ganglia and brain stem can result from involvement of perforator vessels as well. Areas of alternating narrowing and dilatations of the circle of Willis vessels or focal vessel narrowing or stenosis are seen in DSA and MRA/CTA vascular images [29, 41].

11.3.3 Tuberculosis

Approximately 1% of patients with pulmonary tuberculosis (TB) present with tuberculous meningitis, which is the most common manifestation of CNS involvement. Stroke is a common complication of TB meningitis with an incidence range from 15% to 60% [29, 42]. In addition, tuberculous meningitis is the most common cause of chronic meningitis. Vascular complications of TB meningitis are more common in the setting of chronic evolution than in the promptly treated acute TB meningitis. Infection usually originating from the lungs disseminates hematogenously to the leptomeninges which result in subpial deposits (tubercles) that then rupture into the cerebrospinal fluid (CSF) of the subarachnoid space. The inflammatory exudate predominantly settles in the subarachnoid space of the basilar cisterns and Sylvian fissures; it then infiltrates the traversing vessels producing endarteritis (affected vessels can also present granulomatous proliferative angiitis, fibrinoid necrosis, and caseous necrotizing vasculitis) with stenosis and occlusion of the vessels that may be associated or not with thrombosis [42]. This commonly affects medium-sized and small-caliber vessels, often the middle cerebral artery (MCA) and its branches. The most commonly affected small-size vessels are the lenticulostriate and thalamoperforating arteries. Besides the systemic symptoms associated to TB, patients with cerebrovascular

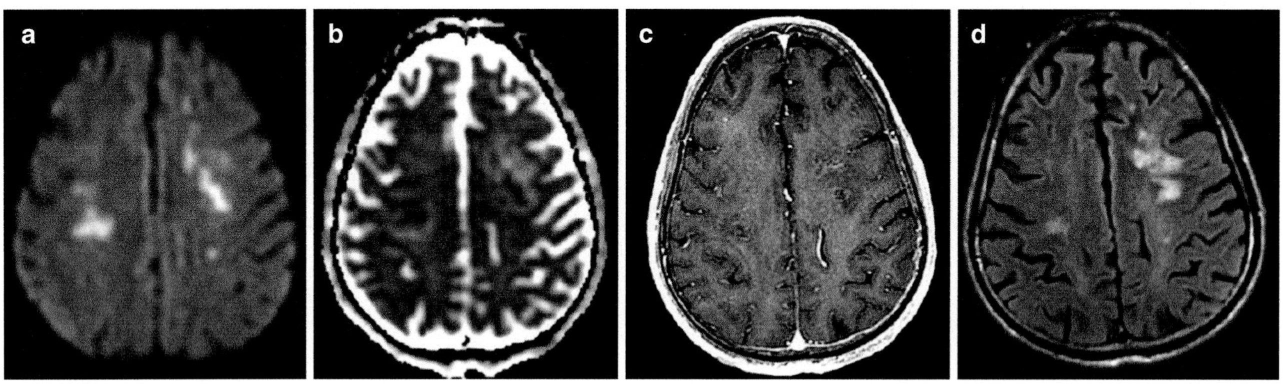

Fig. 11.7 Neurosyphilis in an AIDS patient with watershed acute infarcts. Infectious vasculitis with bilateral multifocal inner zone watershed acute infarcts with DWI (**a**) hyperintensity, ADC map (**b**) hypointensity and on axial T1 + C (**c**) subtle leptomeningeal enhancement, on FLAIR (**d**) hyperintensity in areas of ischemia without subarachnoid hyperintensity (inability to mount a more aggressive inflammatory response, CD4 = 2)

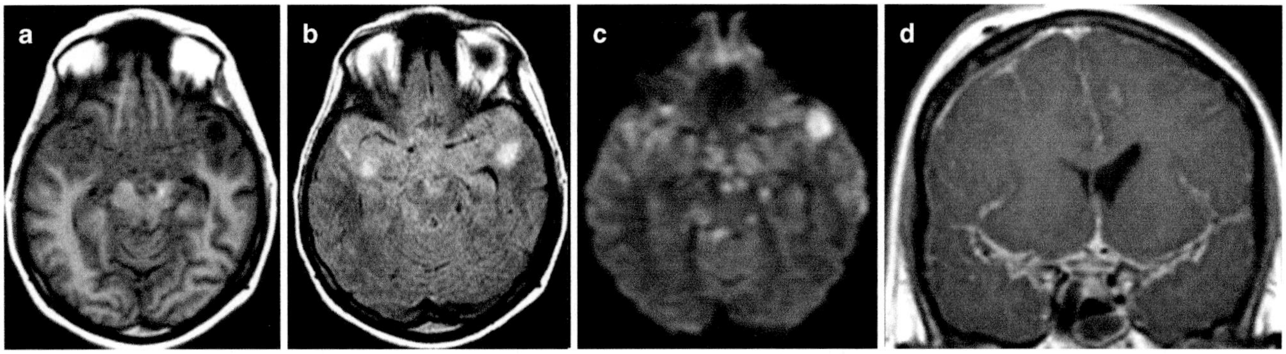

Fig. 11.8 Chronic basilar tuberculous meningitis, initial images without contrast due to pregnancy which also delayed the anti-TB treatment. Widening and filling of the basilar cisterns and Sylvian fissures with T1 (**a**) isointense and FLAIR (**b**) hyperintense exudate; some organized abscesses have mild DWI hyperintensity and restricted diffusion (**c**). Follow-up MRI axial T1 with contrast shows leptomeningeal enhancement along the cisterns, convexal sulci, and perivascular (**d**)

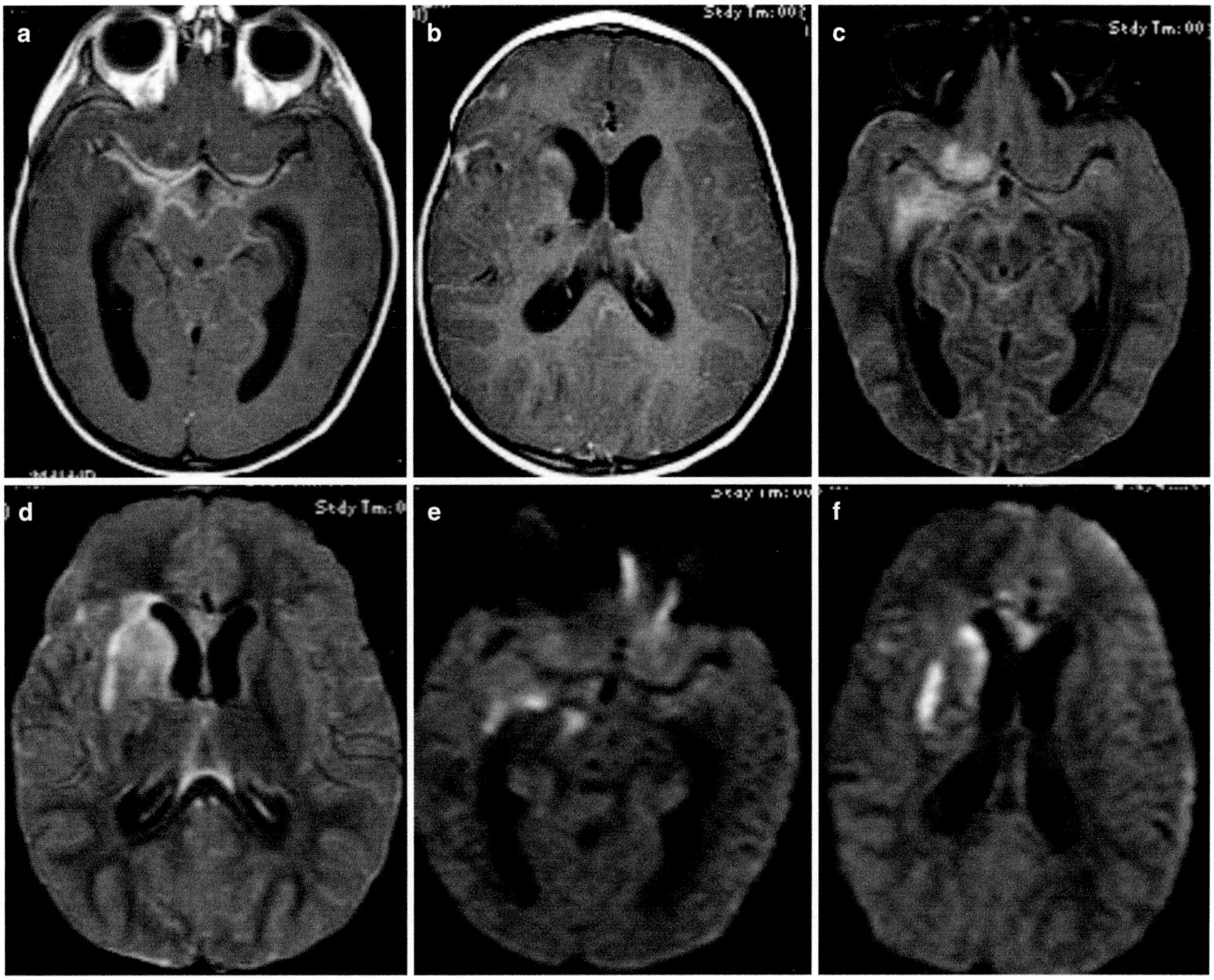

Fig. 11.9 Tuberculous basilar meningitis with basal ganglia infarcts. Axial T1+C (**a**, **b**) with basilar cisterns and right frontal sulci leptomeningeal enhancement, axial FLAIR (**c**, **d**) at the basilar cisterns, and basal ganglia levels show right inferior frontotemporal, striatum nucleus, and callosal hyperintensity with correspondent DWI (**e**, **f**) restricted diffusion consistent with acute infarcts

compromise develop ischemia that evolves insidiously with focal weakness and stroke symptoms that may be obscured by patient's altered level of consciousness caused by the tuberculous meningoencephalitis. Coinfection with HIV increases the risk of tuberculous meningitis [29, 41]. Antituberculous chemotherapy may be ineffective in preventing CNS vascular complications of TB meningitis, which suggest an immune-mediated mechanism [24, 43].

MRI is superior to CT in the detection of the small infarcts. These are seen as areas of T2/FLAIR hyperintensity with restricted diffusion on DWI in the acute stage (Fig. 11.8). Up to 75% of TB-related infarcts are located in the basal ganglia and thalami (Fig. 11.9) [18, 44]. Hemorrhagic transformations of infarcts are particularly conspicuous on susceptibility-weighted images (SWI) [41]. Angiographic images CTA, MRA, and DSA show single or multiple vessel involvement; usually there is segmental irregularity of the vessels, concentric narrowing, beaded appearance, and stenosis or occlusion. The most commonly affected medium-size vessels are the supraclinoid segment of the ICA and proximal portions of the MCA and ACA (almost following a moyamoya-like vascular pattern); additional findings on DSA include delayed circulation in the MCA with paucity of collaterals and early venous drainage [42, 45–47].

11.3.4 Herpesviridae

Herpes simplex virus HSV-1 meningoencephalitis can complicate with intracerebral petechial hemorrhages or hematomas in severe cases, which is due to disruption of the BBB with cerebral edema and necrosis. The dissemination of the infection is from the nasopharyngeal mucosa that then invades sensory lingual branches of the trigeminal nerve and in a retrograde manner reaches the trigeminal ganglion, where it remains latent. The disease is usually expressed in situation of stress, trauma, immunosuppression, or hormonal fluctuations. The infections affect particularly the limbic system, inferomedial-anterior temporal lobes, inferior orbitofrontal gyri, insula, and cingulate cortex (distribution suggests retrograde intracranial dissemination along small branches of the trigeminal nerve). CT in the setting of HSV-1 infection is usually negative or may show areas of hypodensity in the inferior frontal and temporal lobes. This is due to encephalitis with involvement of single or bilateral lobes. The latter is usually asymmetric. MRI findings in patients with HSV-1 include low T1W, high T2/FLAIR signal, and restricted diffusion on DWI (which can last for about 2 weeks) [48]. This is due to edema from encephalitis in the affected areas and from cytotoxic damage. In the post-contrast images, variable cortical and meningeal enhancement can be seen (Fig. 11.10). Characteristic petechial hemorrhage, if present, appears as cortical T1W shortening hyperintensities and blooms of hypointensity on GRE and SWI scans. Fulminant cerebral hemorrhage is rare and usually lethal in spite of aggressive intravenous antiviral therapy [49]. In contrast to other pathogens, HSV-1 CNS infection is not associated with increased risk of stroke [18, 50].

Varicella encephalitis is the most serious CNS complication of varicella zoster virus infection (VSV); the incidence varies depending on the geographic regions and types of studies. The annual incidence in the absence of an outbreak is about 1–2 episodes per 10,000 varicella cases (highest in adults and infants) [51]. VZV can cause intracranial vasculopathy as an acute infection (chickenpox) or as a reactivation of a latent VZV. VZV remains latent in the neuraxis ganglia-trigeminal ganglion (after upper respiratory or conjunctival exposure, given its neurotropic nature); it is reactivated in patients with decreased cell-mediated immunity. The VZV directly infects the adventitia of large and small cerebral vessels, causing arteritis. Immunosuppressed patients are at a higher risk of VZV-associated vasculopathy

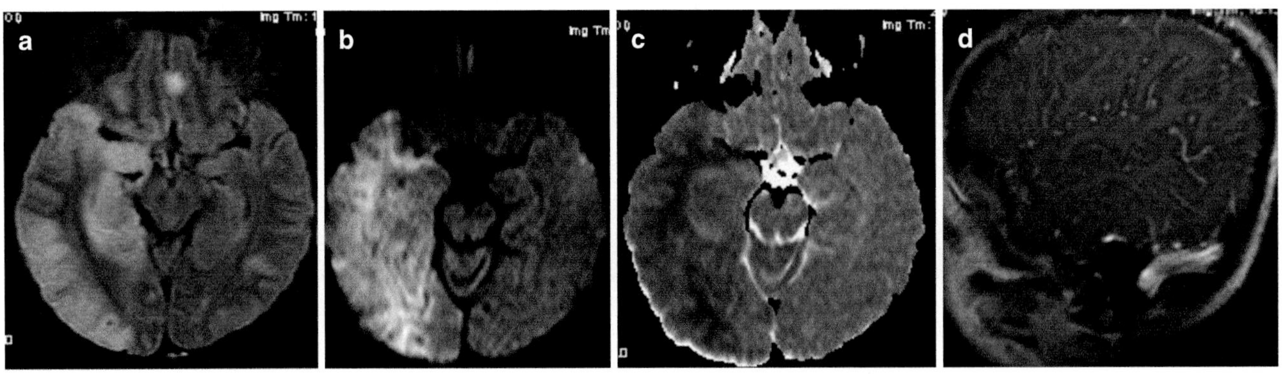

Fig. 11.10 Herpes encephalitis. Multiples areas of FLAIR (**a**) hyperintensity in the right temporo-occipital, left posterior temporal, and left inferior frontal lobes, with corresponding restricted diffusion on DWI/ADC (**b**, **c**) and leptomeningeal enhancement on post-contrast sagittal T1 (**d**)

(HIV and posttransplant patients). VZV vasculopathy is the most common cause of ischemic stroke in children (about one-third of childhood strokes) [52, 53]. Large vessel VZV vasculopathy includes herpes zoster ophthalmicus, granulomatous angiitis, VZV vasculitis, and VZV-associated stroke. Patients with herpes zoster ophthalmicus have a higher risk of stroke; the virus has direct retrograde spread into the ACA, MCA, and ICA [54]. Patients with VZV vasculopathy present with fever, headache, seizures, altered mental status, and focal neurologic deficit from TIA or stroke. Neurological disease may occur months after zoster rash has resolved or even without a history of rash [55]. VZV vasculopathy has a predilection for small-size basal ganglia vessels causing uni- or bilateral deep gray nuclei infarcts. On MR T2/FLAIR, these are seen as hyperintensity with restricted diffusion. When infecting large vessels (granulomatous arteritis), patients present with territorial infarcts, commonly the MCA and ACA distributions. Arterial imaging (CTA, DSA, MRA) shows vessel wall irregularity, segmental narrowing, or occlusion of the vessel. Patients can also present with aneurysms, subarachnoid and parenchymal hemorrhage, and segmental MCA and ACA dissection [29, 53, 56]. Chronic VZV encephalitis presents T2/FLAIR hyperintense demyelinating plaques in the deep white matter and late ischemic or hemorrhagic infarcts in the deep gray nuclei or cortically based. The hemorrhagic component will present prominent blooming on GRE and SWI [51].

11.3.5 Human Immunodeficiency Virus (HIV)

There is a 1.5 higher risk for stroke in patients with human immunodeficiency virus (HIV) infection compared to the general population [18]. This has been attributed to endothelial dysfunction, inflammation, and subclinical atherosclerosis. There are additional factors that increase the risk of stroke in patients with HIV. This includes the coagulopathy/atherogenesis associated with antiretroviral therapy, the increase in inflammatory markers from HIV infection, and the coexisting opportunistic infections (particularly synergistic with concurrent VZV infection [57]). The HIV-infected patients may have increased risk due to a clinical history of drug abuse, hypercoagulable states, or cardiovascular comorbidities. Between 10% and 50% of patients with AIDS with a coagulopathy develop a stroke [58]. These patients present with altered mental status, cognitive impairment, and acute focal deficits. Advance-stage HIV infection mainly in young population (less often adults) can affect directly large-size vessels. There is thinning of the medial layer of the vessel wall that results in fusiform aneurysmal and non-aneurysmal arterial dilatation. Transient ischemic attacks (TIAs) and strokes may present as a result of distal embolization from unruptured aneurysms [18, 57, 59, 60]. The HIV can also affect small-size penetrating intracerebral vessels. For example, infective vasculopathy in adults has been described with wall thickening, dilatation of the perivascular spaces, vessel wall mineralization, perivascular inflammatory cell infiltrates, and vessel occlusion with patchy distribution in different territories [61].

MRI can detect acute subcortical and territorial cortical infarcts seen as areas with restricted diffusion [57, 62]. MRI can help exclude other diagnosis, such as abscess and focal lesions from opportunistic infections that can also present with clinical symptoms of stroke (Fig. 11.11). Angiographic imaging can demonstrate irregularity of the vessel wall and caliber variations. CTA, MRA, and DSA may show fusiform aneurysmal dilatations that are usually multiple (Fig. 11.12). These may be located at the circle of Willis, supraclinoid ICA, proximal MCA, and ACA; rarely small infective aneurysms are seen peripherally in the distal branches, similar to other infectious aneurysms [18, 57, 60, 62, 63].

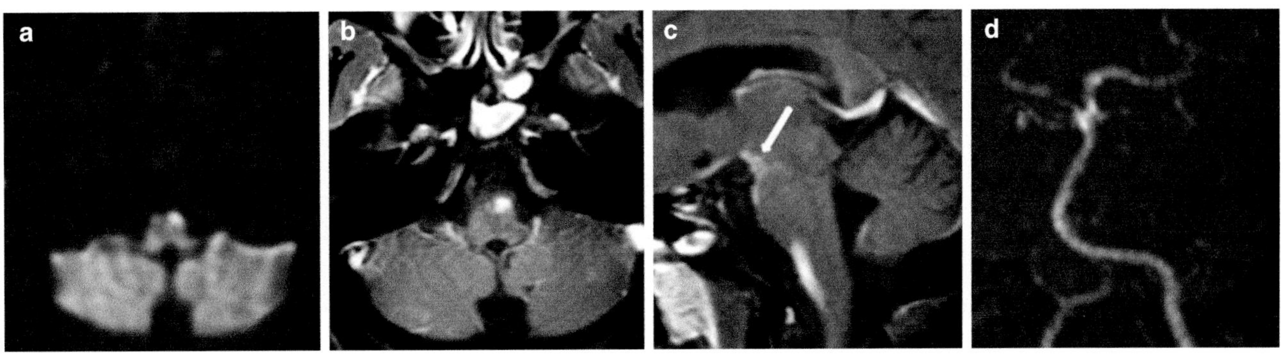

Fig. 11.11 HIV patients with meningoencephalitis and acute pyramidal stroke. Left pyramidal subacute infarct with mild restricted diffusion on DWI (**a**), enhancement on post contrast axial and sagittal T1 (**b**, **c**); also weak leptomeningeal enhancement (CD4 = 4) in the interpeduncular cistern (arrow c). MRA (**d**) beaded appearance of the posterior circulation, mainly the bilateral PCAs with narrowing and poor visualization of the bilateral AICAs and PICAs, from infective vasculitis

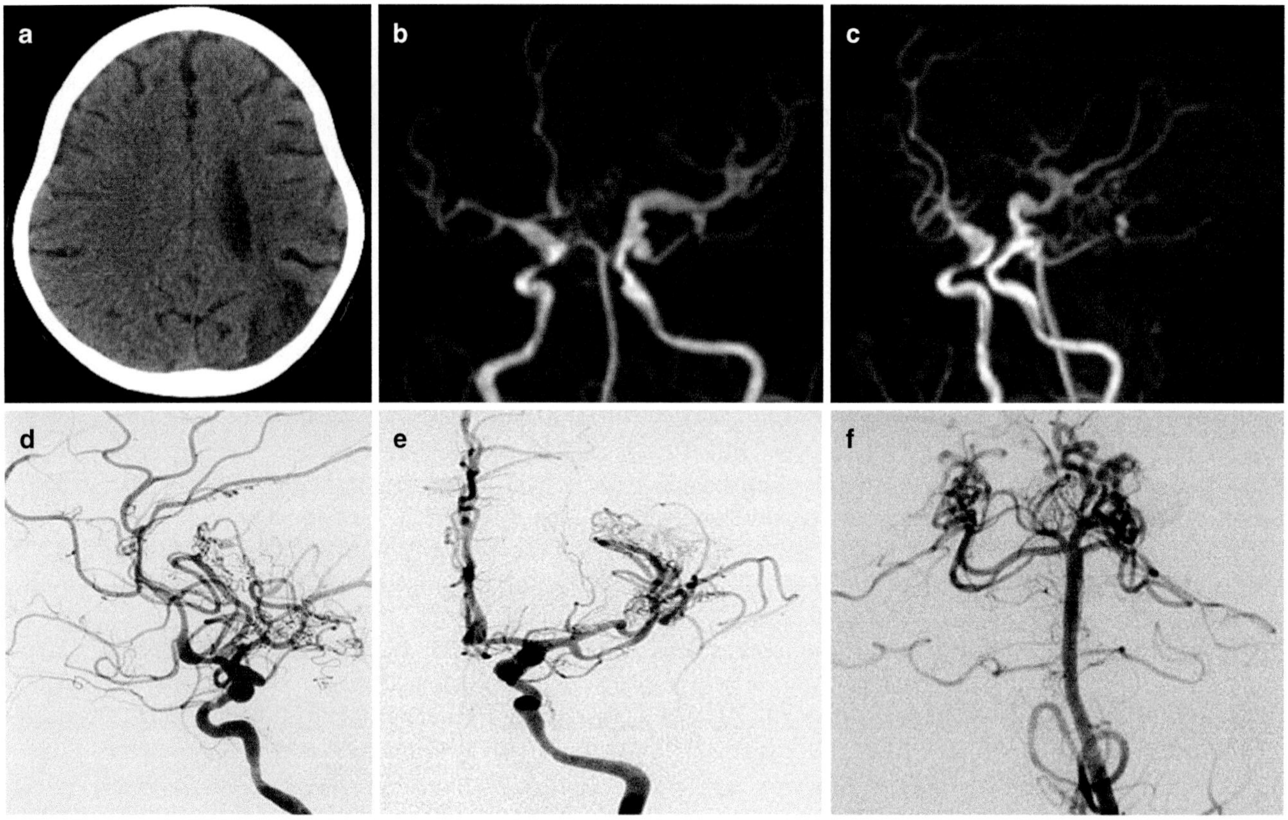

Fig. 11.12 HIV-related aneurysmal dilatation of the COW. Axial head CT (**a**) on a 7-year-old girl with chronic left posterior MCA infarct. Frontal PA and oblique MRA images (**b**, **c**) show multifocal large vessel fusiform aneurysmal (bilateral supraclinoid ICAs, bilateral carotid terminus, and diffusely ACA, MCA M1, and M2 segments) and non-aneurysmal (proximal cavernous ICAs) dilatation of the COW vessels. Also segmental areas of narrowing of the bilateral petrous and distal cavernous ICAs. DSA left ICA injection lateral (**d**) and frontal (**e**) projections confirm aneurysms and show left MCA occlusive changes and small arterial-arterial collaterals with slow flow within its distal territory. Left VA injection DSA (**f**) shows multiple arterial occlusion changes (such as AICA) and multiple arterial-arterial collaterals (Courtesy Brandon Tran, M.D TCH, Houston, TX)

11.3.6 Fungal

Cryptococcus spp. is the most common CNS fungal infections and usually affects HIV and other immunocompromised patients. Cryptococcosis is the most common CNS fungal infection in HIV patients and is the third most common CNS infection on AIDS patients behind HIV demyelination and toxoplasmosis. It occurs in 6–10% of HIV-AIDS patients [64]. Frequently patients with CNS cryptococcal infection lack the characteristic fever and meningism seen in other infectious meningitis. This makes the prospective diagnosis even more challenging [65]. Patients may present with subacute meningoencephalitis, headache, low-grade fever, and slowly and progressive altered sensorium. They usually occur as a hematogenous dissemination from lung infection after inhalation of the spores. Dissemination to the CNS reaches the subarachnoid space and meninges and then spreads along the perivascular (Virchow-Robins) subarachnoid spaces (PVS), which will eventually dilate and collect gelatinous pseudocysts filled with yeasts [66]. The meninges are the most commonly affected location. Basilar meningitis can cause irritation of the subarachnoid traversing basilar vessel that can then cause vasospasm or infective endarteritis with vessel stenosis resulting in the deep gray nuclei, midbrain, and cerebellar ischemic insults and hemorrhages. On MRI the meningeal enhancement is scant [66]. Better depicted on MRI are the dilated PVS that appear as clusters of "soap bubble" non-enhancing cysts that are isointense to CSF on T1 and T2. They are usually located in the basal ganglia, thalami, and midbrain (Fig. 11.13).

Aspergillus spp. *hyphae* are the most important mold associated to stroke. Most cases occur in immunocompromised patients. Approximately 10–20% of patients that have received chemotherapy and/or immunosuppressive therapy after solid organ or bone marrow transplant will develop invasive intracranial dissemination of aspergillosis [65]. Patients present with fever, headache, altered mental status, cranial nerve deficits, seizures, and focal neurologic deficits. There are two forms of CNS aspergillosis: cerebrovascular aspergillosis that occurs through hematogenous dissemination (from lung infection after inhalation of the spore) and

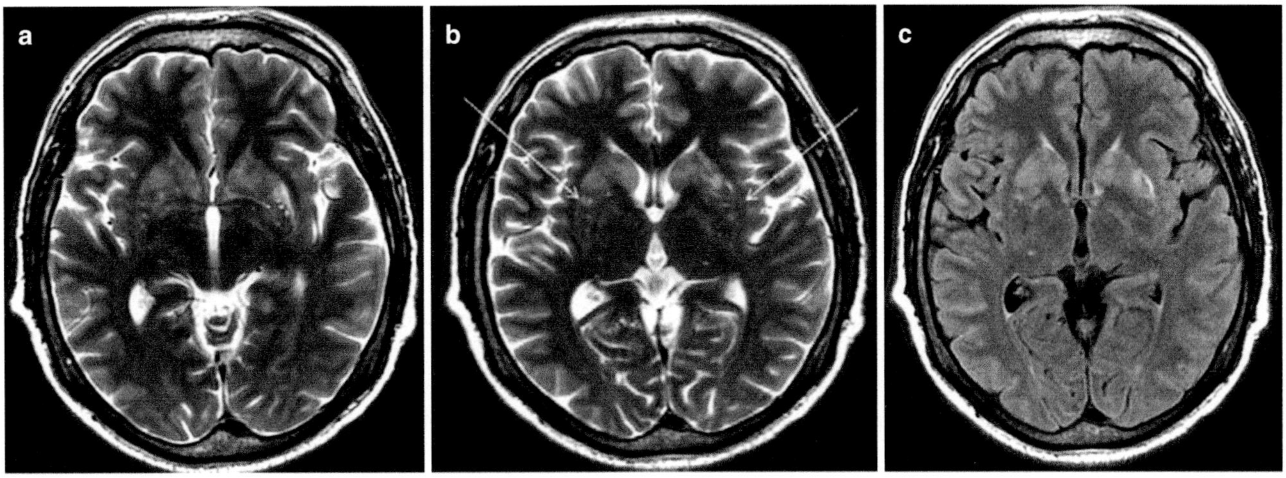

Fig. 11.13 Cryptococcal meningitis on an HIV patient. Axial T2 (**a**, **b**) and FLAIR (**c**) with increased bilateral basal ganglia (striatum nuclei) signal intensity from gelatinous pseudocyst along the basilar perivascular spaces

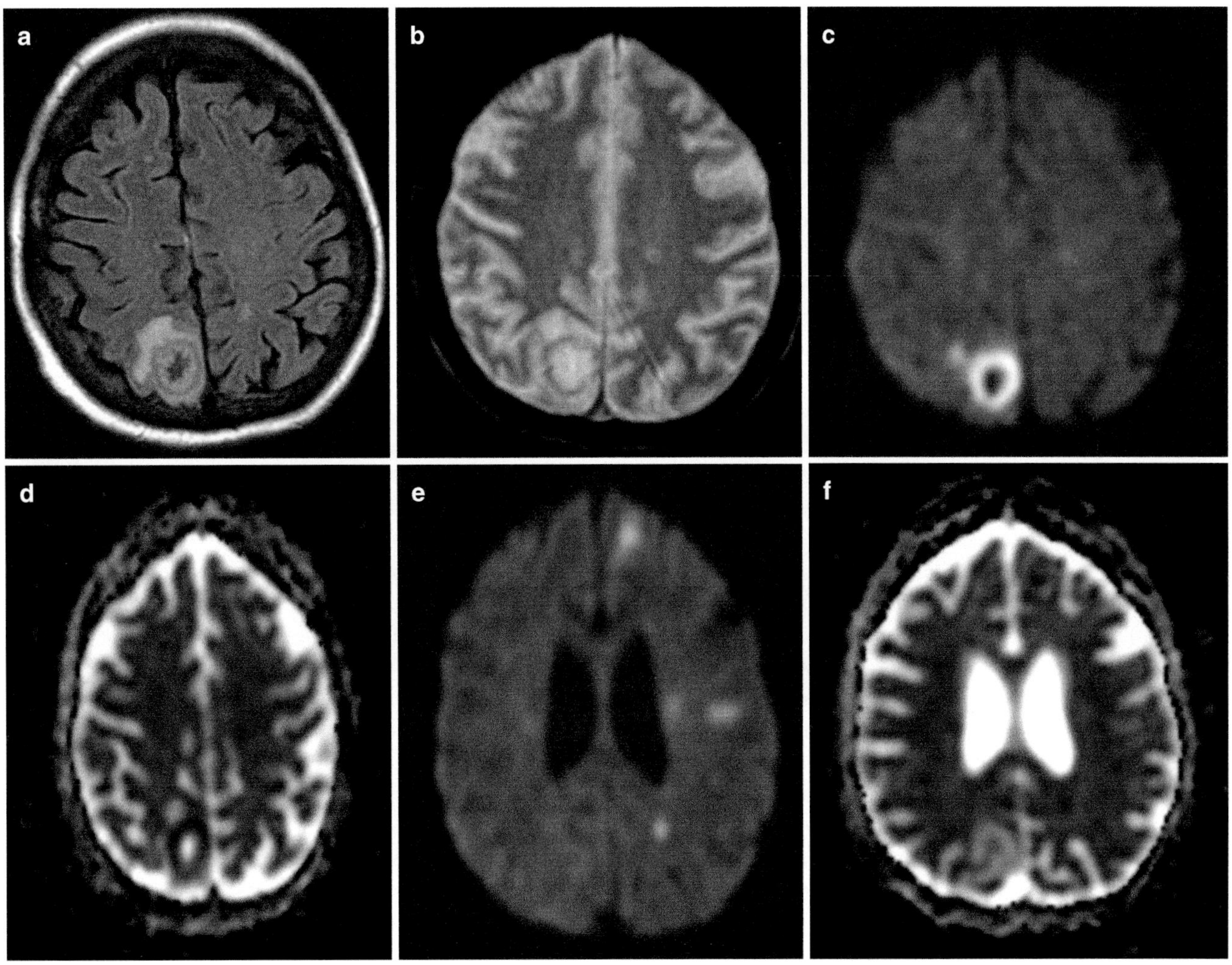

Fig. 11.14 CNS aspergillosis with abscesses and embolic infarcts. Diabetic patient on chronic steroid use with pulmonary aspergillosis and focal fungal abscess in the right superior parietal juxtacortical region with FLAIR (**a**) hyperintense rim, T2* (**b**) hypointense rim, and mural restricted diffusion on DWI/ADC (**c**, **d**) only in the periphery of the abscess. Additional scatter cortico-subcortical solid restricted diffusion correspond to acute embolic lacunar infarcts (**e**, **f**)

rhinocerebral invasion directly from the paranasal sinuses and orbits. Angioinvasion of large- and medium-size vessels results in infective arteritis with vessel occlusion with usually single large territorial stroke or multiple embolic ischemic lacunar infarcts (usually peripherally located in the gray-white junction and in the basal ganglia). They can also develop single or multiple hemorrhagic infarcts and mycotic aneurysms. These result in an increased risk of subarachnoid and parenchymal hemorrhage [18, 67]. Infarctions of the deep gray nuclei, thalami, and corpus callosum are also common and likely the result of secondary involvement of perforating arteries after angioinvasion of the parent larger ACA and MCA arteries. These may be seen in association to a corticomedullary junction lesion but not always [67]. On non-contrast CT there are areas of cortico-subcortical hypodensity with variable hyperdense hemorrhage. MRI shows acute basal ganglia infarcts and territorial vascular insults commonly along the MCA and ACA [65]. On MRI the infarctions will present as areas of homogeneous restricted diffusion of the entire lesion as oppose to just peripheral restricted diffusion. The latter is commonly seen in the fungal abscess counterparts that are also present in these patients. In fact areas of ischemia can evolve to cerebritis and subsequent abscess formation. Abscess has T2*GRE (SWI if available) hypointense rim, mural restricted diffusion in the periphery of the abscess and peripheral rim enhancement on T1 postcontrast images (Fig. 11.14). MR spectroscopy (MRS) may help differentiate between these two entities. Abscesses have disaccharide trehalose peaks between 3.6 and 3.8 ppm, as well as cytosolic amino acids, lipids, and lactate peaks [68, 69]. Angiographic images will demonstrate a pattern of vasculitis and characteristics of infectious-mycotic aneurysms. Additional information on aspergillosis related cavernous sinus thrombosis and mycotic aneurisms in the sinus thrombophlebitis and infectious aneurysms sections, respectively.

Rhinocerebral mucormycosis is a craniofacial infection caused by the *Mucor* spp. or *Rhizopus* spp. *hyphae*. This mostly affects immunocompromised (leukemia, hematopoietic stem cell transplantation, IV drug use, iron overload states, or deferoxamine chelation) and uncontrolled diabetic patients. Delayed diagnosis results in significantly higher mortality rates particularly commonly seen in the setting of diabetic ketoacidosis and stem cell transplant [65, 70]. Patients have juxta-cranial sites of infection, and so they usually have symptoms of sinusitis, facial numbness, pain, oculocranial nerve palsy, visual disturbances, and focal neurologic deficits. *Microorganisms* enter via the nasopharynx and paranasal sinuses. Given the strong angioinvasive nature, it can have cerebrovascular extension reaching the cavernous sinuses. The organism invades the vessel wall causing severe necrotizing vasculitis, with vascular dissection and thrombotic occlusion in major branches of the circle of Willis (COW) at the skull base and vertebrobasilar circulation that result in large territorial infarcts; they can also present with mycotic aneurysms and hemorrhagic infarcts. As the infection extends into the cavernous sinuses, it can cause septic thrombophlebitis with additional narrowing of the cavernous segments of the ICA [69, 71]. Additional information on mucormycosis related cavernous sinus thrombosis and mycotic aneurysms in the sinus thrombophlebitis and infectious aneurysms sections, respectively.

Coccidioidomycosis is caused by the *Coccidioides immitis*; it occurs in the endemic zones of California, Arizona, Mexico, and Central-South America. The disease is usually a mild febrile illness; severe pulmonary or disseminated forms are rare. Approximately 1–5% of patients have extrapulmonary disseminated disease, which carries a higher morbidity and mortality [72]. The CNS involvement is the most serious form, particularly dismal in patients with stroke; CNS infection if left untreated is always fatal [72, 73]. In a large series of patients in the United States, 3.1% of patients with coccidioidomycosis presented with CNS involvement [72]. In the same group of patients, reoccurrence of coccidioidomycosis occurred in 24% of patients; the highest risk (71%) was among patients with CNS disease, which is why these patients require antifungal lifelong treatment [72]. Population at risk for disseminated coccidioidomycosis includes elderly persons, pregnant women, certain ethnic groups, prisoners, and immunocompromised patients with HIV-AIDS, diabetes, and chronic corticosteroid or alcohol use. Besides the pulmonary and systemic coccidioidomycosis-related symptoms, patients present with headache, cranial nerve deficits related to chronic basilar meningitis, changes in mental status, TIA, and stroke symptoms. The fungus infects the lungs and disseminates hematogenously to the CNS usually weeks or months after the initial infection. Ischemic vasculitis may complicate up to 40% of patients months later [65]. The mechanism of stroke is similar to other chronic meningitides, medium- and small-size vessels traveling through the basilar cistern meningitis and subarachnoid space exudate containing pyogranulomatous and fibroblastic inflammation that involves the vessels, and leads to endarteritis obliterans with subsequent thrombosis, brain infarctions, and necrosis. Cerebral ischemia can also result from septic emboli. MRI finding includes leptomeningeal enhancement along the basilar cisterns and Sylvian fissures, territorial cortical strokes, and peripheral corticomedullary embolic infarcts (Fig. 11.15). Peripheral rim of enhancement and restricted diffusion in parenchymal lesions correspond to abscesses and not infarct. Infarcts have diffuse-complete restricted diffusion and only enhance in the subacute phase (Fig. 11.16). Additionally, on MRS, abscesses have disaccharide trehalose peaks between 3.6 and 3.8 ppm, as well as cytosolic amino acids, lipids, and lactate peaks [68, 69]. MRA shows diffuse vascular

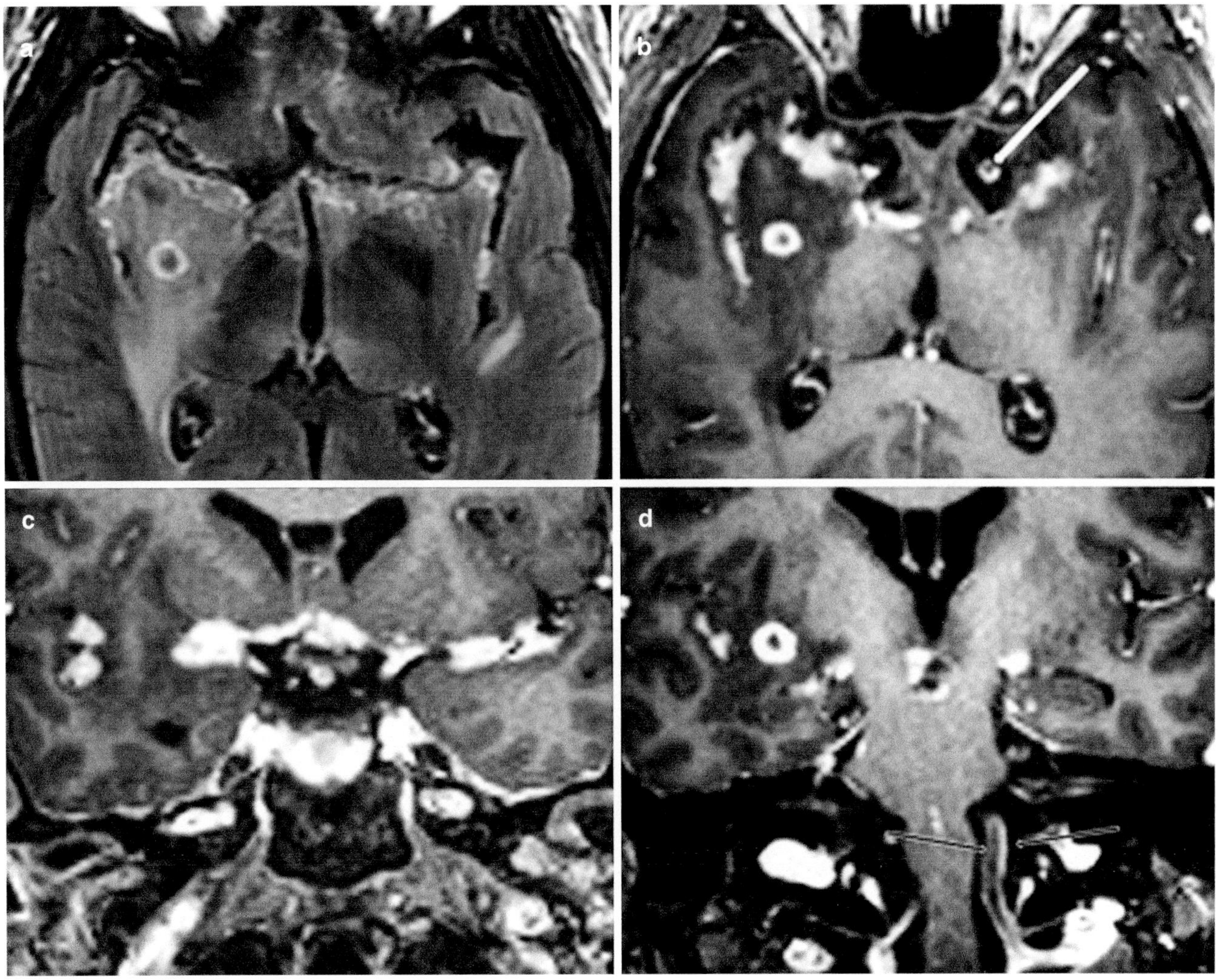

Fig. 11.15 Disseminated Coccidiodomycosis meningoencephalitis and infective vasculitis. Axial FLAIR (**a**) shows irregularity of the bilateral MCAs M1 segments as they cross the basilar cisterns exudate. Axial T1 post contrast (**b**) with prominent enhancing exudate in the basilar cisterns and Sylvian fissures, enhancement of the ICAs wall due to infectious vasculitis (white arrows). Coronals T1 post contrast (**c**, **d**) show leptomeningeal enhancement in the basilar cisterns and Sylvian fissures and enhancement of the left vertebral artery wall (arrows d)

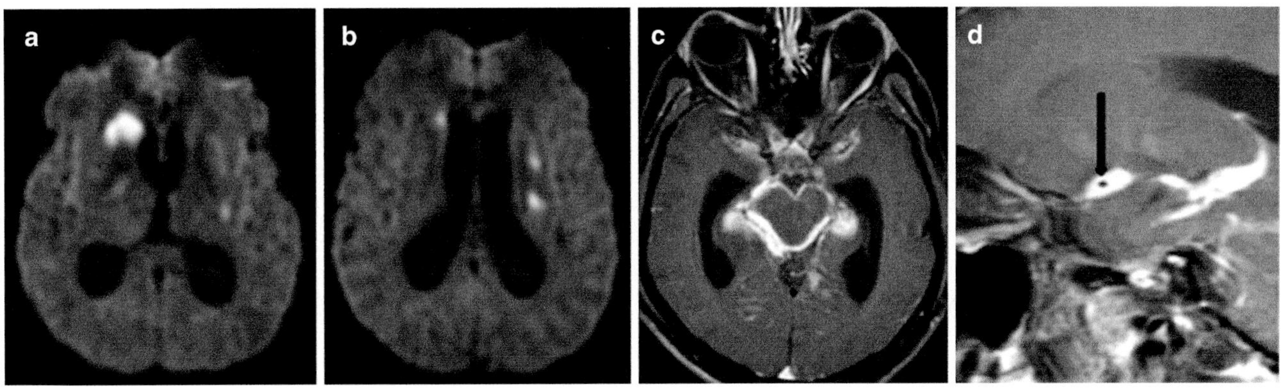

Fig. 11.16 Disseminated Coccidiodomycosis with acute infarcts. Axial DWI (**a**, **b**) with hydrocephalus and right basal ganglia (striatum nucleus) and smaller bilateral corona radiata acute lacunar infarcts. Post-contrast axial T1 (**c**) shows severe leptomeningeal enhancement along the basilar cisterns and Sylvian fissures, sagittal postcontrast T1 (**d**) shows the MCA embedded within the exudate and associated narrowing of the vessel (black arrow)

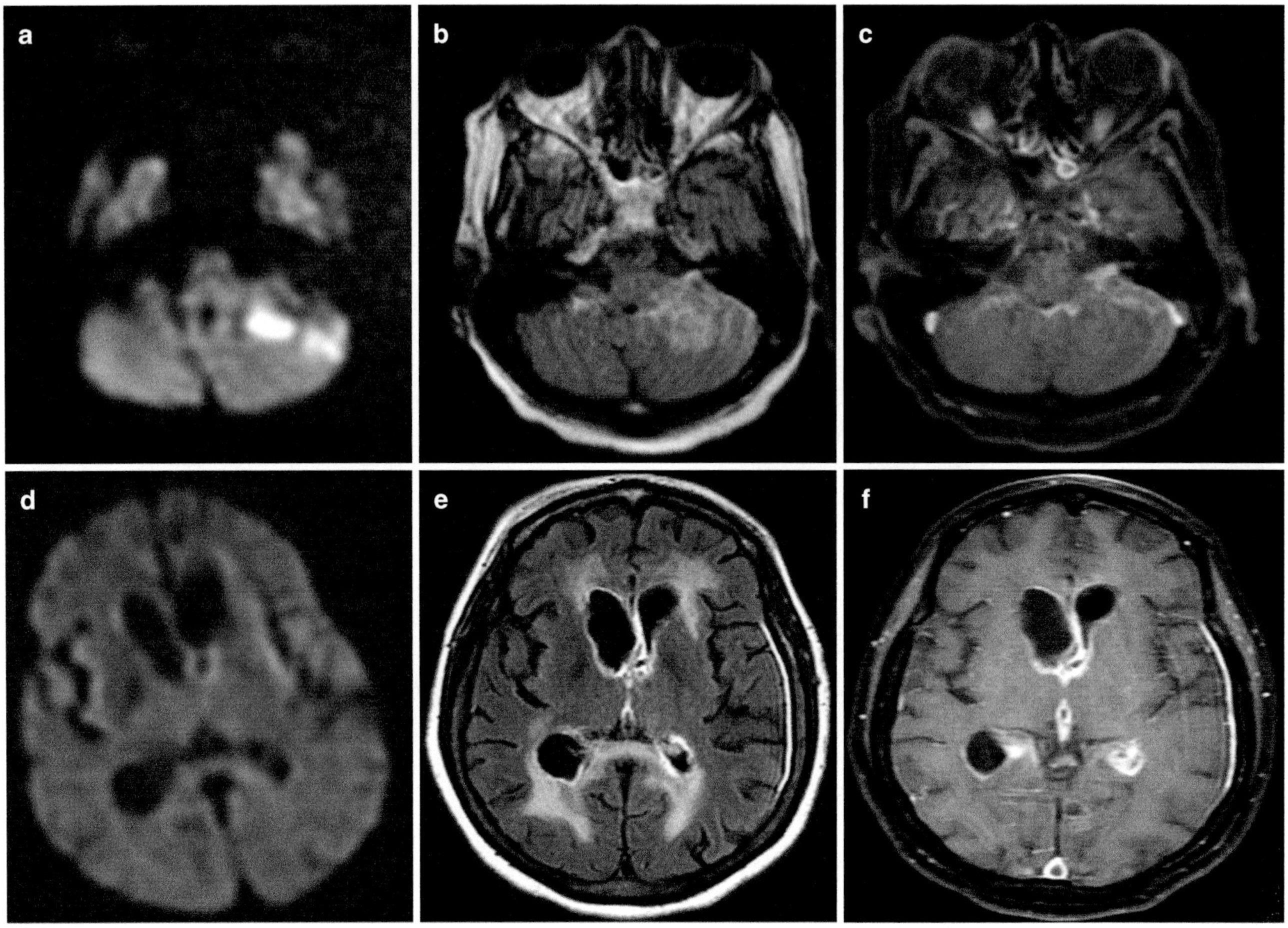

Fig. 11.17 AIDS patient with disseminated histoplasmosis and infarcts. Axial DWI (**a**) with acute embolic infarct with restricted diffusion in the left inferior cerebellum, corresponding FLAIR (**b**) hyperintensity and left CPA cistern leptomeningeal enhancement on post-contrast T1 (white arrows) (**c**). A higher ventricular level shows ventriculitis and hydrocephalus with transependymal CSF spread (**d**–**f**)

narrowing and irregularity of the COW vessels, particularly the supraclinoid ICA/carotid terminus, as well as the ACA, MCA, and PCA with various degrees of stenosis and/or occlusion [74, 75].

Histoplasmosis is caused by the *Histoplasma capsulatum* fungus; it usually presents as a subclinical infection; however it can result in chronic pulmonary infection and/or as a disseminated disease in immune-incompetent patients with deficient cellular immunity, such as patients on chemotherapy and immunosuppressive therapy after solid organ or bone marrow transplant, HIV infection, and chronic steroid use. CNS disease may occur in 5–10% of patients with disseminated disease but can also present as an isolated illness [65]. The infection spreads hematogenously to the CNS after the inhalation of the spores from contaminated soil, bat, and bird guano in endemic areas (along the St. Lawrence River valley, Ohio, and Mississippi and less frequently in selected areas in Africa, Central-South America, and the Middle East). The diagnosis is usually not suspected and difficult to confirm in the isolated CNS form (requires CSF, meninges, or brain tissue evaluation), conducting to chronic infection and delay treatment. Symptoms include headache, altered mental status, seizures, encephalitis, and focal neurologic deficits. Cerebral strokes are usually the consequence of septic emboli from infective endocarditis; these small acute infarcts present with restricted diffusion on MRI and can be located in the basal ganglia, brain stem, or peripheral cerebral corticomedullary junction. Chronic meningoencephalitis and small vessel vasculitis with or without infarcts can also occur (Fig. 11.17) [65, 76–78].

11.3.7 Parasites

Neurocysticercosis (NCC) is caused by the infection with the larval stage of the *Taenia solium*; after fecal-oral

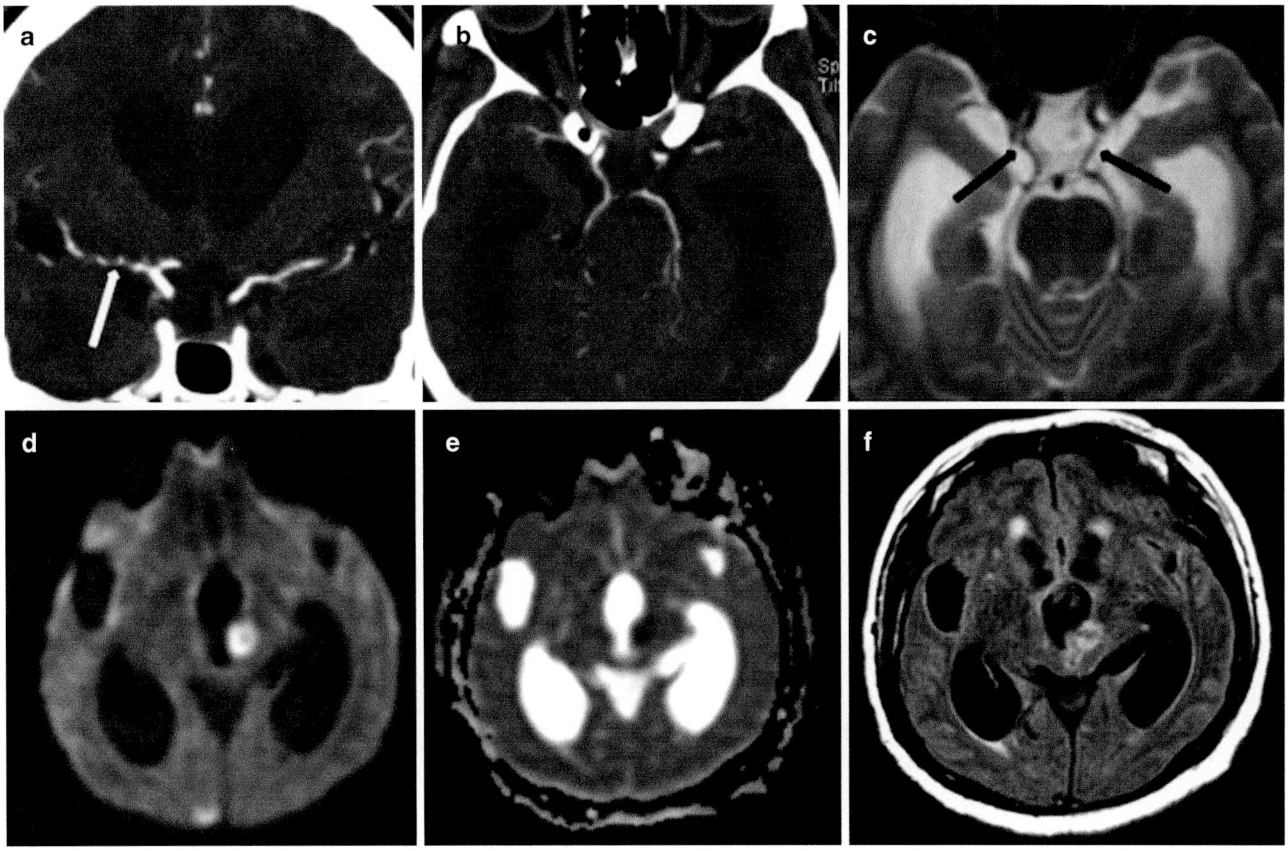

Fig. 11.18 Neurocisticercosis with acute infarcts. Coronal and axial CTA (**a**, **b**) shows hydrocephalus and mildly narrow and irregular right MCA (white arrow). Axial T2 (**c**) the COW vessels are traversing the basilar cisterns and Sylvian fissures cysts (arrows). Axial DWI/ADC map (**d**, **e**) with small acute right posterior occipital and left medial thalamus lacunar infarcts with corresponding FLAIR (f) hyperintensity

contamination and ingestion of the eggs, it disseminates hematogenously to the CNS. NCC is the most common parasitic infection of the CNS in the developing world; most cases in developed countries are related to travel and immigration. Seizures are caused by perilesional inflammation in degenerating cysts but can also be caused by cysticercoid-related nodular calcified lesion or from vasculitis [79]. High clinical suspicion and imaging are essential in making the diagnosis of NCC-related strokes. Cerebrovascular complications are well known but usually underrecognized; they are present in 3–12 % of patients with NCC, and about 50% of patients with subarachnoid space disease will have angiographic evidence of vasculitis [29, 80]. Cerebrovascular complications are more common in subarachnoid cysticercosis, also referred as "racemose," which is usually located in the cerebellopontine angle and suprasellar and perimesencephalic cisterns, along the Sylvian fissures, and less common in the hemispheric convexities (Fig. 11.18). The wall of the vessels within the subarachnoid exudate is inflamed and results in focal cysticercoid angiitis and occlusion (Fig. 11.19). Small-size vessels are preferentially involved, particularly penetrating arteries to the midbrain and lenticulostriate arteries, which result in midbrain and basal ganglia lacunar infarcts, respectively. Severe forms of leptomeningitis (arachnoiditis) can cause circle of Willis vessel arteritis, and so large territorial infarcts, usually affecting the MCA, ACA, and PCA, are also seen (Fig. 11.20). Angiographic imaging demonstrates a pattern of vasculitis with beaded appearance, tapering of the vessels with obstruction or abrupt interruption [81]. NCC can also weaken the wall and develop infective aneurysm with the potential for subarachnoid and parenchymal hemorrhage. Treatment requires antiparasitic antibiotic (praziquantel and albendazole) and steroid to minimize the accelerated parasite destruction and associate subarachnoid inflammatory response that increases the risk of cerebrovascular complications [29, 80–83].

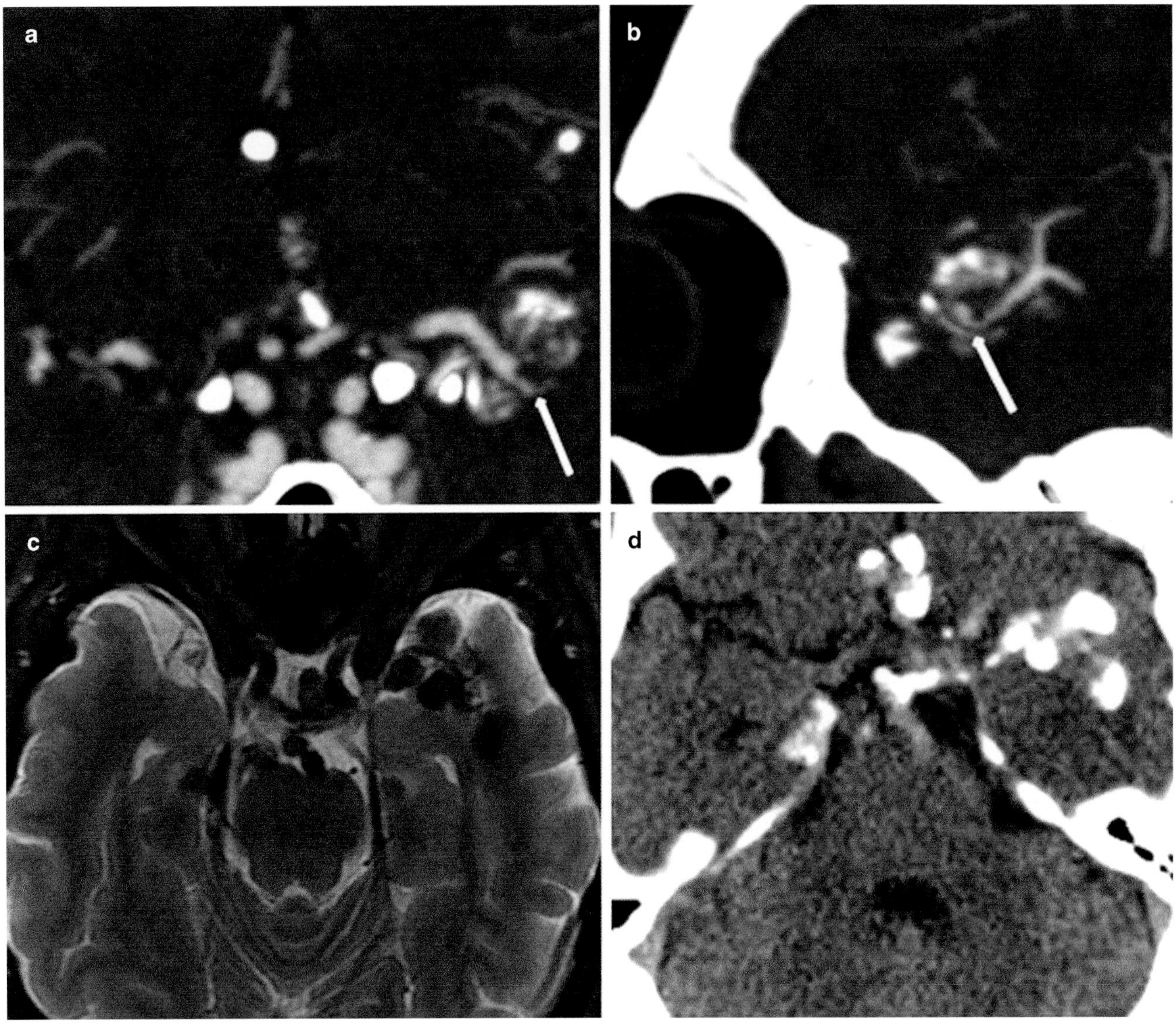

Fig. 11.19 NCC with vascular involvement. Coronal and sagittal CTA (**a**, **b**) shows narrowing of the left MCA, M2 segment with beaded appearance (arrows). Axial T2 (**c**) and axial non-contrast CT (**d**) with multiple racemose subarachnoid calcified cysts

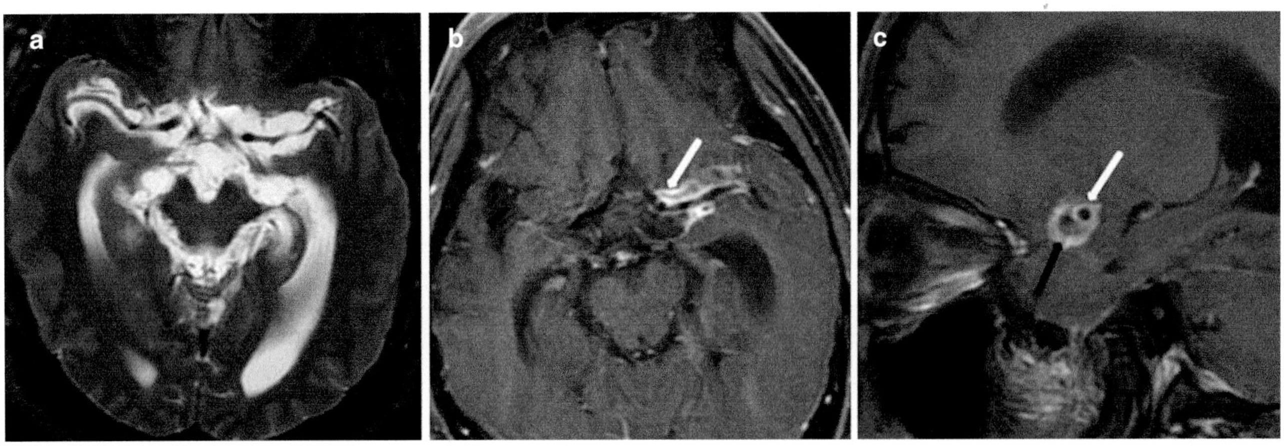

Fig. 11.20 NCC with infectious vasculitis. Axial T2 (**a**) depicts hydrocephalus, and bilateral basilar cisterns and Sylvian fissures cysts surrounding the COW vessels. Axial (**b**), and sagittal (**c**) T1 post-contrast show left Sylvian fissure enhancing cysts (black arrow) surrounding the left Supraclinoid-carotid terminus and proximal A1 and M1 segments (white arrows). Wall enhancement along the ICA, left A1 and M1 (white arrows)

11.4 Infectious Thrombophlebitis

11.4.1 Epidemiology

The term cerebral venous thrombosis (CVT) refers to thrombosis of the dural venous sinuses and/or of the cerebral veins. CVT is responsible for 0.5–1.0% of all strokes. This incidence increases to as high as 5% of all strokes in the younger population [84, 85].

Septic thrombophlebitis refers to the combination of thrombosis with an infection of the sinus-affected vein or sinus. The most common microorganism associated with septic thrombophlebitis is *Staphylococcus aureus* followed by streptococcal species, rarely gram negatives, anaerobes, viruses, and angioinvasive fungal agents. CVT/thrombophlebitis most commonly affects the cavernous sinus (CS) and to a lesser extent the lateral transverse-sigmoid sinus (LTS). There is a propensity for retrograde infection extension from the paranasal sinuses, orbit, mouth, face, and neck into the CS and from the middle ear/mastoids into the LTS. This is due to the valveless nature of the central nervous system (CNS) venous structures and the anatomic proximity.

Infectious CVT is responsible for about 6–12% of patients with dural sinus thrombosis [86, 87]. This is significantly less common than non-septic CVT, which is usually associated to prothrombotic conditions, pregnancy/puerperium, and oral contraceptives. Most of which are young female of childbearing age which has related risk factors; up to 70% of CVT are reported in this population [87]. Up to 44% of patients have more than one predisposing factors, for instance, approximately 30% of cases have an underlying inherited or acquired prothrombotic conditions [84, 88]. In the pediatric population, septic CVT is more common than non-septic CVT (up to 56%), particularly associated to mastoiditis and meningitis [89, 90].

11.4.2 Presentation and Natural History

Patients with infectious CVT usually present very sick and septic. The time period between initial onset of symptoms related to CVT and the diagnosis is usually about a week [88]. The diagnosis of CVT requires a high clinical suspicion and is confirmed with neuroimaging. The clinical manifestations of CVT are nonspecific and can be grouped into four types: (1) related to raise intracranial pressure from venous hypertension, particularly headache, which is present in 90% of the patients, papilledema, and diplopia (from cranial nerve VI palsy); (2) constitutional symptoms such as fever, vomiting, impaired consciousness, encephalopathy, and focal or generalized seizures that occur in approximately 40% of patents; (3) focal neurologic deficits, such as stroke or transient ischemic attacks (TIA), usually related to parenchymal edema, venous infarction, and/or hemorrhage either from dural sinus thrombosis or cortical vein thrombosis, which may be present in 25–40% of patients [85]; and (4) site-specific symptoms that vary depending on the infection site and location and extension of the thrombosed sinus.

Early recognition is the main factor on clinical outcome of patients with CVT: (1) lateral transverse-sigmoid sinus thrombophlebitis related to otomastoiditis presents with ear and mastoid pain, local tenderness, external auditory canal discharge, and possibly aphasia [91]. Cavernous sinus thrombophlebitis may be the result of ethmoidal/sphenoid sinusitis, dental abscess, facial-orbital soft tissue infection-cellulitis, beesting, or septic thrombosis of the internal jugular vein. Patients may present with cranial nerve impairment, narrowing of the carotid artery with brain infarcts, and orbital symptoms of venous congestion (exophthalmos, diplopia, visual impairment, ophthalmoplegia, ptosis, chemosis, and eyelid edema) (Fig. 11.21) [92].

Infectious superior sagittal sinus (SSS) thrombophlebitis is rare, usually the consequence of meningitis, subdural or epidural abscess. Patients present with focal symptom associated to commonly bilateral vertex region brain parenchyma venous infarctions and/or hemorrhage.

Established treatment includes high-dose parental broad-spectrum antibiotics, anticoagulation, and surgical evacuation of the abscess. The use of anticoagulation is controversial; this treatment may start with intravenous heparin followed by oral anticoagulation [88]. Early diagnosis and prompt medical and radical surgical treatment of immunocompromised patients with fungal angioinvasive sinusitis are the main prognostic indicators to predict survival and minimize morbidity. Failure to do so will result in rapid osseous destruction and extension of the disease to the orbits and intracranially to include the CS.

11.4.3 Pathophysiology

The cavernous sinuses (CSs) are the most commonly affected sinuses in adult septic CVT. The CSs are anatomically highly septated and contain the cavernous segment of the internal carotid artery (ICA) and cranial nerve VI (CN VI) centrally within it. The CS lies lateral to the sella turcica. The CN III, CN IV, and V1 and V2 divisions of CN V run within the lateral dural wall of the CS. The tributaries to the CS are the facial veins via the superior and inferior ophthalmic veins (allowing facial and periorbital cellulitis retrograde infection dissemination) as well as the sphenoparietal sinus. The CS communicates with each other through a rich network of intercavernous sinuses plexus, which allows the transmission of pressure-driven flow and infection from one CS to another and to other connecting draining sinuses. The CS drains into the pterygoid venous plexuses, clival venous plexus, and inferior and superior petrosal sinuses and finally ends in the internal jugular veins (JV).

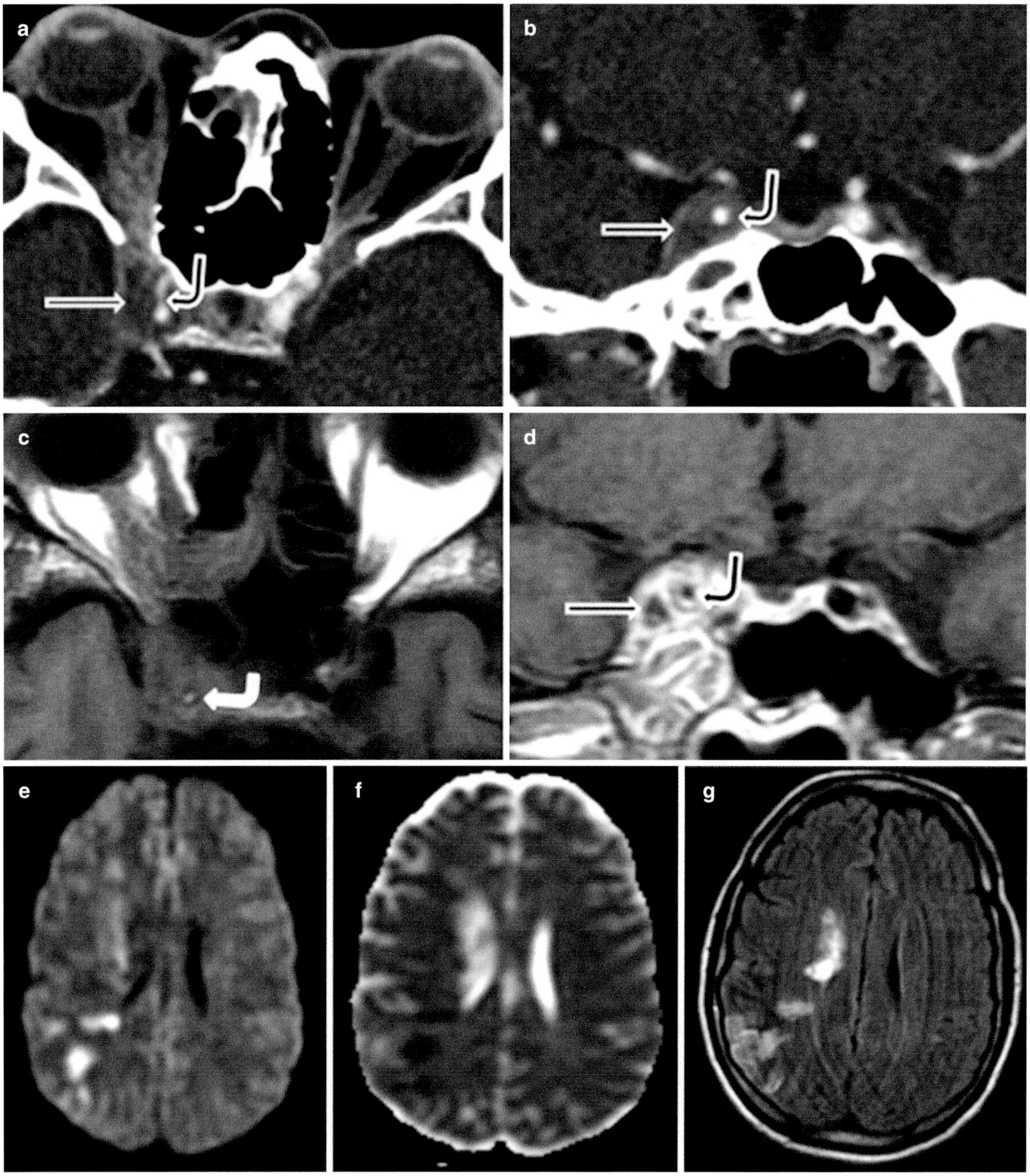

Fig. 11.21 Acute right orbit cellulitis with right cavernous sinus thrombosis. Axial and coronal CTA (**a**, **b**) images with fullness and concavity of the right cavernous sinus lateral wall; diffuse non-enhancing filling defects (straight arrows) and severe narrowing of the cavernous ICA (curved arrow). Noncontract orbits axial T1 (**c**) show lack of right cavernous ICA flow void (compare left) with T1 hyperintense hemorrhage within the wall of the vessel (curved solid white arrow) and near complete occlusion, coronal T1 post-contrast (**d**) shows prominent thickening and enhancement of the vessel wall on (curved arrow) and cavernous sinus thrombus (straight arrow). Axial DWI/ADC/FLAIR (**e–g**) with acute right inner and cortical watershed corona radiata and temporoparietal ischemic infarcts respectively

Septic thrombosis/thrombophlebitis can be initiated by direct bacterial infection of the dural sinus or as septic embolus to the sinus by bacteria located within the sinus. The thrombus itself is a good growth medium for bacteria [88]. Once the thrombus is formed into the sinus, it produces venous congestion, flows venous obstruction, and raises the venous pressure with disruption of the blood-brain barrier (BBB). This may lead to intracranial infection dissemination. The raised intracranial pressure would reduce the cerebral blood flow and the cerebral perfusion pressure. These changes will lead to parenchyma venous infarction [93].

11.4.4 Imaging

CT

The non-enhanced CT is usually negative. It is abnormal in approximately 30% of the cases. Specific findings associated with CVT include hyperdense thrombus (usually more than 70 HU) within a cortical vein or in the dural sinus (cord sign) and a diffusely hyperdense, completely filled thrombosed sinus (dense delta sign). This is seen usually along the posterior aspect of the superior sagittal sinus (SSS). Indirect imaging findings include hypodense areas of brain parenchyma crossing different arterial vascular territories with or without hemorrhagic component. This is suggestive of a venous infarction or infectious cerebritis [94–96]. Parenchymal hemorrhage may be seen in patients with CVT; rarely convexal subarachnoid hemorrhage may also be present in 0.5–0.8% of CVT [85]. CVT is a common cause of nontraumatic intracranial hemorrhage in young population, and adults who present with atypical lobar or atypical subarachnoid hemorrhage should raise the suspicion for this diagnosis. The bone window allows localization of the potential source for infection, i.e., paranasal sinusitis causing CS thrombophlebitis as well as otomastoiditis producing lateral transverse-sigmoid thrombophlebitis. The bone window also is useful in evaluating the integrity of the osseous margins; osseous destruction is seen in invasive fungal infections.

In the post-contrast CT, the dural wall of the affected sinus enhances. The lateral wall of the CS is bulging out laterally. The lateral margin of the CS will demonstrate a convexity instead of its normal concave morphology. There is inhomogeneous opacification of the sinus, with filling defects within the CS (Fig. 11.22). This is equivalent to the "empty delta sign" usually described for the posterior aspect of the SSS. This empty delta sign corresponds to a central non-enhancing thrombus within the sinus. This can be seen in the setting of LTS thrombophlebitis [96]. Orbital findings on post-contrast CT include distension of the superior

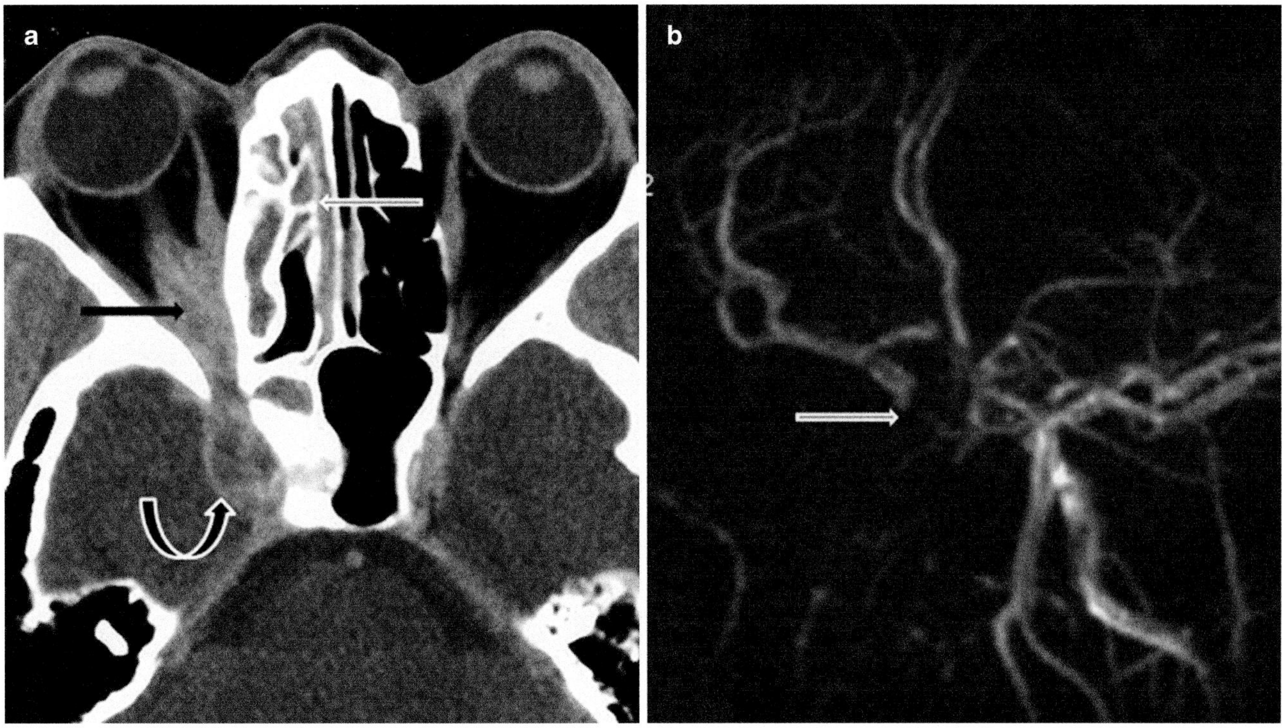

Fig. 11.22 Mucormycosis sinusitis/orbit cellulitis with cavernous sinus thrombosis. Axial post-contrast CT (**a**) shows right intra-conal cellulitis (black arrow) and etmoido-sphenoid sinusitis (white arrow), enlarged non-opacifying right cavernous sinus due to thrombus (curved arrow) compare to the normal left. MRA (**b**) shows complete occlusion of the right intracranial ICA, only partial distal reconstitution of carotid terminus (straight arrow)

ophthalmic vein with or without thrombus, stranding of the retrobulbar intraconal fat with proptosis, and periorbital soft tissue swelling (Fig. 11.22). Sinusitis may be seen with opacification of the paranasal sinuses. In cases of ethmoidal sinusitis, there may be a medial orbital wall subperiostic abscess. Described imaging findings of post-contrast CT for early detection of invasive fungal sinusitis include lack of normal osseous enhancement of the nasal walls, nasal septum, and turbinates due to tissue necrosis, extension of inflammatory changes to the periantral fat, orbit, and intracranially with dural thickening and enhancement [97–99].

Magnetic Resonance Imaging

Acute thrombus (occurring within the first week) is isointense to the brain on T1 and hypointense on T2. This is due to an increase intracellular deoxyhemoglobin. In subacute thrombus (second week), the thrombus is hyperintense on T1 and on T2. This is due mostly to extracellular methemoglobin. Chronic thrombus (after 2 weeks) becomes isointense on T1 and hyperintense on T2. At this time recanalization starts to occur and normal flow void may be restored [100]. On gradient-echo and susceptibility-weighted images (SWI), the thrombus appears mostly hypointense on all acute, subacute, and chronic thrombi phases [85, 101]. On post-contrast T1-weighted images, there is enlargement of the cavernous sinus with a convex lateral wall and non-enhancing filling defects (thrombi) (Fig. 11.23). Non-enhancing thrombi in the orbital veins may be present as well.

Brain parenchyma changes associated with CVT include venous ischemia (Fig. 11.24), abscess, or arterial infarction when associated with arterial compromise (vessels luminal narrowing or occlusion due to mass effect from dural sinus thrombosis, concomitant infectious vasculitis, direct infection extension, or wall hemorrhage) (Figs. 11.21, 11.22 and 11.23). Focal lesions, a result of venous infarction, have variable signal. These are mostly low on T1 in the nonhemorrhagic cases and hyperintense on the T2 and FLAIR series without restricted diffusion on DWI (Fig. 11.24). This signal pattern corresponds to vasogenic edema but non-infarcted, viable tissue. Restricted diffusion may be seen in few patients in the setting of actual cytotoxic edema (up to 30% of patients with CVT complicated by intraparenchymal abnormalities) (Fig. 11.21) [102]. The ADC values fail to predict sequela on follow-up MR images on these patients [84, 93, 103]. Classically and in contrast to arterial infarct, venous infarcts follow a venous drainage region and not the arterial vascular distribution (Fig. 11.24). This may result in crossing of typical arterial vascular territories. Venous infarctions tend to be irregular and no wedge shape and tend to involve the subcortical white matter with sparing of the cortex, and the initial area of T2/FLAIR/DWI abnormality does not correspond with the final size of the permanently injured parenchyma [104]. Often the findings of venous infarction are reversible. This explains the relatively better prognosis [103]. Parenchymal hemorrhage often presents as multiple focal areas of T1 hyperintensity and T2/SWI hypointensity or as a frank lobar hematoma. Parenchymal hemorrhage is present in approximately 30–40% of patients with CVT [85], which can result from further increase in venous and capillary pressure within areas of vasogenic edema. Hemorrhage prevents adequate interpretation of the ADC because of the signal loss induced by blood products [85, 93].

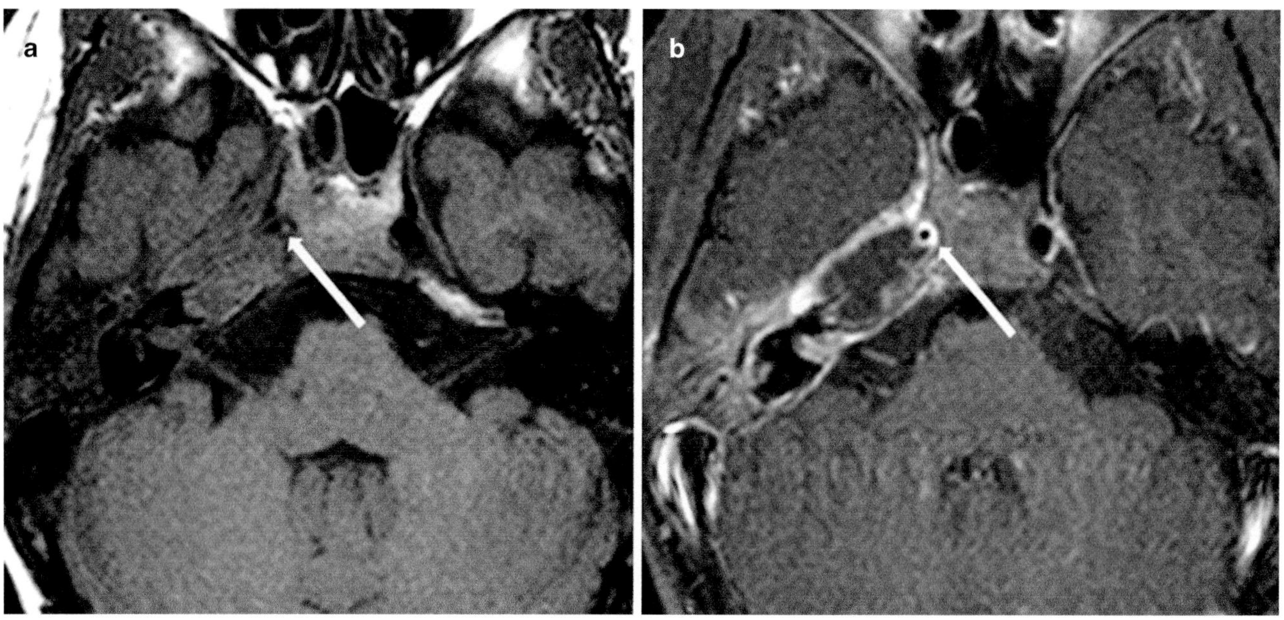

Fig. 11.23 Right oto-mastoiditis with petrous apex abscess and right ICA infectious vasculitis. Axial T1 pre-contrast (**a**) show opacification of the right mastoid-middle ear and narrow cavernous ICA (arrow), post-contrast T1 FS (**b**) shows peripherally enhancing petrous apex abscess, thickened and enhancing right ICA wall and narrow lumen (arrow) compare to the normal left side

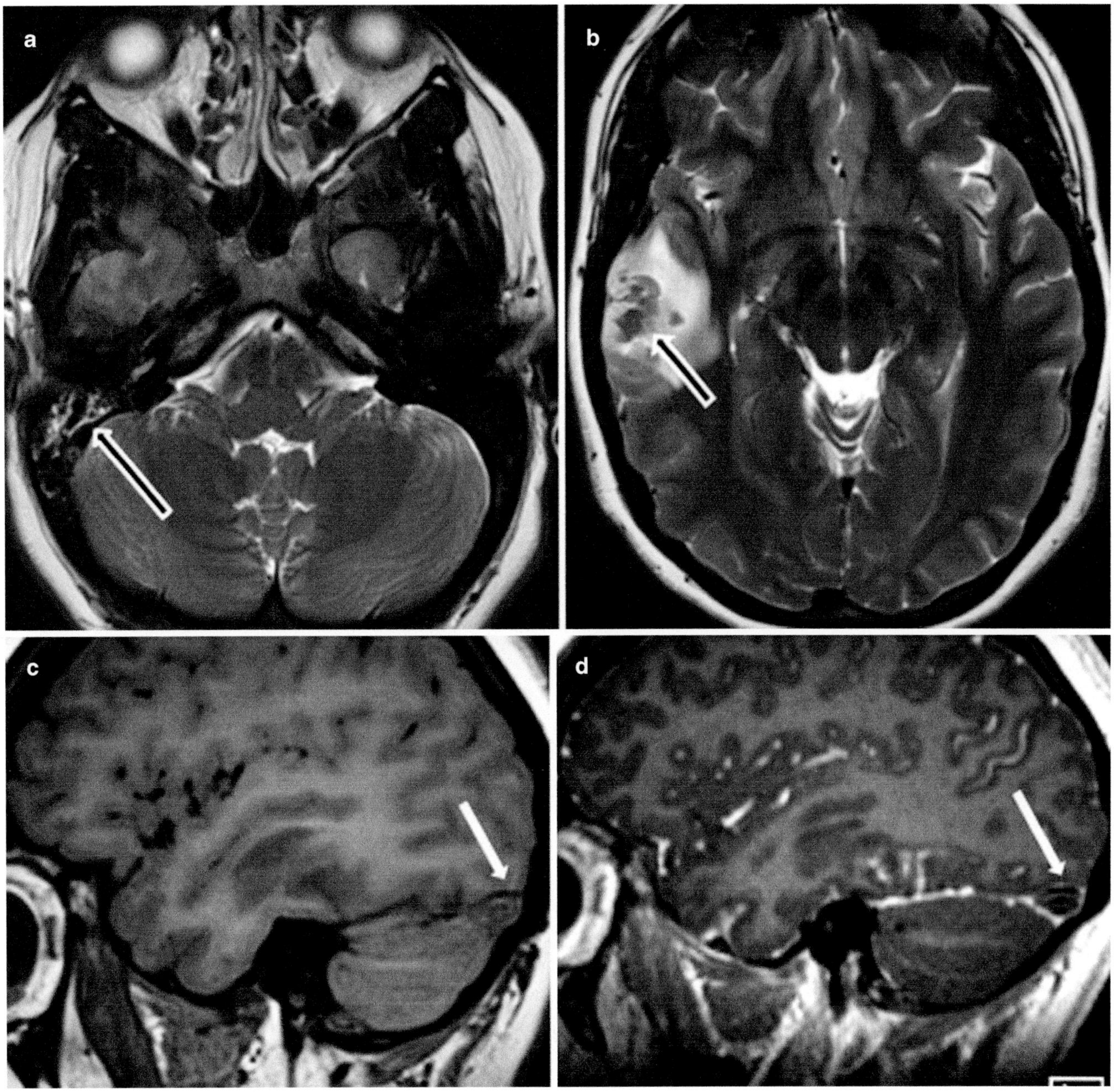

Fig. 11.24 Right lateral transverse-sigmoid sinuses thrombophlebitis and inferior temporal venous infarct. Axial T2 (**a**, **b**) images show partial opacification of the right mastoiditis with T2 hyperintense effusion (arrow) and right inferior temporal gyrus white matter hyperintensity with areas of hypointense hemosiderin from hemorrhage (arrow), note predominant involvement of the white matter and no restricted diffusion (not shown). Sagittal T1 pre gad (**c**) shows T1 isointense filling on the right transverse-sigmoid sinus and inferior temporal lobe edema, on postcontrast T1 (**d**) "delta sign" corresponds to the filling defect from the thrombus (arrow) and mild associated inferior temporal lobe leptomeningeal enhancement

Computed Tomography Venogram (CTV) and Magnetic Resonance Venogram (MRV)

Enhanced CTV and MRV are considered the most reliable examinations for the confirmation of the diagnosis of cerebral venous thrombosis. CTV allows direct visualization of the thrombus as a filling defect. CTV is better in the detection of thrombi in smaller sinuses and in detecting partial venous thrombosis (Figs. 11.21 and 11.25). The disadvantages of CTV include the radiation exposure, contrast allergy, and limitations in the setting of poor renal function. The main advantages of CTV are that it is noninvasive and has fewer artifacts leading to fewer false-positive results [105–107]. The utilization of multiphase CTA in the evaluation of collateral vessels may also have a value on detecting CVT, particularly the evolution of incomplete recanalization.

Time-resolved MR angiography of the intracranial venous system allows a dynamic evaluation of the venous system. This is limited due to the suboptimal spatial resolution.

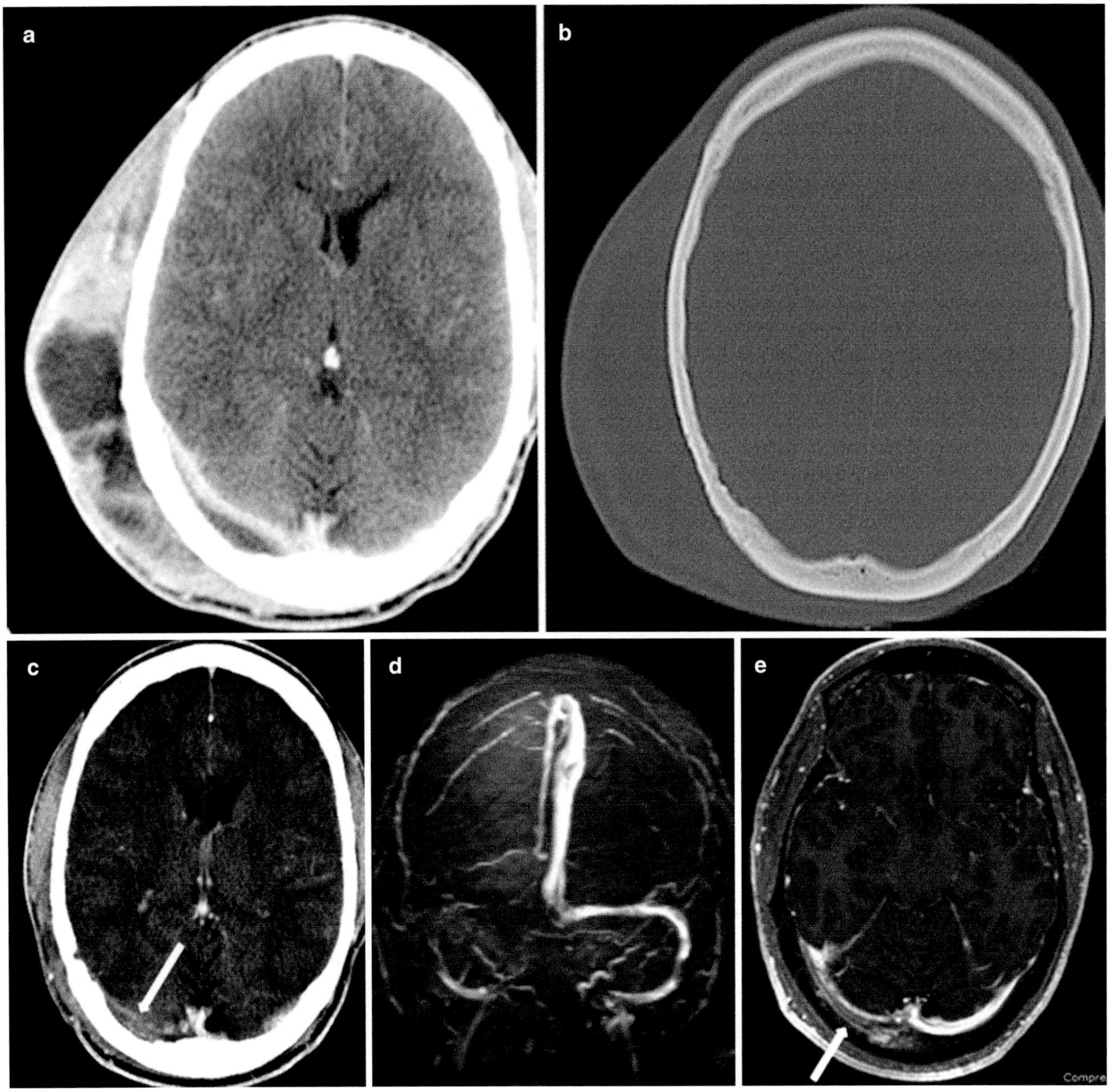

Fig. 11.25 Right occipito-temporal scalp abscess and right lateral transverse-sigmoid sinuses thrombosis. Axial CT postcontrast (**a**, **b**) shows scalp cellulitis and abscess with intracranial epidural extension and anterior displacement of the right transverse sinus, also right parietal bone irregularity. Post evacuation patient presented with worsening headaches, follow up CTV (**c**) shows filling defect in the right transverse sinus consistent with thrombosis (arrow), enhanced MRV 3D reconstruction (**d**) and axial source images (**e**) confirm right transverse and sigmoid sinuses thrombosis

A combination of contrast-enhanced 3D MRV and dynamic acquisition has been proposed as a more sensitive technique to evaluate CVT [108, 109]. Subtraction MRV acquired from time-resolved contrast-enhanced MRA is also an alternate technique that allows dynamic evaluation of the cerebral venous system [109, 110]. Contrast-enhanced 3D MRV is superior to non-enhanced 2D time-of-flight (TOF) MRV; however organizing thrombus may enhance (Fig. 11.25), which lowers the accuracy of the contrast-enhanced techniques; contrast-enhanced MRV sensitivity/specificity is 90%/96% compared to 2D TOF MRV 63%/48% [111–113]. A more recent MR approach to venous imaging is wall vessel imaging. This is a promising technique that allows visualization of small canalizing channels in resolving CVT.

11.4.5 Dural Sinus Thrombosis Mimics/Pitfalls

The sensitivity of CT and MRI for the diagnosis of dural sinus thrombosis is reduced because acute thrombus may appear isointense to the brain parenchyma on T1WI and hypointense on T2WI, imaging features that simulate normal flow void. Additionally, false negatives can result from enhancing chronic thrombus on T1 contrast-enhanced MRI which will obscure the thrombus and also from intense dural sinus enhancement related to collateral vessels associated to thrombosis which can be mistaken for meningitis [96].

The specificity of CT and MRI for the diagnosis of CVT is reduced in patients with hyperdense sinuses on noncontract CT, which can be caused by elevated hematocrit and not thrombus. In these cases, however, the density of the arteries will also be increased and help in making the correct interpretation. Hyperdense sinus is also frequently seen in children and in patients with right to left cardiac shunt and polycythemia vera.

On contrast-enhanced CT, giant arachnoid granulations may mimic a thrombus. These are commonly seen in the lateral aspect of the transverse sinus and tend to be rounded, short segment, and isodense to CSF. Another cause for decreased specificity is the artifacts associated with slow flow, in-plane flow, and entry slice phenomena that may be seen on spin-echo MRI sequences and non-contrast magnetic resonance venogram (MRV). Another artifact on MRI is the flow gap artifact that is commonly seen on the transverse-sigmoid sinus. This artifact can be confirmed by the detection of flow in the source images [96, 104].

Asymmetry of the transverse sinuses is common and may be misinterpreted as thrombosis of the smaller hypoplastic sinus. This occurs more commonly in the left transverse sinus. The hypoplastic transverse-sigmoid sinus has small osseous jugular foramen, which is better depicted on CT bone window. Sometimes, lateral transverse-sigmoid sinus thrombophlebitis may be related to otomastoiditis or cerebellar abscess, in which conditions one should observe the sinus carefully to prevent overlooking the thrombosis (Fig. 11.26).

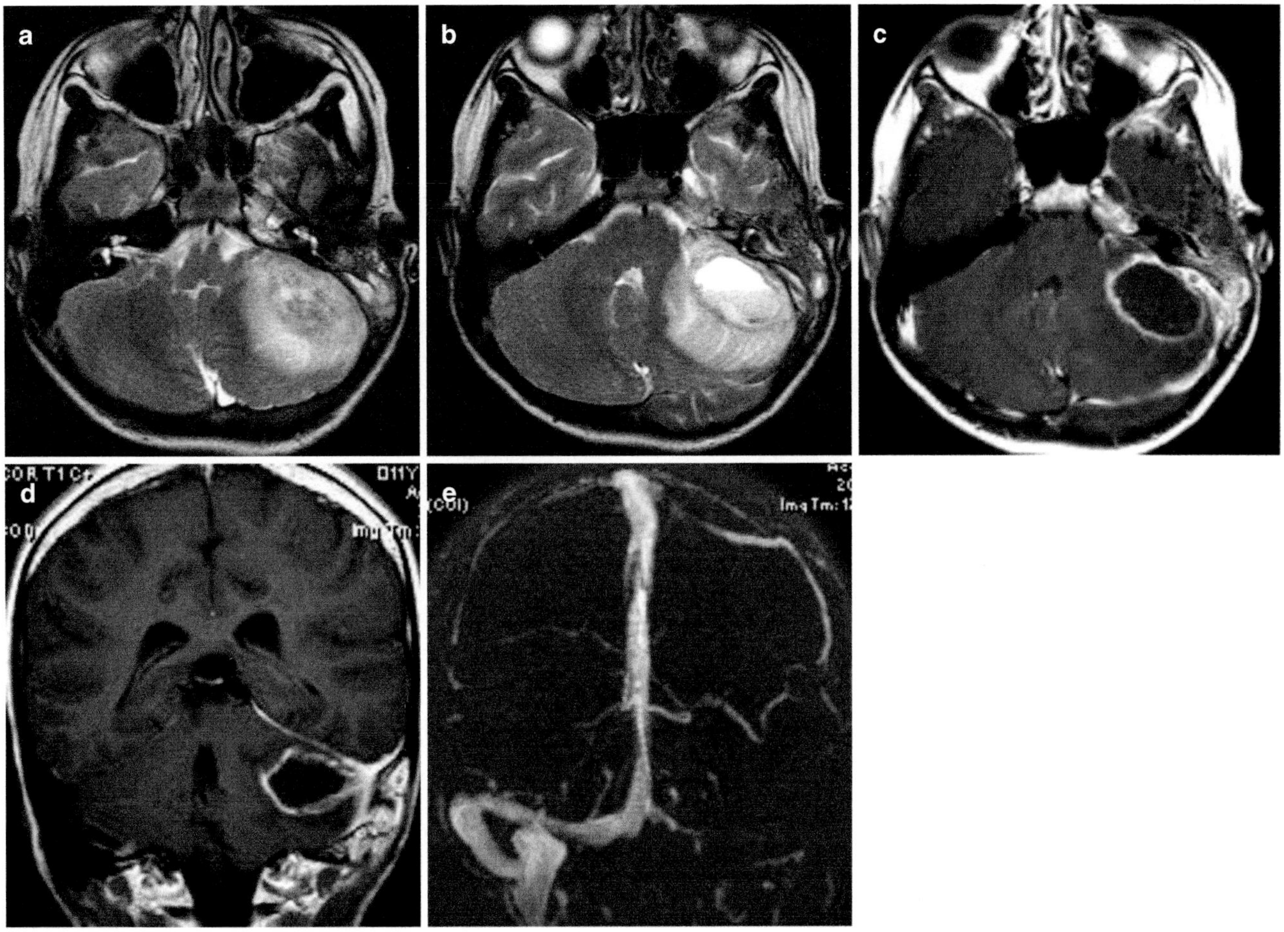

Fig. 11.26 Left transverse-sigmoid (LTS) sinus thrombophlebitis and left cerebellar abscess. Axial T2 (**a**, **b**) shows hyperintense opacification of the left petrous apex, left mastoid/middle otomastoiditis, and abscess in the left cerebellum. Axial and coronal T1 post-contrast (**c**, **d**) demonstrate the left cerebellar abscess, enhancement of the left otomastoid region, and the dura about the left LTS sinuses due to thrombophlebitis. Coronal enhanced MRV (**e**) shows complete occlusion of the left LTS sinuses and proximal IJ

11.5 Conclusions

Systemic and local infections can result in CNS cerebrovascular complications of these diseases. Among the most common and dreadful complications is the development of cerebral infarctions. The correct diagnosis of the cause of the stroke is challenging as these cerebrovascular events secondary to infection may be indistinguishable from more common causes of stroke. In addition, clinical signs and symptoms of infection may not always be present or clear at the time of diagnosis. The role of imaging in the management of patients with CNS complications of infections includes the confirmation of the diagnosis of infarction and helps exclude other pathologies that can present with stroke symptoms such as brain tumors and toxic-metabolic disorders. The added value of imaging in the setting of a stroke is to characterize the stroke as ischemic or hemorrhagic and its origin venous or arterial. Imaging of the vessels with CTA/CTV, MRA/MRV, and DSA technique allows direct visualization of the vessels and detects the underlying pathology that leads to the CNS complication. Imaging can also play a role in distinguishing acute versus chronic type of infections. This, for example, may be applied in the setting of acute pyogenic meningitis compared to chronic tuberculous and fungal basilar meningitis. CT and MR images can also better localize the disease and the extension. The latter can be useful to distinguish between various pathogens. For example, herpes encephalitis affects distinct areas when compared to more generalized involvement in the setting of pyogenic meningitis. In conclusion, imaging plays an essential role in the evaluation of CNS complications of infection. This information is critical for much needed prompt medical treatment of these patients. Delay in the diagnosis and treatment will most likely result in an unfavorable outcome.

References

1. Ducruet AF, Hickman ZL, Zacharia BE, et al. Intracranial infectious aneurysms: a comprehensive review. Neurosurg Rev. 2010;33(1):37–46.
2. Krings T, Geibprasert S, ter Brugge KG. Pathomechanisms and treatment of pediatric aneurysms. Childs Nerv Syst. 2010;26(10):1309–18.
3. Flores BC, Patel AR, Braga BP, et al. Management of infectious intracranial aneurysms in the pediatric population. Childs Nerv Syst. 2016;32(7):1205–17.
4. Peters PJ, Harrison T, Lennox JL. A dangerous dilemma: management of infectious intracranial aneurysms complicating endocarditis. Lancet Infect Dis. 2006;6(11):742–8.
5. Kannoth S, Thomas SV, Nair S, et al. Proposed diagnostic criteria for intracranial infectious aneurysms. J Neurol Neurosurg Psychiatry. 2008;79(8):943–6.
6. Bartakke S, Kabde U, Muranjan MN, et al. Mycotic aneurysm: an uncommon cause for intra-cranial hemorrhage. Indian J Pediatr. 2002;69(10):905–7.
7. Clare CE, Barrow DL. Infectious intracranial aneurysms. Neurosurg Clin N Am. 1992;3(3):551–66.
8. Allen LM, Fowler AM, Walker C, et al. Retrospective review of cerebral mycotic aneurysms in 26 patients: focus on treatment in strongly immunocompromised patients with a brief literature review. AJNR Am J Neuroradiol. 2013;34(4):823–7.
9. Zanaty M, Chalouhi N, Starke RM, et al. Endovascular treatment of cerebral mycotic aneurysm: a review of the literature and single center experience. Biomed Res Int. 2013;2013:151643.
10. Fusco MR, Stapleton CJ, Griessenauer CJ, et al. Endovascular treatment of intracranial infectious aneurysms in eloquent cortex with super-selective provocative testing: case series and literature review. Interv Neuroradiol. 2016:22(2):148–52.
11. Singla A, Fargen K, Blackburn S, et al. National treatment practices in the management of infectious intracranial aneurysms and infective endocarditis. J Neurointerv Surg. 2016;8(7):741–6.
12. Ghali MG, Ghali EZ. Intracavernous internal carotid artery mycotic aneurysms: comprehensive review and evaluation of the role of endovascular treatment. Clin Neurol Neurosurg. 2013;115(10):1927–42.
13. Lee WK, Mossop PJ, Little AF, et al. Infected (mycotic) aneurysms: spectrum of imaging appearances and management. Radiographics. 2008;28(7):1853–68.
14. Baddour LM, Wilson WR, Bayer AS, et al. Infective endocarditis: diagnosis, antimicrobial therapy, and management of complications: a statement for healthcare professionals from the Committee on Rheumatic Fever, Endocarditis, and Kawasaki Disease, Council on Cardiovascular Disease in the Young, and the Councils on Clinical Cardiology, Stroke, and Cardiovascular Surgery and Anesthesia, American Heart Association: endorsed by the Infectious Diseases Society of America. Circulation. 2005;111(23):e394–434.
15. Murdoch DR, Corey GR, Hoen B, et al. Clinical presentation, etiology, and outcome of infective endocarditis in the 21st century: the International Collaboration on Endocarditis-Prospective Cohort Study. Arch Intern Med. 2009;169(5):463–73.
16. Novy E, Sonneville R, Mazighi M, et al. Neurological complications of infective endocarditis: new breakthroughs in diagnosis and management. Med Mal Infect. 2013;43(11-12):443–50.
17. Schut ES, Lucas MJ, Brouwer MC, et al. Cerebral infarction in adults with bacterial meningitis. Neurocritical Care. 2012;16(3):421–7.
18. Fugate JE, Lyons JL, Thakur KT, et al. Infectious causes of stroke. Lancet Infect Dis. 2014;14(9):869–80.
19. Paganini-Hill A, Lozano E, Fischberg G, et al. Infection and risk of ischemic stroke: differences among stroke subtypes. Stroke. 2003;34(2):452–7.
20. Smeeth L, Thomas SL, Hall AJ, et al. Risk of myocardial infarction and stroke after acute infection or vaccination. N Engl J Med. 2004;351(25):2611–8.
21. Cooper HA, Thompson EC, Laureno R, et al. Subclinical brain embolization in left-sided infective endocarditis: results from the evaluation by MRI of the brains of patients with left-sided intracardiac solid masses (EMBOLISM) pilot study. Circulation. 2009;120(7):585–91.
22. Duval X, Iung B, Klein I, et al. Effect of early cerebral magnetic resonance imaging on clinical decisions in infective endocarditis: a prospective study. Ann Intern Med. 2010;152(8):497–504, W175.
23. Ferro JM, Fonseca AC. Infective endocarditis. Handb Clin Neurol. 2014;119:75–91.
24. Sheu JJ, Chiou HY, Kang JH, et al. Tuberculosis and the risk of ischemic stroke: a 3-year follow-up study. Stroke. 2010;41(2):244–9.
25. Klein M, Koedel U, Pfefferkorn T, et al. Arterial cerebrovascular complications in 94 adults with acute bacterial meningitis. Crit Care. 2011;15(6):R281.
26. Kastenbauer S, Pfister HW. Pneumococcal meningitis in adults: spectrum of complications and prognostic factors in a series of 87 cases. Brain. 2003;126(Pt 5):1015–25.

27. Schut ES, de Gans J, van de Beek D. Community-acquired bacterial meningitis in adults. Pract Neurol. 2008;8(1):8–23.
28. Eisenhut M. Vasospasm in cerebral inflammation. Int J Inflam. 2014;2014:509707.
29. Chow FC, Marra CM, Cho TA. Cerebrovascular disease in central nervous system infections. Semin Neurol. 2011;31(3):286–306.
30. Pfister HW, Borasio GD, Dirnagl U, et al. Cerebrovascular complications of bacterial meningitis in adults. Neurology. 1992;42(8):1497–504.
31. Obusez EC, Hui F, Hajj-Ali RA, et al. High-resolution MRI vessel wall imaging: spatial and temporal patterns of reversible cerebral vasoconstriction syndrome and central nervous system vasculitis. AJNR Am J Neuroradiol. 2014;35(8):1527–32.
32. Choi YJ, Jung SC, Lee DH. Vessel Wall Imaging of the Intracranial and Cervical Carotid Arteries. J Stroke. 2015;17(3):238–55.
33. Mossa-Basha M, Hwang WD, De Havenon A, et al. Multicontrast high-resolution vessel wall magnetic resonance imaging and its value in differentiating intracranial vasculopathic processes. Stroke. 2015;46(6):1567–73.
34. Zhu XJ, Wang W, Liu ZJ. High-resolution Magnetic Resonance Vessel Wall Imaging for Intracranial Arterial Stenosis. Chin Med J (Engl). 2016;129(11):1363–70.
35. Chien LN, Chi NF, Hu CJ, et al. Central nervous system infections and stroke-a population-based analysis. Acta Neurol Scand. 2013;128(4):241–8.
36. Katchanov J, Siebert E, Endres M, et al. Focal parenchymal lesions in community-acquired bacterial meningitis in adults: a clinico-radiological study. Neuroradiology. 2009;51(11):723–9.
37. Clark EG, Danbolt N. The Oslo study of the natural history of untreated syphilis; an epidemiologic investigation based on a restudy of the Boeck-Bruusgaard material; a review and appraisal. J Chronic Dis. 1955;2(3):311–44.
38. Brightbill TC, Ihmeidan IH, Post MJ, et al. Neurosyphilis in HIV-positive and HIV- negative patients: neuroimaging findings. AJNR Am J Neuroradiol. 1995;16(4):703–11.
39. Johns DR, Tierney M, Felsenstein D. Alteration in the natural history of neurosyphilis by concurrent infection with the human immunodeficiency virus. N Engl J Med. 1987;316(25):1569–72.
40. Czarnowska-Cubala M, Wiglusz MS, Cubala WJ, et al. MR findings in neurosyphilis--a literature review with a focus on a practical approach to neuroimaging. Psychiatr Danub. 2013;25(Suppl 2):S153–7.
41. Patkar D, Narang J, Yanamandala R, et al. Central nervous system tuberculosis: pathophysiology and imaging findings. Neuroimaging Clin N Am. 2012;22(4):677–705.
42. Misra UK, Kalita J, Maurya PK. Stroke in tuberculous meningitis. J Neurol Sci. 2011;303(1–2):22–30.
43. Lammie GA, Hewlett RH, Schoeman JF, et al. Tuberculous cerebrovascular disease: a review. J Infect. 2009;59(3):156–66.
44. Nair PP, Kalita J, Kumar S, et al. MRI pattern of infarcts in basal ganglia region in patients with tuberculous meningitis. Neuroradiology. 2009;51(4):221–5.
45. Rojas-Echeverri LA, Soto-Hernandez JL, Garza S, et al. Predictive value of digital subtraction angiography in patients with tuberculous meningitis. Neuroradiology. 1996;38(1):20–4.
46. Singh B, Garg RK, Singh MK, et al. Computed tomography angiography in patients with tuberculous meningitis. J Infect. 2012;64(6):565–72.
47. Kalita J, Prasad S, Maurya PK, et al. MR angiography in tuberculous meningitis. Acta Radiol. 2012;53(3):324–9.
48. Kuker W, Nagele T, Schmidt F, et al. Diffusion-weighted MRI in herpes simplex encephalitis: a report of three cases. Neuroradiology. 2004;46(2):122–5.
49. Argyriou AA, Tsota I, Solomou E, et al. Intracerebral haemorrhage as a rare complication of HSV-1 meningoencephalitis: case report and review of the literature. Scand J Infect Dis. 2006;38(1):63–6.
50. Alexandri NM, Tavernarakis A, Potagas C, et al. Ischemic stroke and herpes simplex virus type-1 associated meningoencephalitis. Rev Neurol. 2004;160(5 Pt 1):579–81.
51. Gnann JW Jr. Varicella-zoster virus: atypical presentations and unusual complications. J Infect Dis. 2002;186(Suppl 1):S91–8.
52. Askalan R, Laughlin S, Mayank S, et al. Chickenpox and stroke in childhood: a study of frequency and causation. Stroke. 2001;32(6):1257–62.
53. Kramer AH. Viral encephalitis in the ICU. Crit Care Clin. 2013;29(3):621–49.
54. Lin HC, Chien CW, Ho JD. Herpes zoster ophthalmicus and the risk of stroke: a population-based follow-up study. Neurology. 2010;74(10):792–7.
55. Gilden DH, Mahalingam R, Cohrs RJ, et al. The protean manifestations of varicella-zoster virus vasculopathy. J Neurovirol. 2002;8(Suppl 2):75–9.
56. Chiang F, Panyaping T, Tedesqui G, et al. Varicella zoster CNS vascular complications. A report of four cases and literature review. Neuroradiol J. 2014;27(3):327–33.
57. Patsalides AD, Wood LV, Atac GK, et al. Cerebrovascular disease in HIV-infected pediatric patients: neuroimaging findings. AJR Am J Roentgenol. 2002;179(4):999–1003.
58. Ionita CC, Siddiqui AH, Levy EI, et al. Acute ischemic stroke and infections. J Stroke Cerebrovasc Dis. 2011;20(1):1–9.
59. Goldstein DA, Timpone J, Cupps TR. HIV-associated intracranial aneurysmal vasculopathy in adults. J Rheumatol. 2010;37(2):226–33.
60. Gutierrez J, Glenn M, Isaacson RS, et al. Thinning of the arterial media layer as a possible preclinical stage in HIV vasculopathy: a pilot study. Stroke. 2012;43(4):1156–8.
61. Connor MD, Lammie GA, Bell JE, et al. Cerebral infarction in adult AIDS patients: observations from the Edinburgh HIV Autopsy Cohort. Stroke. 2000;31(9):2117–26.
62. Gutierrez J, Ortiz G. HIV/AIDS patients with HIV vasculopathy and VZV vasculitis: a case series. Clin Neuroradiol. 2011;21(3):145–51.
63. Corr PD. Imaging of cerebrovascular and cardiovascular disease in AIDS patients. AJR Am J Roentgenol. 2006;187(1):236–41.
64. Mitchell TG, Perfect JR. Cryptococcosis in the era of AIDS--100 years after the discovery of Cryptococcus neoformans. Clin Microbiol Rev. 1995;8(4):515–48.
65. Panackal AA, Williamson PR. Fungal infections of the central nervous system. Continuum. 2015;21(6 Neuroinfectious Disease):1662–78.
66. Klock C, Cerski M, Goldani LZ. Histopathological aspects of neurocryptococcosis in HIV-infected patients: autopsy report of 45 patients. Int J Surg Pathol. 2009;17(6):444–8.
67. DeLone DR, Goldstein RA, Petermann G, et al. Disseminated aspergillosis involving the brain: distribution and imaging characteristics. AJNR Am J Neuroradiol. 1999;20(9):1597–604.
68. Luthra G, Parihar A, Nath K, et al. Comparative evaluation of fungal, tubercular, and pyogenic brain abscesses with conventional and diffusion MR imaging and proton MR spectroscopy. AJNR Am J Neuroradiol. 2007;28(7):1332–8.
69. Khandelwal N, Gupta V, Singh P. Central nervous system fungal infections in tropics. Neuroimaging Clin N Am. 2011;21(4):859–66, viii.
70. Raman SR. Fungal infections of the nervous system: current perspective and controversies in management. Int J Surg. 2010;8(8):591–601.
71. Saini J, Gupta RK, Jain KK. Intracranial infections: key neuroimaging findings. Semin Roentgenol. 2014;49(1):86–98.
72. Crum NF, Lederman ER, Stafford CM, et al. Coccidioidomycosis: a descriptive survey of a reemerging disease. Clinical characteristics and current controversies. Medicine (Baltimore). 2004;83(3):149–75.

73. Arsura EL, Johnson R, Penrose J, et al. Neuroimaging as a guide to predict outcomes for patients with coccidioidal meningitis. Clin Infect Dis. 2005;40(4):624–7.
74. Wrobel CJ, Meyer S, Johnson RH, et al. MR findings in acute and chronic coccidioidomycosis meningitis. AJNR Am J Neuroradiol. 1992;13(4):1241–5.
75. Lammering JC, Iv M, Gupta N, et al. Imaging spectrum of CNS coccidioidomycosis: prevalence and significance of concurrent brain and spinal disease. AJR Am J Roentgenol. 2013;200(6):1334–46.
76. Zalduondo FM, Provenzale JM, Hulette C, et al. Meningitis, vasculitis, and cerebritis caused by CNS histoplasmosis: radiologic-pathologic correlation. AJR Am J Roentgenol. 1996;166(1):194–6.
77. Nguyen FN, Kar JK, Zakaria A, et al. Isolated central nervous system histoplasmosis presenting with ischemic pontine stroke and meningitis in an immune-competent patient. JAMA Neurol. 2013;70(5):638–41.
78. Saccente M. Central nervous system histoplasmosis. Curr Treat Options Neurol. 2008;10(3):161–7.
79. Del Brutto OH. Neurocysticercosis. Handb Clin Neurol. 2014;121:1445–59.
80. Barinagarrementeria F, Cantu C. Frequency of cerebral arteritis in subarachnoid cysticercosis: an angiographic study. Stroke. 1998;29(1):123–5.
81. Abdel Razek AA, Watcharakorn A, Castillo M. Parasitic diseases of the central nervous system. Neuroimaging Clin N Am. 2011;21(4):815–41, viii.
82. Hauptman JS, Hinrichs C, Mele C, et al. Radiologic manifestations of intraventricular and subarachnoid racemose neurocysticercosis. Emerg Radiol. 2005;11(3):153–7.
83. Kimura-Hayama ET, Higuera JA, Corona-Cedillo R, et al. Neurocysticercosis: radiologic-pathologic correlation. Radiographics. 2010;30(6):1705–19.
84. Bousser MG, Ferro JM. Cerebral venous thrombosis: an update. Lancet Neurol. 2007;6(2):162–70.
85. Saposnik G, Barinagarrementeria F, Brown RD Jr, et al. Diagnosis and management of cerebral venous thrombosis: a statement for healthcare professionals from the American Heart Association/American Stroke Association. Stroke. 2011;42(4):1158–92.
86. Ferro JM, Canhao P, Stam J, et al. Prognosis of cerebral vein and dural sinus thrombosis: results of the International Study on Cerebral Vein and Dural Sinus Thrombosis (ISCVT). Stroke. 2004;35(3):664–70.
87. Stam J. Thrombosis of the cerebral veins and sinuses. N Engl J Med. 2005;352(17):1791–8.
88. Khatri IA, Wasay M. Septic cerebral venous sinus thrombosis. J Neurol Sci. 2016;362:221–7.
89. Wasay M, Dai AI, Ansari M, et al. Cerebral venous sinus thrombosis in children: a multicenter cohort from the United States. J Child Neurol. 2008;23(1):26–31.
90. Vieira JP, Luis C, Monteiro JP, et al. Cerebral sinovenous thrombosis in children: clinical presentation and extension, localization and recanalization of thrombosis. Eur J Paediatr Neurol. 2010;14(1):80–5.
91. Sitton MS, Chun R. Pediatric otogenic lateral sinus thrombosis: role of anticoagulation and surgery. Int J Pediatr Otorhinolaryngol. 2012;76(3):428–32.
92. Smith DM, Vossough A, Vorona GA, et al. Pediatric cavernous sinus thrombosis: A case series and review of the literature. Neurology. 2015;85(9):763–9.
93. Ducreux D, Oppenheim C, Vandamme X, et al. Diffusion-weighted imaging patterns of brain damage associated with cerebral venous thrombosis. AJNR Am J Neuroradiol. 2001;22(2):261–8.
94. Linn J, Pfefferkorn T, Ivanicova K, et al. Noncontrast CT in deep cerebral venous thrombosis and sinus thrombosis: comparison of its diagnostic value for both entities. AJNR Am J Neuroradiol. 2009;30(4):728–35.
95. Roland T, Jacobs J, Rappaport A, et al. Unenhanced brain CT is useful to decide on further imaging in suspected venous sinus thrombosis. Clin Radiol. 2010;65(1):34–9.
96. Provenzale JM, Kranz PG. Dural sinus thrombosis: sources of error in image interpretation. AJR Am J Roentgenol. 2011;196(1):23–31.
97. Silverman CS, Mancuso AA. Periantral soft-tissue infiltration and its relevance to the early detection of invasive fungal sinusitis: CT and MR findings. AJNR Am J Neuroradiol. 1998;19(2):321–5.
98. Safder S, Carpenter JS, Roberts TD, et al. The "Black Turbinate" sign: an early MR imaging finding of nasal mucormycosis. AJNR Am J Neuroradiol. 2010;31(4):771–4.
99. Middlebrooks EH, Frost CJ, De Jesus RO, et al. Acute invasive fungal rhinosinusitis: a comprehensive update of CT findings and design of an effective diagnostic imaging model. AJNR Am J Neuroradiol. 2015;36(8):1529–35.
100. Renowden S. Cerebral venous sinus thrombosis. Eur Radiol. 2004;14(2):215–26.
101. Idbaih A, Boukobza M, Crassard I, et al. MRI of clot in cerebral venous thrombosis: high diagnostic value of susceptibility-weighted images. Stroke. 2006;37(4):991–5.
102. Mullins ME, Grant PE, Wang B, et al. Parenchymal abnormalities associated with cerebral venous sinus thrombosis: assessment with diffusion-weighted MR imaging. AJNR Am J Neuroradiol. 2004;25(10):1666–75.
103. Rottger C, Trittmacher S, Gerriets T, et al. Reversible MR imaging abnormalities following cerebral venous thrombosis. AJNR Am J Neuroradiol. 2005;26(3):607–13.
104. Poon CS, Chang JK, Swarnkar A, et al. Radiologic diagnosis of cerebral venous thrombosis: pictorial review. AJR Am J Roentgenol. 2007;189(6 Suppl):S64–75.
105. Khandelwal N, Agarwal A, Kochhar R, et al. Comparison of CT venography with MR venography in cerebral sinovenous thrombosis. AJR Am J Roentgenol. 2006;187(6):1637–43.
106. Leach JL, Fortuna RB, Jones BV, et al. Imaging of cerebral venous thrombosis: current techniques, spectrum of findings, and diagnostic pitfalls. Radiographics. 2006;26(Suppl 1):S19–41. discussion S2-3.
107. Linn J, Ertl-Wagner B, Seelos KC, et al. Diagnostic value of multidetector-row CT angiography in the evaluation of thrombosis of the cerebral venous sinuses. AJNR Am J Neuroradiol. 2007;28(5):946–52.
108. Meckel S, Reisinger C, Bremerich J, et al. Cerebral venous thrombosis: diagnostic accuracy of combined, dynamic and static, contrast-enhanced 4D MR venography. AJNR Am J Neuroradiol. 2010;31(3):527–35.
109. Yigit H, Turan A, Ergun E, et al. Time-resolved MR angiography of the intracranial venous system: an alternative MR venography technique. Eur Radiol. 2012;22(5):980–9.
110. Jang J, Kim BS, Sung J, et al. Subtraction MR venography acquired from time-resolved contrast-enhanced MR angiography: comparison with phase-contrast MR venography and single-phase contrast-enhanced MR venography. Korean J Radiol. 2015;16(6):1353–63.
111. Fu JH, Lai PH, Hsiao CC, et al. Comparison of real-time three-dimensional gadolinium-enhanced elliptic centric-ordered MR venography and two-dimensional time-of-flight MR venography of the intracranial venous system. J Chin Med Assoc. 2010;73(3):131–8.
112. Liang L, Korogi Y, Sugahara T, et al. Evaluation of the intracranial dural sinuses with a 3D contrast-enhanced MP-RAGE sequence: prospective comparison with 2D-TOF MR venography and digital subtraction angiography. AJNR Am J Neuroradiol. 2001;22(3):481–92.
113. Kirchhof K, Welzel T, Jansen O, et al. More reliable noninvasive visualization of the cerebral veins and dural sinuses: comparison of three MR angiographic techniques. Radiology. 2002;224(3):804–10.

12 Infections of the Spinal Cord

Chenglong Ren

12.1 Anatomy of the Spinal Cord

The spinal cord is located in the spinal canal, which was cylindrical and slightly flat. The length of the spinal cord varies. There are two swellings, that is, cervical enlargement and lumbar enlargement. From the waist to the lower spinal cord gradually shifts to be thin, which come into being conus medullaris. Filum terminale is distributed below the conus terminalis. Each spinal nerve is formed from the combination of nerve fibers from its dorsal and ventral roots. The spinal nerve emerges from the spinal column through an opening (intervertebral foramen) between adjacent vertebrae. There are eight pairs of cervical nerves, twelve pairs of thoracic nerves, five pairs of lumbar nerves, five pairs of sacral nerves, and one pair of coccygeal nerves. The spinal nerves are part of the peripheral nervous system.

The cauda equina (Latin for horsetail) is a bundle of spinal nerves and spinal nerve roots, which arise from the lumbar enlargement and the conus medullaris. The spinal gray matter is H-shaped in the spinal cord in the axial anatomy, which extends to the anterior part and was called the spinal anterior and posterior crus, the horizontal part of the gray matter with a central tube. The central tube passes upward through the fourth ventricle, the lower end of the spinal cord in the expansion of the formation of the final room. Blood supply of spinal cord sources from the spinal artery which includes the anterior and posterior spinal artery of the vertebral artery and the deep cervical artery, the intercostal artery, the lumbar artery, and the sacral artery.

12.2 Epidural and Intramedullary Cord Abscess

Epidural Abscess

Epidural abscess is an important form of infection that needs to be quickly diagnosed and managed due to the risk of cord compression. Spinal epidural abscess can typically be traced to contiguous spread of infection from the skin or other soft tissue or complications post-procedure. Rarer cases are due to abscesses originating from a remote site via the blood flow. The most common pathogen is *Staphylococcus aureus*, accounting for up to two thirds of all cases. Other pathogens in order of decreasing probability include gram-negative bacilli, *Streptococci*, coagulase-negative staph, and anaerobes [1]. Risk factors for a spinal epidural abscess include diabetes mellitus, alcoholism, trauma, hemodialysis, IV drug use, HIV infection, and concurrent other infections [2]. Damage to the spinal cord is propagated by direct compression, interruption of the arterial blood supply, thrombosis of local veins, and from bacterial toxins and inflammation. The acute abscess contains pus, but within weeks, granulation tissue is the primary finding during surgical drainage. The average extent of spine involvement is three to five vertebral segments, but in rare severe cases, the entire spine can be involved. However, the extent of involvement does not correlate directly with the severity of symptoms. The typical clinical triad is pain, fever, and neurologic deficits. However, not all cases will present with all symptoms. Thus, imaging is key to rapid diagnosis, and MRI is the preferred modality.

C. Ren (✉)
Department of Radiology, Affiliated Hospital of Shaanxi University of Chinese Medicine, Xianyang, China

B. Gao et al. (eds.), *Imaging of CNS Infections and Neuroimmunology*, https://doi.org/10.1007/978-981-13-6904-9_12

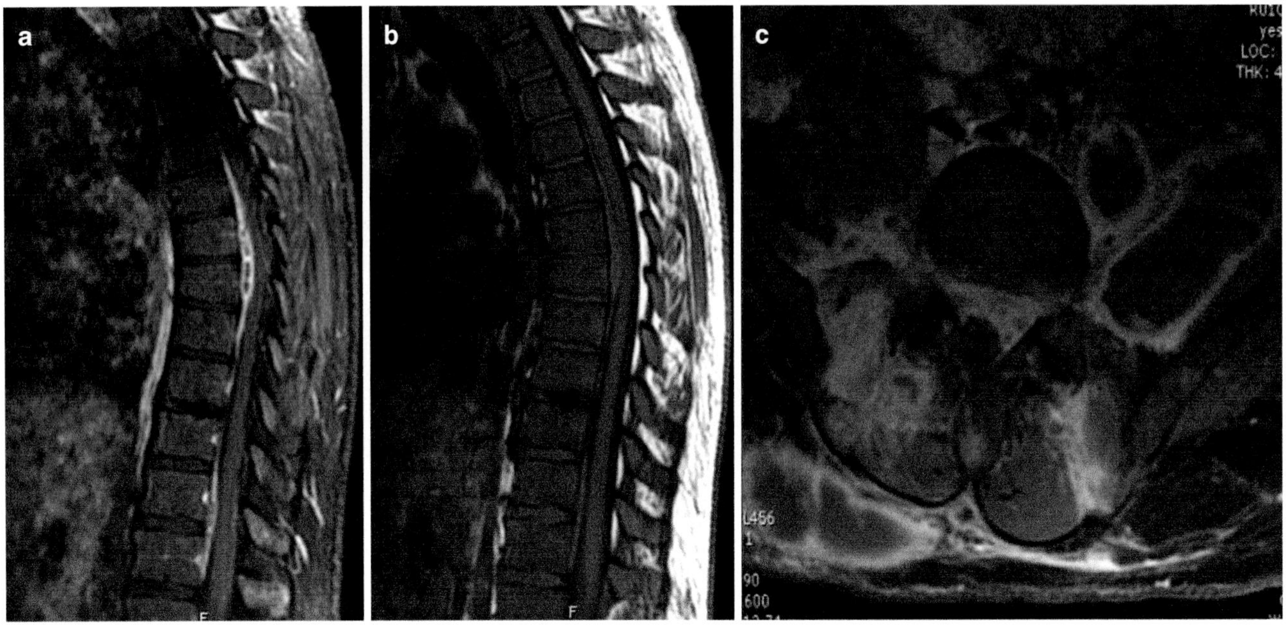

Fig. 12.1 Ventral thoracic epidural abscesses. Noncontrast (**a**) and contrast-enhanced (**b**) sagittal T1-weighted images show peripherally enhancing ventral epidural abscesses extending from T3-T4 to T7-T8 and T10-T11 through T12, compressing the cord at T6-T7 level. (**c**) Axial contrast-enhanced fat suppressed T1-weighted image shows multiple pelvic intramuscular and soft tissue abscesses and ventral epidural phlegmon at L5 level (Courtesy of Kirt Gill MD., Keck School of Medicine, University of Southern California, USA)

Imaging of the entire cord is recommended. Abscesses visualized on MRI demonstrate T2 hyperintensity equivalent to fluid with rim enhancement around a hypointense center (Fig. 12.1). Soft tissue edema will present as diffuse hypointensity on TI and hyperintensity on T2WI with contrast enhancement in adjacent soft tissue and epidural space [1]. Once an abscess has been identified on MR imaging, then the diagnostic algorithm can progress to finding the type and source of the infection.

Intramedullary Abscess

Intramedullary spinal cord abscess (ISCA) is a rare condition, especially in children; developmental anomalies such as infected dermal sinus tract are a common source of ISCA, whereas in adults, most cases are cryptogenic or hematogenous. Although uncommon, these infections are associated with significant mortality and morbidity, especially in the preantibiotic. The other reason infected by the surrounding tissue infection could bring about it. In very rare cases, intramedullary abscess can form affecting spinal cord tissue directly. Under normal conditions, the spinal cord is exceptionally resilient to infection, but in a compromised state due to an underlying condition, abscesses can form [3]. Due to the paucity of cases, a clear association delineating pathogenesis is not available. Underlying causes may include infections elsewhere, penetrating trauma, and congenital dermal sinuses. Case reports have detailed instances of intramedullary abscess following wide range of presentations and histories, including endocarditis, a history of radiation therapy for Hodgkin's lymphoma, concurrent epidural abscess, chronic tuberculosis, and complications secondary to stab wounds or spinal puncture [4]. Congenital dermal sinuses are excess layers of tissue that can be found in the midline between the nasal bone and the tailbone, and a number of pediatric cases have detailed intramedullary abscess formation within congenital dermal sinuses.

Upon imaging, intramedullary abscesses can be viewed as a heterogeneous T2 hyperintense lesion with cord enlargement (Fig. 12.2). Rim enhancement may be visualized on T1 [3, 5]. An oval regular sharpened edged area could be presented as abscess on MR image. Signal of the pus on T1-weighted image is lower than that of the spinal cord but higher than cerebrospinal fluid; the signal is usually homogeneous but also slightly heterogeneous. The abscess wall on the T1-weighted image is similar to the signal intensity of the spinal cord. Pus on T2-weighted images displays homogeneous hyperintensity. Spinal abscess is usually combined with bleeding, which is characterized by hyperintensity on T1-weighted image and also can be deposited in the side of abscess with T1 hyperintensity. T1 post-contrast image presents significantly contrast enhanced for the abscess; however, pus does not enhance (Fig. 12.3) [6].

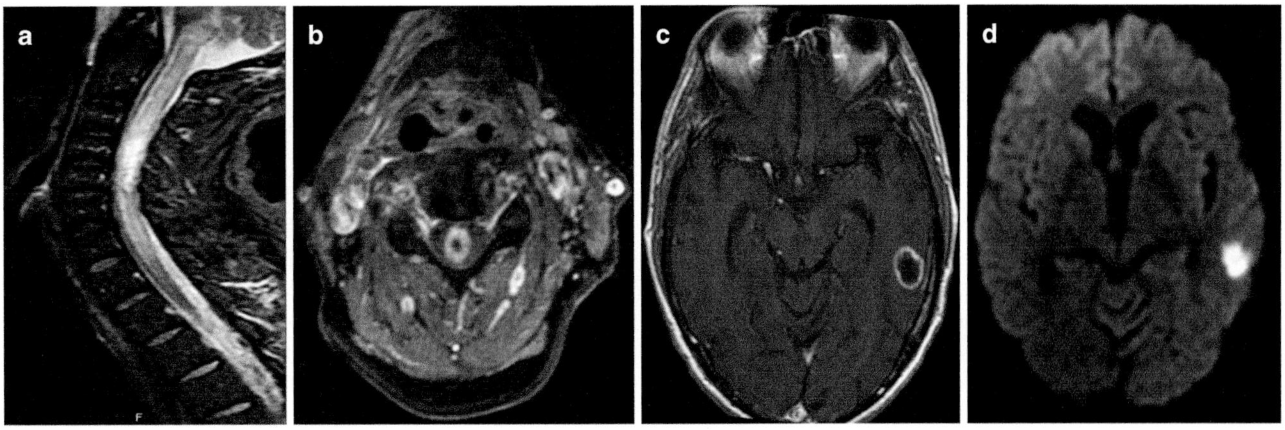

Fig. 12.2 Intramedullary abscess of the cervical cord in immunocompromised patient. Sagittal STIR image (**a**) demonstrates a T2 hyperintense lesion extending from the medulla to the cervical cord at C5/C6 level. There is associated cord edema and expansion. Post contrast T1-weighted axial image (**b**) demonstrates peripheral ring enhancement consistent with intramedullary abscess. Contrast-enhanced axial T1-weighted image of the brain (**c**) shows a ring-enhancing lesion in the left temporal lobe. Axial DWI (**d**) demonstrates hyperintensity due to diffusion restriction (confirmed on ADC map which is not shown) consistent with abscess (Courtesy of Alexander Lerner MD., Keck School of Medicine, University of Southern California, USA)

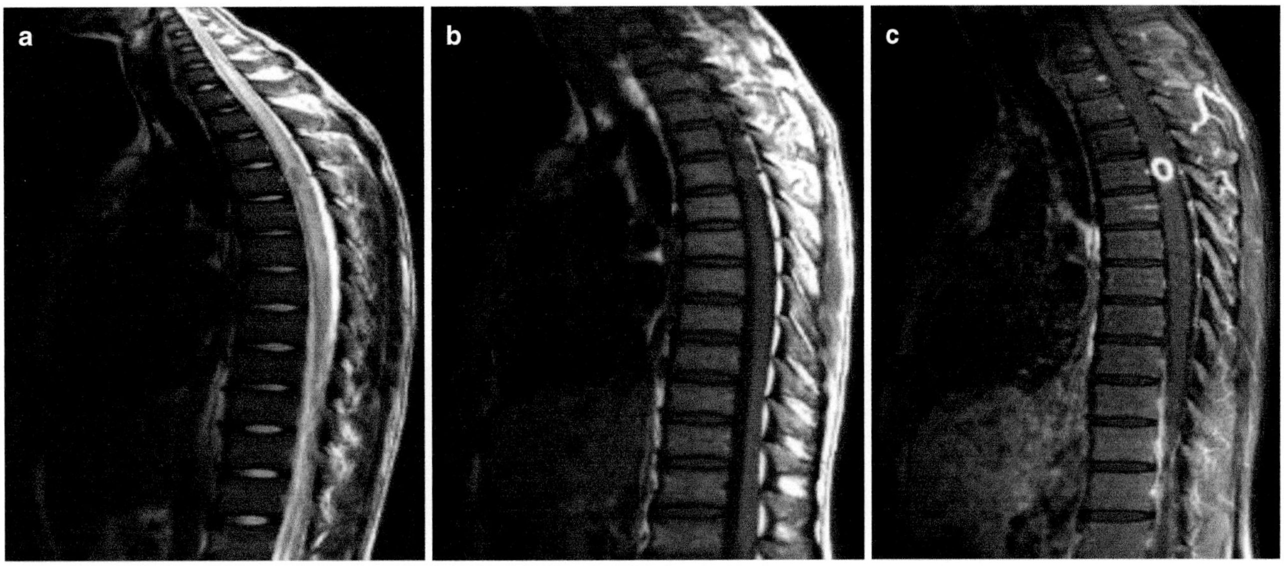

Fig. 12.3 Intramedullary abscess. (**a**) T2-weighted image shows abscess is mildly high signal in the thoracic spinal cord, (**b**) T1-weighted image shows abscess is similar to the spinal cord signal in the thoracic spinal cord, and (**c**) shows ring-shaped enhancement of abscess in the thoracic spinal cord

12.3 Viral Myelitis

Viral myelitis is divided into two groups based on how the spinal cord is involved:

1. Acute viral disease targets the gray matter of the spinal cord resulting in lower motor neuron disease. Viruses that fall into this group include *Flaviviruses* (West Nile virus, Japanese encephalitis virus) and *Enteroviruses* (poliovirus, coxsackievirus). These viruses invade the anterior horn producing asymmetric flaccid weakness. MRI shows T2 hyperintensity in the anterior horn [7–9].
2. Viral myelitis is those viruses affecting the spinal cord similar to the presentation of transverse myelitis. This group of viruses includes herpes simplex virus, varicella virus, cytomegalovirus, Epstein-Barr virus, and hepatitis C [10]. This type of viral myelitis can manifest either post-infectious or directly due to viral damage.

12.4 AIDS Myelopathy

HIV infection can lead to a vacuolar myelopathy seen in up to half of all AIDS patients on autopsy. Pathological features focus on spinal cord demyelination changes caused by HIV virus directly invading spinal cord nerve cells, similar to subacute combined degeneration. Only 25% of those cases will present with clinical symptoms while alive. AIDS myelopathy typically occurs in the later stages of the disease with most patients dying within 6 months of diagnosis. The typical clinical presentation is a progressive spastic paraparesis with sensory deficits and urinary symptoms [11]. Imaging findings vary depending on the stage and extent of the myelopathy, but a common underlying similarity is visualization of cord atrophy on MRI. MRI T2-weighted images show hyperintensity in the demyelination region, and T1 post-contrast images could show abnormal contrast [12]. Cord changes are typically localized in the thoracic cord and to a lesser degree the cervical cord. Additionally, symmetric bilateral dorsal column involvement may be seen, reminiscent of findings seen in subacute combined degeneration [13].

12.5 Neurocysticercosis

Neurocysticercosis (NCC) is one of the most common causes of epilepsy in endemic regions around the world. Caused by the larval stage of the pork tapeworm *Taenia solium*, neurocysticercosis primarily manifests as parenchymal lesions. The clinical presentation of neurocysticercosis can be nonspecific and variable depending on the location and number of lesions. Diagnostic neuroimaging not only plays a critical role in categorizing CNS involvement in patients presenting for seizures and epilepsy, but it also provides the essential information for the diagnostic criteria of NCC by detection of enhancing lesions, multilobulated cystic lesions, parenchymal brain calcifications, or cystic lesions with or without a discernible scolex among other minor or confirmatory criteria [14].

However, spinal cord involvement occurs in an estimated 1% of cases. Intramedullary spinal cysticercosis was considered extremely rare, with only a few cases described in the literatures up to the 1970s [15]. Spinal cysticerci are typically located in the subarachnoid space where they lead to secondary inflammatory and demyelinating change in the cord. The rarer findings of intramedullary cysticerci are associated with edema similar to transverse myelitis (Fig. 12.4). The neurological deficits vary based on the site of spinal cord involvement.

12.6 Neurosyphilis

Neurosyphilis involving the spinal cord is also rare, which can be divided into three types according to the different parts involved—meningovascular syphilis, spinal cord parenchymal syphilis, and syphilitic pachymeningitis. Meningovascular syphilis on MRI shows the spinal cord thickening with scattered patchy lesions. T1 post-contrast image has slightly enhancement. Spinal parenchymal syph-

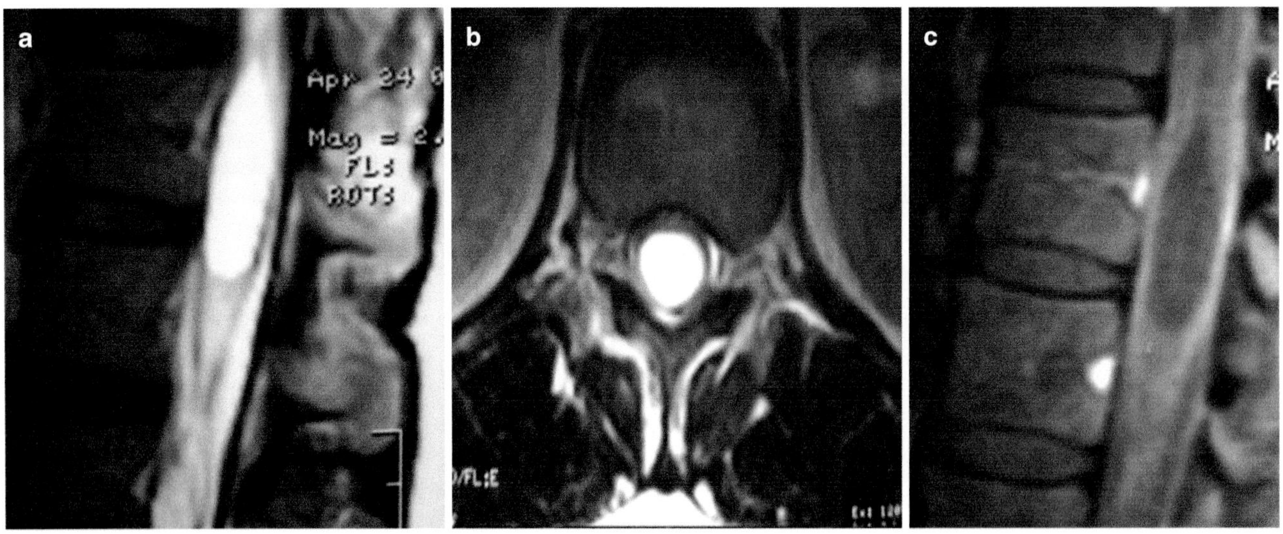

Fig. 12.4 Neurocysticercosis of the spinal cord. Sagittal (**a**) and axial (**b**) T2-weighted images demonstrate a large cystic ovoid intramedullary cystic lesion in lower thoracic cord with associated cord expansion. Contrast-enhanced sagittal T1 (**c**) demonstrates no significant enhancement in the lesion consistent with a cystic neurocysticercosis lesion. Subtle linear enhancement along dorsal aspect of the cord is due to involvement of subarachnoid space by neurocysticercosis (Courtesy of Meng Law MD., Keck School of Medicine, University of Southern California, USA)

ilis, similar to spinal tuberculosis, mainly presents syphilis granulation and syringomyelia [16]. The MRI characteristic is similar to granuloma and syringomyelia caused by other disease. The diagnosis mainly relies on clinical symptoms.

References

1. Darouiche RO. Spinal epidural abscess. N Engl J Med. 2006;355(19):2012–20.
2. Krishnamohan P, Berger JR. Spinal epidural abscess. Curr Infect Dis Rep. 2014;16(11):436.
3. Vo DT, Cravens GF, Germann RE. *Streptococcus pneumoniae* meningitis complicated by an intramedullary abscess: a case report and review of the literature. J Med Case Rep. 2016;10(1):290.
4. da Silva PS, de Souza Loduca RD. Intramedullary spinal cord abscess as complication of lumbar puncture: a case-based update. Childs Nerv Syst. 2013;29(7):1061–8.
5. Kurita N, Sakurai Y, Taniguchi M, et al. Intramedullary spinal cord abscess treated with antibiotic therapy--case report and review. Neurol Med Chir (Tokyo). 2009;49(6):262–8.
6. Sinha P, Parekh T, Pal D. Intramedullary abscess of the upper cervical spinal cord. Unusual presentation and dilemmas of management: case report. Clin Neurol Neurosurg. 2013;115(9):1845–50.
7. Chen CY, Chang YC, Huang CC, et al. Acute flaccid paralysis in infants and young children with enterovirus 71 infection: MR imaging findings and clinical correlates. AJNR Am J Neuroradiol. 2001;22(1):200–5.
8. Jeha LE, Sila CA, Lederman RJ, et al. West Nile virus infection: a new acute paralytic illness. Neurology. 2003;61(1):55–9.
9. Kraushaar G, Patel R, Stoneham GW. West Nile Virus: a case report with flaccid paralysis and cervical spinal cord: MR imaging findings. AJNR Am J Neuroradiol. 2005;26(1):26–9.
10. Kincaid O, Lipton HL. Viral myelitis: an update. Curr Neurol Neurosci Rep. 2006;6(6):469–74.
11. Dal Pan GJ, Glass JD, McArthur JC. Clinicopathologic correlations of HIV-1-associated vacuolar myelopathy: an autopsy-based case-control study. Neurology. 1994;44(11):2159–64.
12. Thurnher MM, Post MJ, Jinkins JR. MRI of infections and neoplasms of the spine and spinal cord in 55 patients with AIDS. Neuroradiology. 2000;42(8):551–63.
13. Quencer RM. AIDS-associated myelopathy: clinical severity, MR findings, and underlying etiologies. AJNR Am J Neuroradiol. 1999;20(8):1387–8.
14. Del Brutto OH, Nash TE, White AC Jr, et al. Revised diagnostic criteria for neurocysticercosis. J Neurol Sci. 2017;372:202–10.
15. Del Brutto OH, Garcia HH. Intramedullary cysticercosis of the spinal cord: a review of patients evaluated with MRI. J Neurol Sci. 2013;331(1–2):114–7.
16. Yang C, Li G, Fang J, et al. Gumma: an unusual presentation of neurosyphilis. World Neurosurg. 2016;95:622.e17–23.

Infections in Childhood

13

Vivek Yedavilli, Vivek Pandey, and Delilah Burrowes

13.1 Introduction

Congenital infections and infections in the perinatal period can result in overwhelming effects to the developing brain and are dependent on several factors: (1) the maturity of the brain, at what period of developing brain the infection was introduced, and (2) the dose of the offending pathogen to the host central nervous system that is particularly susceptible to infection usually during the period of maximum growth from fetal life to early childhood [1]. Early intrauterine exposure to infection can result in severe malformations of the brain, while exposure later in uterine development results in encephaloclastic/destructive lesions [2]. The goal is for early recognition and treatment to avoid this long-term neurologic sequela [3].

Beyond the perinatal period in children, there are four main routes in the spread of infection: (1) hematogenous dissemination from a distant focus, most common route (i.e., infected emboli); (2) direct implantation, usually traumatic sometimes iatrogenic (i.e., during surgery or lumbar puncture); (3) direct extension from infected source (i.e., sinusitis, osteomyelitis, otitis, infected encephalocele); and (4) spread via the peripheral CNS as seen with certain viruses such as herpes simplex.

Imaging is utilized as a tool in the evaluation of suspected CNS infection and is crucial in assisting with the diagnosis. Ultrasound is typically the first line of defense [3] in evaluating the neonate within the first few months of life for suspected injury. It acts as a good screening tool while the fontanelle remains open, however has its limitations due to its lack of specificity [2]. Computed tomography (CT) is an alternative imaging choice, providing greater special resolution and ideal for evaluating for calcifications commonly found with congenital infections [2]. CT however has fallen out of favor in the more recent years given the more recent concern of radiation exposure ([3]—look up ACR info on radiation exposure). Magnetic resonance imaging, however, is the imaging modality of choice. It is the most sensitive of the neuroimaging modalities providing optimal tissue contrast when evaluating for pediatric infection of the pediatric brain. Current magnet strengths for clinical use range from 0.2 T to 3.0 T with increased sensitivity with the higher strength magnets. MRI not only provides anatomic information but with advanced MRI can also provide functional data with the use of diffusion imaging, perfusion, tractography, spectroscopy, and functional imaging, requiring the higher strength magnets (i.e., 1.5 T or greater). A limitation, however, is that it takes more time to acquire images, and therefore there is an increased risk of imaging degradation due to patient motion. Children, therefore, more often require sedation in order to obtain a successful scan, which is an added risk for children [1]. Newer techniques are now available and evolving with reduced scan time, thereby mitigating the need for sedation in this younger population; however, improving and optimizing image quality are currently being investigated [3].

Many CNS infections demonstrate age-dependent susceptibility with increased incidence, susceptibility, and severity in the very young due to multiple factors including an immature immune system [1, 4–6]. Genetic factors affecting the host resistance tend to manifest during the child's development as they are progressively introduced to various pathogens, some of which may cause disease. There are also certain imaging features that share similar common features with the adult counterpart; however, their complications can be quite different [3].

V. Yedavilli · V. Pandey
Advocate Illinois Masonic Medical Center, Chicago, IL, USA

D. Burrowes (✉)
Division of Neuroradiology, Ann & Robert H. Lurie Children's Hospital of Chicago, Chicago, IL, USA
e-mail: dburrowes@luriechildrens.org

B. Gao et al. (eds.), *Imaging of CNS Infections and Neuroimmunology*, https://doi.org/10.1007/978-981-13-6904-9_13

13.2 Pediatric CNS Infection

13.2.1 Bacterial Cerebritis/Meningitis

Incidence and Clinical Presentation

Bacterial cerebritis/meningitis and its associated high morbidity and mortality are crucial to diagnose for timely management in children. These are the most common form of CNS infections within the pediatric population with a mortality rate of 50% when left untreated [1]. In developing countries, where there are limited resources due to poor socioeconomic status with malnutrition and lack of clean water sources and overcrowding conditions, their rates of infection are higher.

The clinical presentation of bacterial cerebritis/meningitis is varied depending on the age and immune state of the child. Classically the child will present with fever, headache, neck stiffness, seizures, and focal deficits with fever being the single most specific symptom for bacterial cerebritis [7]. There are, however, other nonspecific prodromal symptoms such as altered mental status and lethargy that can often make a prompt diagnosis challenging. Oftentimes, pediatric patients will not have meningeal signs, which could lead to delayed or incorrect diagnoses. Cerebritis can occur once the bacteria invade the brain parenchyma through hematogenous spread.

Bacterial Organisms

The most common organisms worldwide are *Streptococcus pneumoniae*, *Haemophilus influenzae*, and *Neisseria meningitidis*. With the advent of vaccination, *H. influenzae* infection has decreased considerably. In certain Asian countries, other bacteria have a higher prevalence. For example, in Hong Kong, *M. tuberculosis*, a mycobacterium, is a commonly implicated organism. Gram-negative bacilli, such as *Klebsiella*, are often the cause of bacterial cerebritis in Taiwan. Meningoccus has a similarly high rate of infection in Vietnam. Other common organisms seen in Asian countries include *Salmonella* and *Acinetobacter* [8].

Imaging

Imaging plays an important role in early diagnosis and treatment of complications. CT is the initial modality of choice; however a normal CT exam is common during the initial presentation. It is generally used to exclude other possible diagnoses presenting with nonspecific symptoms. Early findings that may be seen on CT are mild ventriculomegaly and effacement of cortical sulci, both of which are related to increased intracranial pressures and are seen in fewer than half of such cases [1]. Magnetic resonance imaging (MRI) is the gold standard for diagnosing bacterial cerebritis and its complications, with T1-weighted post-contrast imaging being the most specific. Enhancement of the leptomeninges is the main feature of acute cerebritis accompanied by meningeal enhancement and can range from subtle increased enhancement of the meninges to frank intense enhancement of the meninges and leptomeninges (Fig. 13.1). In more severe cases, there are more pronounced and often asymmetric leptomeningeal enhancement greater than physiological limits. FLAIR imaging can also play a role detecting subtle leptomeningeal enhancement by demonstrating increased signal in the affected areas of abnormal enhancement.

13.2.2 Complications of Bacterial Cerebritis/Meningitis

Hydrocephalus

Bacterial cerebritis is often complicated by hydrocephalus due to changes in the intracranial pressure from invasion of the bacteria into subarachnoid spaces. It can lead to either a

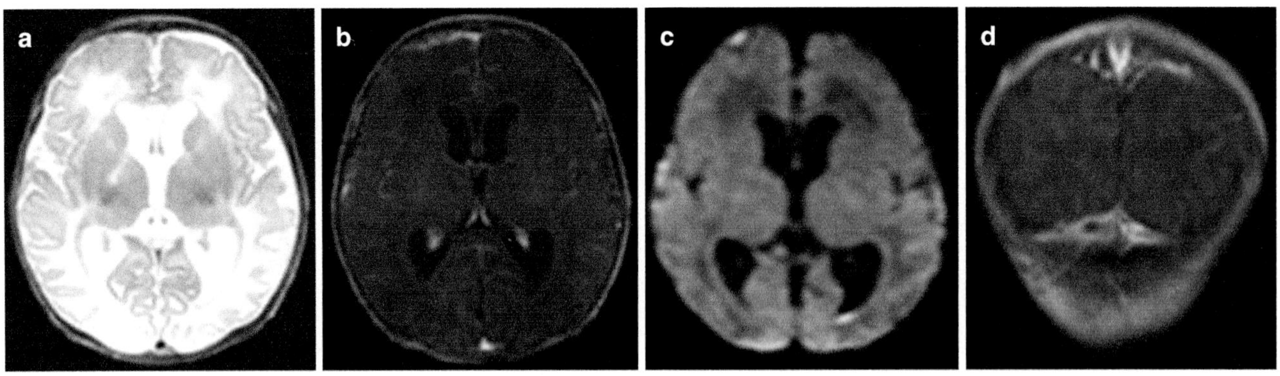

Fig. 13.1 *E. coli* meningitis with hydrocephalus and thrombosis. A 12-day-old newborn infant with mild hydrocephalus and abnormal increased signal in the bilateral occipital lobes and frontal white matter despite incomplete myelination on axial T2 (**a**). Bilateral leptomeningeal enhancement with enhancement in the right frontal extradural space on axial T1 post (**b**) and corresponding diffusion restriction on DWI (**c**) consistent meningitis with a purulent small epidural empyema. Diffusion restriction is also noted in the left occipital horn consistent with ventriculitis (**c**). Focal defect is seen in the right transverse sinus indicating partial thrombosis on coronal T1 post-contrast images (**d**)

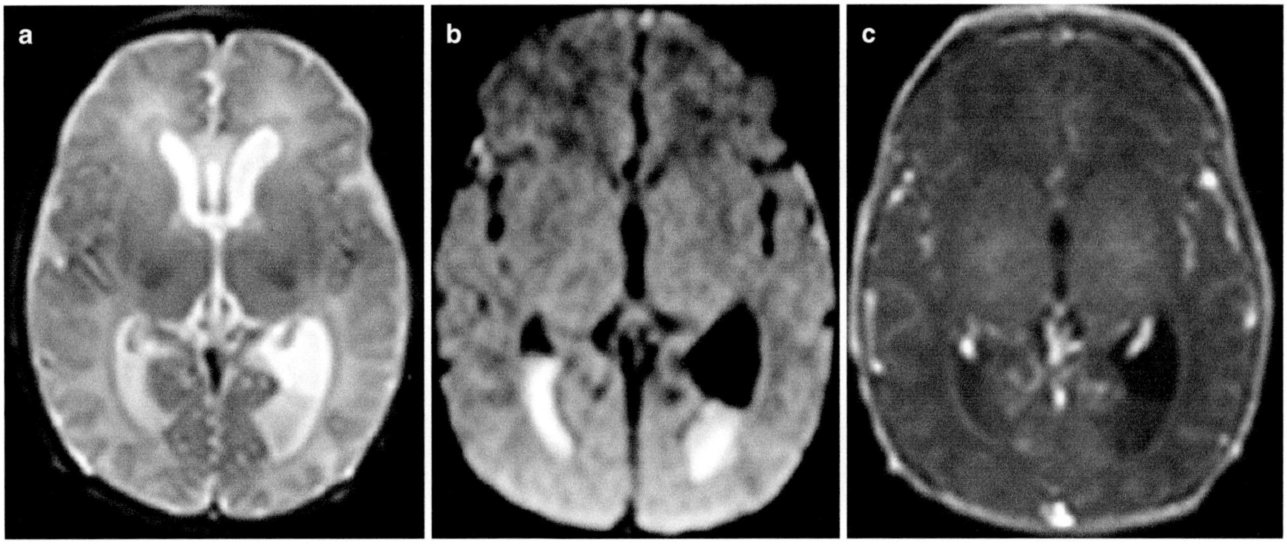

Fig. 13.2 Infected hydrocephalus and ventriculitis. An 11-day-old female axial T2 with hydrocephalus and abnormal signal in the occipital horns (**a**) which restrict on DWI (**b**) consistent with purulent debris. Axial T1 post-contrast shows mild enhancement along the ventricular lining on axial T1(**c**) seen with ventriculitis along with leptomeningeal enhancement seen along the temporal and frontal regions

communicating or non-communicating hydrocephalus. Parenchymal cavitation can lead to obstructing (non-communicating) hydrocephalus through direct blockage of normal CSF flow. Communicating hydrocephalus is often a combination of increased CSF production and decreased absorption by arachnoid villi from the inflammation [1]. MRI is often superior to CT in detecting early hydrocephalus and localization of sites of obstruction (Fig. 13.2).

Cerebral Abscess

Cerebral abscess is one of the common complications of bacterial meningitis and cerebritis. *Streptococcus pneumoniae* and *Staphylococcus* are the most common bacteria found in cerebral abscesses, although gram-negative bacteria have also been implicated. Cerebral abscesses can be found anywhere in the brain but tend to have a predilection for the supratentorial brain parenchyma. Brain abscesses evolve from cerebritis in four distinct stages. Once bacteria invade the meninges, it can quickly spread into the brain parenchyma by causing vascular inflammation resulting in a focal cerebritis, the first stage of an evolving abscess development lasting up to 5 days. The second stage, considered late cerebritis, is an ill-defined unencapsulated fluid collection comprised of congested, edematous vessels secondary to a neutrophilic reaction that begins to form, eventually leading to liquefactive necrosis which can last up to 14 days. This ill-defined collection appears heterogeneous on both T1- and T2-weighted sequences with associated patchy enhancement. The third stage is early encapsulation consisting of collagen and reticulum fibers that begin to organize around inflamed and necrotic tissue. The late capsular stage is the fourth and final component. In this stage, there is thickening of the fibrous capsule, more pronounced near the cortical side due to the increased overall vascularity. The early and late capsular stages together can last for several months. Once the capsule forms during the last stages, it appears more homogeneously high on T1, low on T2, and heterogeneous in the necrotic core with intense capsule enhancement. Diffusion-weighted imaging (DWI) is useful for demonstrating diffusion restriction within the cystic collection due to its purulent content (Fig. 13.3). Magnetic resonance spectroscopy (MRS) can add value when evaluating an abscess showing an elevated lactate peak due to the anaerobic metabolism. Often there is an increased risk of ventriculitis from capsular rupture into the ventricle due to proximity to the ventricular system. This can lead to a poor outcome due to the dissemination of the offending agent throughout the ventricular system.

Empyema

Effusions are non-enhancing CSF fluid collections which are often extra-axial presenting in either the subdural or epidural spaces. If these collections become infected, they become empyemas. Effusions and empyemas are most often seen along the cerebral convexities and less commonly along the falx. Effusions often appear low on T1 and high on T2 with no peripheral enhancement. Empyemas, on the other hand, can present heterogeneously on both T1- and T2-weighted sequences (due to internal purulent content). Marked rim enhancement is demonstrated due to vascular inflammation and subsequent fibrosis (Fig. 13.4). DWI will also help differentiate empyemas given its purulent content as seen with an abscess and thereof lacking with a simple effusion. This restricted diffusion is also important in distinguishing empyemas not only from effusions but from other cystic collections such as hematomas and hygromas (Fig. 13.5). Inflammation from empyemas can often lead to venous thrombosis due to the vascular inflammation with possible adjacent cerebritis. For that reason, MR venography (MRV) is indicated when empyemas are diagnosed (Fig. 13.4).

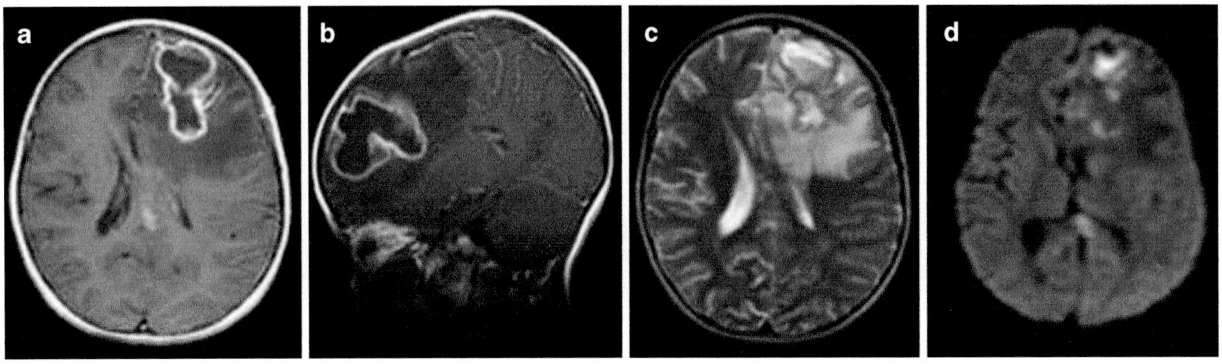

Fig. 13.3 Cerebral abscess TB. A 2-year-old male axial and sagittal T1 post shows ring enhancement in left frontal lobe (**a**, **b**) with fluid-fluid level on axial T2 (**c**) and restricted diffusion on DWI (**d**) consistent with and a left frontal lobe abscess from tuberculosis. Extensive surrounding edema is also seen on T2- and T1-weighted images

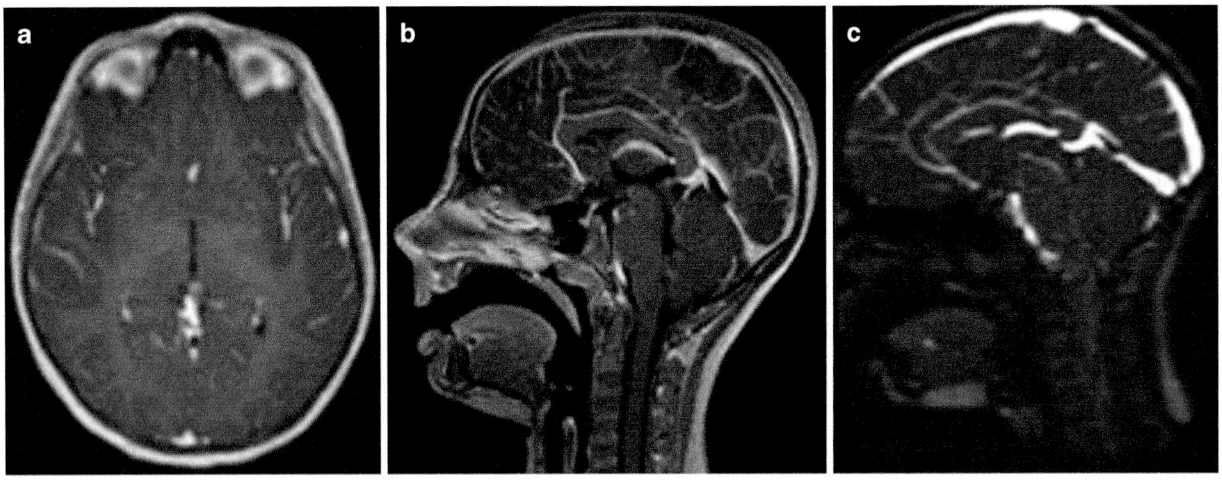

Fig. 13.4 Meningoencephalitis with thrombosis. A 7-year-old female axial T1 post-contrast showing leptomeningeal enhancement on axial (**a**) and sagittal T1 post-contrast (**b**) from meningitis. Sagittal T1 post-contrast images also show focal thrombus in the proximal straight sinus (**b**) confirmed on sagittal MR venogram (**c**)

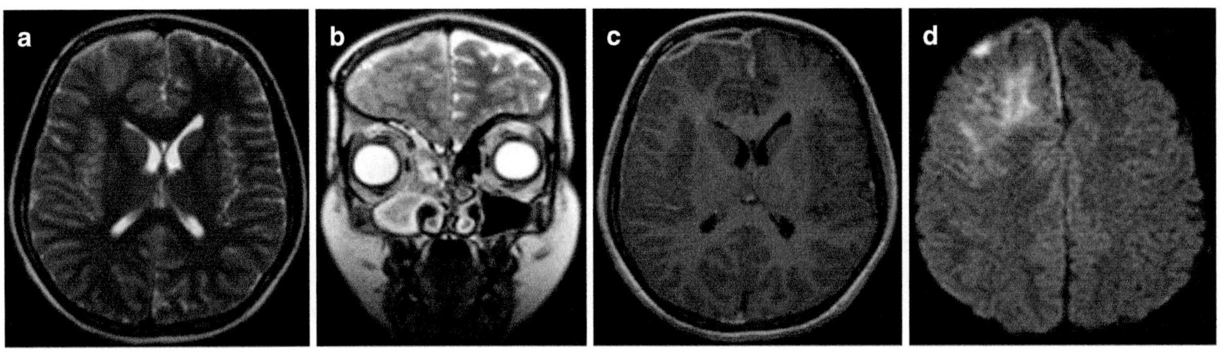

Fig. 13.5 Right frontal subdural empyema. An 11-year-old male with small extra-axial collection right frontal region on axial and coronal T2 (**a**, **b**) with mild mass effect and mild cortical swelling. Rim enhancement is seen on axial T1 post-contrast with enhancement along anterior interhemispheric fissure (**c**) with corresponding diffusion restriction (**d**) consistent with subdural empyema. Diffusion restriction is also seen in the right frontal lobe white matter consistent with a cerebritis (**d**). Coronal T2 also shows extensive sinus disease involving the right paranasal sinuses (**b**), a common source for epidural empyema

13.2.3 Viral Encephalitis

13.2.3.1 Herpes Simplex Virus

Incidence and Clinical Presentation

Herpes simplex virus (HSV) is a debilitating DNA virus that results in significant morbidity in the pediatric population. There are two main strands of the virus, HSV 1 and HSV 2. It is essential to distinguish these subtypes as each afflicts a different demographic with distinct modes of transmission. The neonatal subtype of HSV encephalitis is thought to be due to the HSV 2 strand (HSV2), while the sporadic encephalitis is secondary to the HSV 1 infection. The neonatal form of HSV encephalitis caused by HSV 2 is discussed in the neonatal section of this chapter.

Non-neonatal HSV encephalitis (HSV1) is the most common cause of fatal focal encephalitis in the world [9]. The virus can be seen in older pediatric patients and primarily affects those less than 18 years of age, comprising roughly 30% of total HSV1 cases [10]. Of note, HSV1 is also a major cause of adult encephalitis. HSV1 is thought to be secondary to reactivation of the latent virus and affects 1 in every 250,000–500,000. Without antiviral therapy, the mortality rate exceeds 70%. Patients who receive the appropriate antiviral therapy have approximately a 3% chance of full neurological recovery [1].

Patients who are infected with HSV1 often present with a nonspecific prodrome. Symptoms include fever, lethargy, irritability, focal deficits, and headache [1]. Generalized and focal seizures have also been reported in a third of patients. Its nonspecific prodrome makes it essential to utilize various diagnostic tools, such as lumbar puncture with polymerase chain reaction (PCR) analysis, in achieving a timely diagnosis.

Imaging

HSV1 have a greater predilection to affect the temporal and inferior frontal cortices as opposed to more diffuse involvement affecting gray and deep white matter seen in neonatal HSV2 encephalitis. CT is typically the initial imaging study and is often normal. Occasionally, CT will demonstrate nonspecific hypodensity in the frontal and temporal lobes. MRI, however, is the diagnostic study of choice for the imaging diagnosis of HSV1. It generally shows asymmetric involvement of the temporal and inferior frontal lobes manifesting as geographic regions of low T1 and high T2 signal abnormalities secondary to edema. Hemorrhagic involvement is common and may result in high T1 signal due to subacute blood products. It is of note that there are no periventricular white matter abnormalities in HSV1, which are often seen in the neonatal form (HSV2). Gradient sequences demonstrate blooming artifact secondary to the hemorrhage. Positive diffusion restriction can also be seen on DWI due to the cytotoxic edema from the neuronal spread from the viral infection, which can lead to necrosis. It is typical to also see enhancement of the cortex and meninges, a feature also seen in HSV2 (Fig. 13.6). Given the blooming artifact and restricted diffusion seen on gradient echo MR imaging and DWI, HSV1 can mimic a hemorrhagic stroke; however, it differs in that it does not follow a vascular distribution as stroke would and tends to affect the insular cortex of the frontal lobes. Antiviral therapy, such as acyclovir, has been shown to decrease mortality to roughly 10–20%.

13.2.3.2 Japanese Encephalitis/West Nile Virus

Japanese encephalitis (JE) is an RNA flavivirus-mediated encephalitis and the leading cause of viral encephalitis in Asia according to the World Health Organization [1]. It is the most common epidemic viral encephalitis in the world, resulting in nearly 50,000 new cases a year [1]. It is a prevalent disease with an incidence of at least 10 per 100,000. The disease is endemic in Southeast Asia and East Asia, and if left untreated, 30% of cases are noted to result in death [1]. JE is part of the *Flaviviridae*, a serocomplex family of nine genetically and anti-genetically related viruses, the West Nile virus (WNV) being the most widely distributed member of the JE virus complex of flaviviruses.

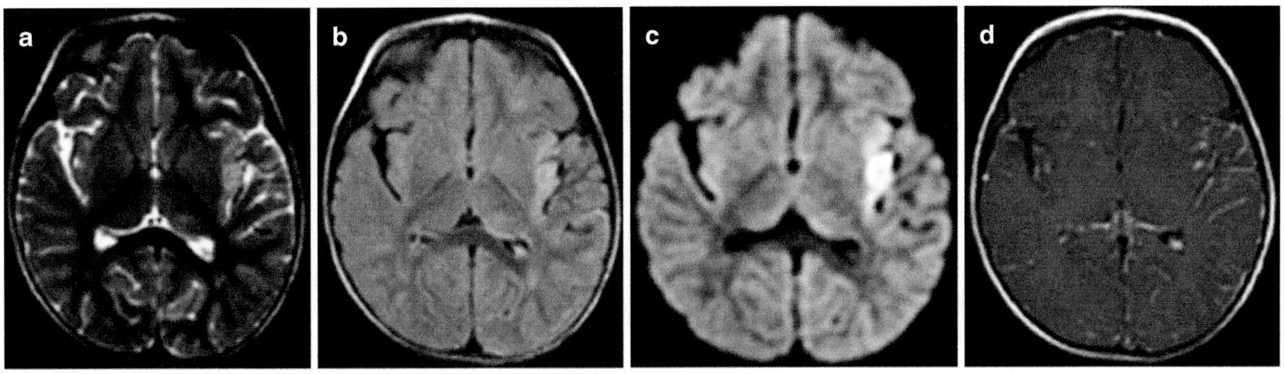

Fig. 13.6 Herpes simplex HSV1. A 20-month-old female with abnormal increase signal in the insular cortex on axial T2 and axial FLAIR (**a**, **b**) with restricted diffusion in the same region (**c**). Post-contrast images show leptomeningeal enhancement in the left Sylvian fissure surrounding the left temporal lobe tip and insular cortex (**d**)

Clinical Presentation

JE and WNV are slow progressively debilitating viruses which present similarly. They are known to have a biphasic course. It can present insidiously with high fever, vomiting, diarrhea, and headache during the initial phase. They are often followed by tonic-clonic seizures and spasming which can further lead to coma in the second phase. The two most specific clinical signs for JE are hyperventilation and extrapyramidal signs, in the form of hemiplegia and dystonia. The WNV was once considered a relatively benign virus; however its importance took notice during outbreaks in the late 1900s [11]. The patients affected range from a broad spectrum of clinical symptoms ranging from nonspecific febrile illnesses to severe meningoencephalomyelitis affecting the brain and spine [11].

Imaging

JE and WNV have similar imaging features. They classically infect the thalami and basal ganglia symmetrically. Because of its slower course, CT is often negative even days after infection but can demonstrate hypodensities in the thalami in the later stages. MRI classically shows low T1 and high T2 signal abnormalities in the thalami, basal ganglia, substantia nigra bilaterally along with cortical involvement of the temporal lobes, and cerebellar regions. Associated hemorrhage is not uncommon and can result in variable blooming artifact on gradient images with restricted diffusion on DWI. Contrast enhancement is also variable depending on the stage of disease and severity of edema (Fig. 13.7). JE can mimic HSV1 due to the overlapping temporal lobe involvement and possibility of hemorrhage. However, JE can be distinguished from other etiologies given its symmetric presentation and involvement of the thalami, basal ganglia, and substantia nigra; these areas are uncommonly affected in HSV1. JE also differs from HSV1 in the temporal lobe. Classically, JE affects the hippocampus, while HSV1 tends to favor the insula [12]. It is essential to differentiate JE from HSV1 as the treatment for JE is supportive, while HSV1 can be treated with antiviral therapy.

13.2.3.3 Enteroviruses

Enteroviruses are a class of RNA viruses that commonly infect the CNS. Subtypes of this family include Coxsackie, polio, and echoviruses. Polio and echoviruses most commonly result in long-term sequelae. The polio vaccine has dramatically reduced the incidence in developed countries. However, the virus is still seen in countries that lack resources and overall infrastructure. EV71, a subtype of

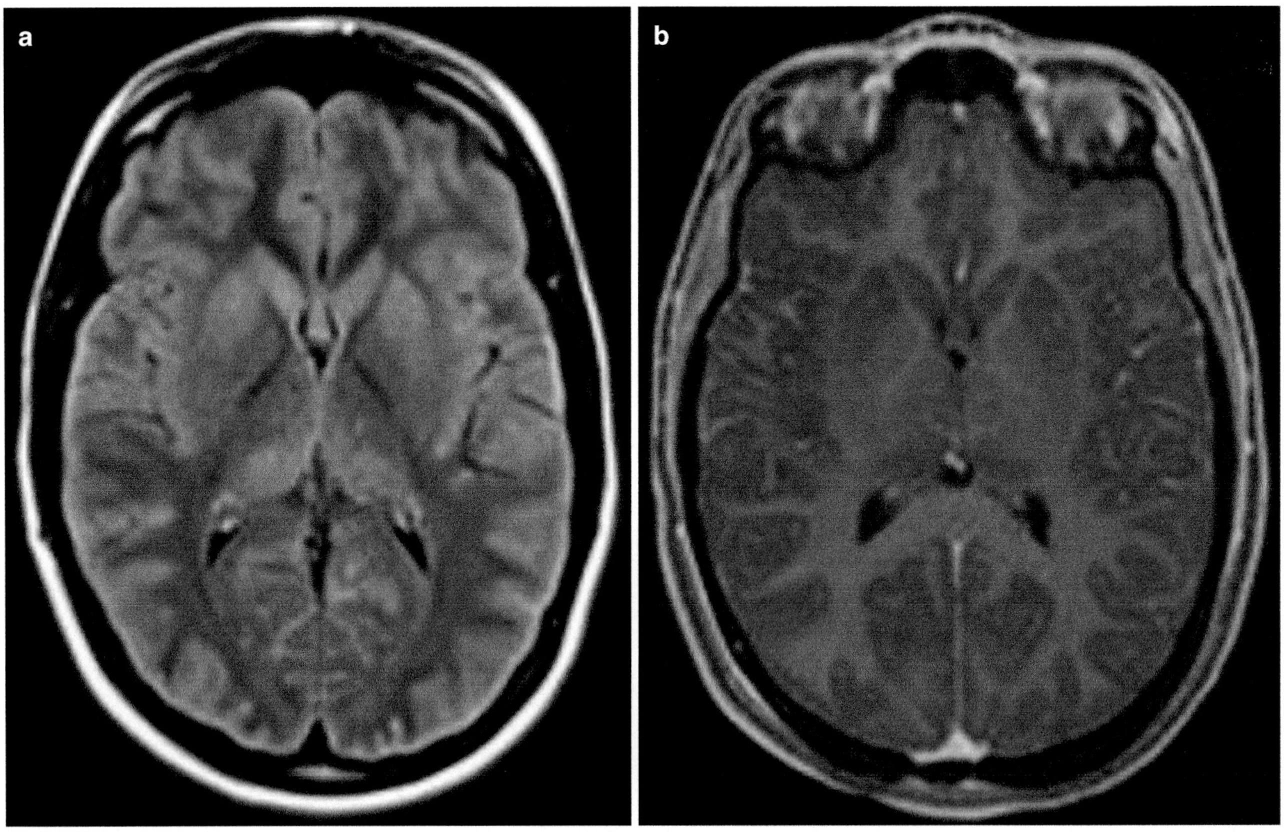

Fig. 13.7 West Nile virus. A 15-year-old female with mild increased FLAIR signal involving the cortical sulci and thalami (**a**). Post-contrast images show diffuse mild leptomeningeal enhancement (**b**)

Coxsackie A virus, has been implicated in cases of fatal rhombencephalitis specifically in Southeast Asia often presenting as hand-foot-and-mouth disease with a complication rate of up to 50% [13]. Mortality rates of nearly 20% in Taiwan have been reported for EV71-induced rhombencephalitis. Coxsackie viruses have also been prevalent in eastern China where multiple strains have been reported to cause encephalitis. Echoviruses have been shown to cause aseptic meningitis and preferentially infect infants and the younger demographics. Most enteroviruses are acquired through ingestion of contaminated food and water sources. As these viruses are often self-limiting, treatment is generally supportive.

Clinical Presentation

Enteroviruses can have varied clinical presentations depending on the subtype. Polio classically presents with acute flaccid paralysis. EV71 presents with high fevers, sore throat, and vesicular lesions on the hands, feet, and gluteal regions resulting in the commonly known hand-foot-and-mouth disease. Ulcerations of the palate, known as herpangina, have also been seen with EV71. This specific virus also causes rapid onset apnea and overall respiratory distress with focal deficits, ataxia, and tremor, which can lead to coma in severe instances [1] of rhombencephalitis. Cardiac arrest can also be seen in severe cases. Echoviruses on the other hand present with seizures, fever, and irritability as it affects infants more commonly.

Imaging

Enteroviruses often can present with no MRI findings. When positive, enteroviruses predominantly affect the brainstem with lesions in the midbrain, posterior pons and medulla, as well as the anterior horns of the spinal cord. The tegmentum of the pons is the most commonly affected area in the brainstem [14]. Supratentorial lesions are rare in enteroviral encephalitis but have been reported in the putamen [14]. Hemorrhage and lack of restricted diffusion are characteristic of these viruses and may help distinguish from stroke and other infectious and inflammatory encephalitis.

Polio presents with high T2 lesions primarily within the substantia nigra and anterior horns of the spinal cord, causing the acute flaccid paralysis. Classically there is lack of supratentorial lesions, hemorrhage, or restricted diffusion excluding differentials such as ischemic infarcts and autoimmune demyelinating disorders such as multiple sclerosis and acute demyelinating encephalomyelitis.

EV71 has the tendency to affect the brainstem with predilection for the posterior pons, medulla, dentate nucleus, and anterior horns of the cervical spinal cord. Isointense T1 and high T2 signal lesions are often identified in these areas. Lesions within the dorsal pons and medulla may not enhance, while enhancement of the cranial nerve roots arising from the brainstem and ventral horns is more commonly seen [14]. Nerve root enhancement can be seen in both enterovirus and Guillain-Barre; however brainstem involvement is the distinguishing feature seen with enteroviruses [14], whereas nerve root enhancement excludes differential of transverse myelitis in the setting of T1 and T2 signal abnormalities found in the spinal cord.

13.2.3.4 Rabies Encephalitis

Rabies is an RNA zoonotic virus that spreads through the saliva of affected animals with bats and dogs as the most common hosts. Dog bites are the most common form of human infection. It can cause a fatal and rapid encephalitis when left untreated. Approximately 55,000 deaths per year results from rabies with 95% of those deaths occurring in Asian and African countries. Many developed countries such as Japan and island countries such as Barbados are rabies-free, which is defined as no reported cases of rabies in a 2-year span [1].

Clinical Presentation

In humans, rabies have two forms, classic and paralytic, the former being the more common type. Rabies begins with a nonspecific viral prodrome of fever, fatigue, sore throat, and headache. Pain at the site of the bite is the most specific early symptom. Patients subsequently present with hydrophobia, aerophobia, hyperreflexia, mydriasis, and hypersalivation from sympathetic overstimulation. Mental status changes, convulsions, and coma tend to be later presentations of the disease as seen in the classic form. The paralytic form presents with bilateral motor weakness with sparing of the sensory nervous system. Without proper treatment, rabies can be fatal within 10 days. Treatment generally involves administration of the rabies vaccine with immunoglobulin therapy [1].

Imaging

Imaging is often not obtained due to the rapid course of the disease; however, rabies characteristically affects the gray matter. It has a predilection for the basal ganglia, hypothalami, hippocampus, pulvinar of the thalamus, and spinal cord and presents as ill-defined hypoattenuation in these areas of the brain on CT. MRI classically demonstrates non-enhancing high T1 and T2/FLAIR lesions within the basal ganglia and thalami secondary to methemoglobin from petechial hemorrhages in the late stages of the classical subtype of the disease. Within the paralytic form, there is more involvement of the spinal cord, but in most cases, the two subtypes that are indistinguishable on MRI lesions seen in the hypothalamus, hippocampus, and spinal cord often enhance. Restricted diffusion is generally not seen with these lesions but has not been adequately investigated [15].

13.2.3.5 Tuberculosis

Tuberculosis (TB), which is caused by *Mycobacterium tuberculosis*, is one of the most common infections worldwide, most commonly seen in the immunocompromised. Involvement of the central nervous system (CNS) is rare in tuberculosis, accounting for less than 5% of the disease manifestations. The rate triples in the immunocompromised, where it affects approximately 15–20% of this population manifesting as CNS abnormalities [16].

Clinical Presentation

Tuberculosis is considered a great mimicker with its varied nonspecific symptoms. In children, it most commonly manifests as meningitis with neck stiffness, paralysis, papilledema from intracranial hypertension, and coma in the most dire situations [16]. Neonates more commonly present with hydrocephalus with bulging fontanelles. In a prior study by Udani et al. of 500 Indian school children, hemiparesis and hemiplegia were the most common presentations of tuberculosis. Late onset of symptoms is also not uncommon, most frequently seen in with paralysis and hydrocephalus.

Imaging

Tuberculous Meningitis

Tuberculous meningitis (TM) is the most common CNS manifestation in both the pediatric and adult populations through hematogenous dissemination. CT is useful for detecting TB as an initial test, generally presenting with leptomeningeal enhancement with enhancement of the subpial and subarachnoid spaces, characteristically affecting basal cisterns.

Contrast MRI, however, is the imaging study of choice for diagnosis of CNS TB meningitis. In the early stage of the disease, there may be no abnormalities on pre-contrast imaging, and for that reason post-contrast imaging is crucial [17]. Leptomeningeal enhancement is better delineated accompanied by T2 and FLAIR abnormalities. Basal cistern involvement can lead to obstruction of CSF flow from the leptomeningeal exudates, leading to Tb's most common CNS complication, communicating hydrocephalus. In a study by Yaramis et al., hydrocephalus was seen in 80% of pediatric cases.

Entrapment of the cranial nerves from leptomeningeal inflammation leading to ischemia and cranial nerve palsy can also be seen as another relatively common complication. This is demonstrated in up to 70% of cases with the second, third, fourth, and seventh cranial nerves most commonly affected in the most severe cases [16].

Cerebral infarction is another dire complication that is seen in up to 40% of patients with CNS TB and most commonly involves the basal ganglia and internal capsule. These infarcts are secondary to necrotizing arteritis which subsequently leads to ischemia. CNS TB can also cause venous infarcts secondary to dural venous sinus thrombosis which can lead to hemorrhagic infarcts.

Tuberculoma

Tuberculomas are the most common intraparenchymal CNS manifestation of TB [16]. They can present as rounded solitary, multifocal, or miliary lesions. On CT, they are often heterogeneously isodense or hyperdense with nodular ring-like enhancement in a targetoid appearance on post-contrast imaging. On post-contrast MRI, these lesions show a low T2/FLAIR rim with a high signal central core corresponding to a region of necrosis. Tuberculomas are the cause of noncaseating granulomas that can eventually caseate in chronic stages. This is an important distinguishable feature on imaging. Noncaseating tuberculomas demonstrate low T1 central cores and peripheral high T2 with nodular but relatively homogenous enhancement [16]. Once caseation occurs, these tuberculomas can have two forms – solid or central necrosis. The solid form demonstrates markedly low T1 and T2 signal on MRI due to granulation tissue formation and hypercellularity. The central necrotic form, representing liquefactive necrosis, demonstrates a low T1, high T2 central core, and peripheral nodular appearance that parallels what is seen on CT as described earlier [16]. Healed tuberculomas appear as foci of calcification on CT.

Tuberculous Cerebral Abscess

TB-related cerebral abscess (TCS) is a rare but severe complication. They appear as rounded hypodensities with surrounding edema which can often cause mass effect. On MRI, they appear as central low T1 signal with a high T1 peripheral rim corresponding to central high T2 signal with a low T2 peripheral rim on T2 and FLAIR sequences with characteristic ring enhancement on post-contrast imaging [17]. These lesions often mimic the necrotic caseating form of tuberculomas but differ in the composition of the central core. This differs from caseating tuberculomas having a central core of liquefactive necrosis as opposed to TCS in which its content is composed of purulent material. These presentations can be diagnostically challenging on imaging as they appear similar and cannot be distinguished on conventional MRI sequences [18]. MR spectroscopy (MRS), however, has played an important role in distinguishing the two entities. Both can also demonstrate similar findings on MRS, demonstrating markedly elevated lipid and lactate peaks; however an elevated cytosolic amino acid peak can help to distinguish TCS from tuberculomas [18].

Miliary Tuberculosis

Miliary TB (MTb) is often seen in severely immunocompromised patients secondary to hematogenous spread. On CT, these lesions appear as punctate scattered hypodensities at the gray-white matter junction. MRI can better delineate

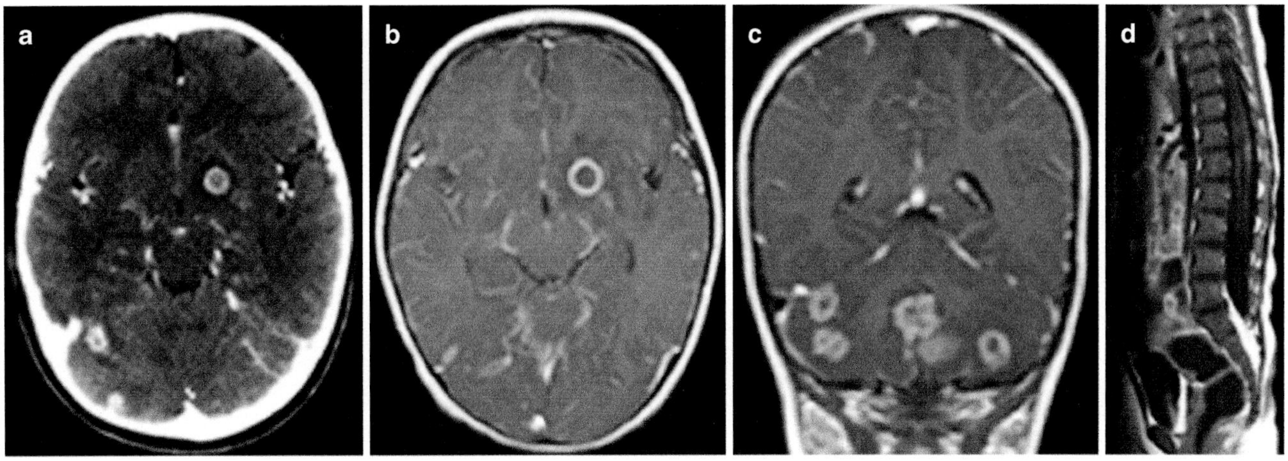

Fig. 13.8 Miliary tuberculosis. A 17-month-old female with history of multiple ring-enhancing lesions of the both right and left cerebellum, left anterior commissure, and left basal ganglia on post-contrast CT and MRI axial and coronal T1 post-contrast images (**a**, **b**, **c**) consistent with multiple intracranial abscesses related to miliary tuberculosis. Sagittal T1 post-contrast image of the spine shows enhancement of the leptomeninges and nerve roots of the cauda equine (**d**) consistent with leptomeningitis

these lesions often only 3 mm in maximal dimension. On MRI they appear as low T1, high T2 rounded lesions which often demonstrate ringlike enhancement on post-contrast studies (Fig. 13.8).

TB Myelitis

TB myelitis is another manifestation that can occur, secondary to spread through the subarachnoid space. Additionally, there is a clumped appearance of nerve roots on post-contrast MR imaging primarily in the lumbar region with diffuse nodular, thickened dural enhancement (Fig. 13.8). Arachnoiditis is a common complication which can further lead to a non-enhancing syringomyelia with CSF intensity on T1 and T2 images.

13.2.4 Fungal Infections

Opportunistic fungi also must be considered among agents which can infect the CNS. These organisms can spread in individuals who are both healthy with an intact immune system and immunocompromised. In immunocompromised hosts, HIV is a common systemic cause linked to such infections. Certain fungal infections are endemic to some Asian countries due to the lack of resources and adequate healthcare. Despite treatment, these infections still carry a high morbidity and mortality. Fungal infections can be stratified into subtypes such as yeasts, molds, and zygomycetes. This review will focus on yeasts and molds given the overall prevalence of these entities.

13.2.4.1 *Aspergillus*

Aspergillus is a type of yeast that is endemic to Asia. It often begins as a pulmonary infection that subsequently invades the CNS through hematogenous spread especially in immunocompromised patients. *Aspergillus* infections begin in the paranasal sinuses and can spread into the extradural space through microvascular invasion with eventual hemorrhagic necrosis. Overall, CNS aspergillosis is seen in 10–15% of invasive aspergillosis cases, frequently manifesting as cerebral abscesses with focal neurological deficits.

Clinical Presentation

Aspergillus, being both a yeast and hyphae, can cause a number of clinical manifestations. Meningitis is the most common cause due to the microvascular invasion which can eventually progress into encephalitis, subsequently leading to focal parenchymal lesions, infarctions, and abscesses. The *Aspergillus* infection can present as a nonspecific constellation of symptoms such as new-onset seizures, fevers, headaches, lethargy, impaired consciousness, and/or focal neurological deficits.

Imaging

CT and MRI can both demonstrate pathology which can expedite diagnosis of *Aspergillus* in conjunction with labs and clinical data, although findings still tend to be nonspecific. Multifocal areas of hypoattenuation primarily within the cortical and subcortical white matter are one of the more common CT manifestations. T2 and FLAIR sequences are of great utility often exhibiting high T2 signal in focal lesions. Post-contrast studies are also beneficial demonstrating both dural enhancement and the more classic appearance of a ring-enhancing lesion predominantly involving the paranasal sinuses, basal ganglia, thalami, and subcortical white matter [19] (Fig. 13.9). Vascular invasion with involvement of the thalamostriate vessels and terminal arteries of the larger branches, via an embolic source, can lead to infarction and abscess formation. Studies have shown that involvement of

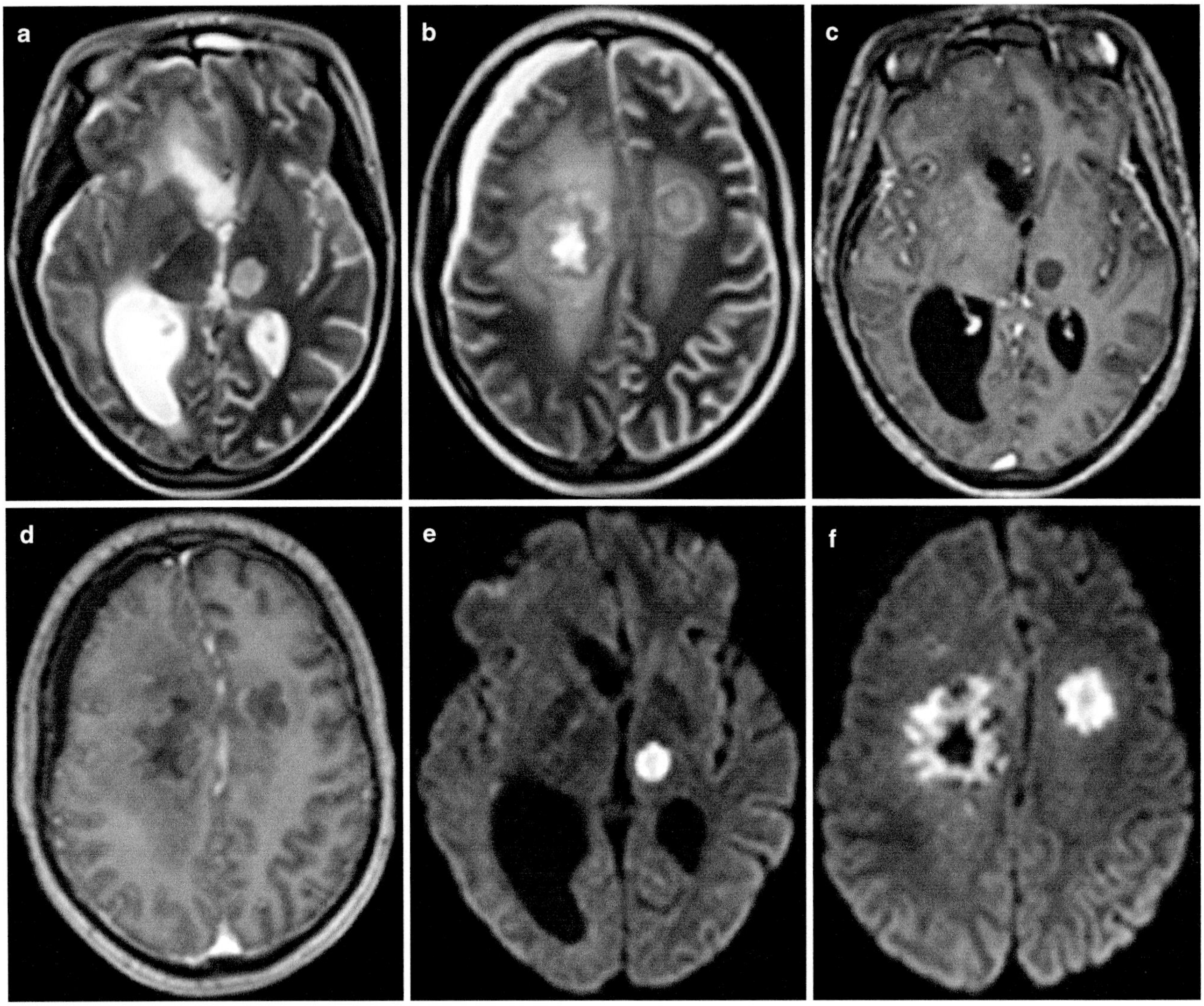

Fig. 13.9 *Aspergillus* meningitis. A 14-year-old female with intraparenchymal aspergillus with lesions involving the left thalamus, and right and left frontal centrum semiovale with extensive surrounding edema on axial T2 (**a**, **b**), mild ring enhancement on axial T1 post-contrast (**c**, **d**) and restricted diffusion on DWI (**e**, **f**)

basal ganglia and thalami when seeking an etiology for an infection should raise suspicion for *Aspergillus* as a potential cause. FLAIR is especially sensitive for detecting subtle lesions with meningeal involvement. Unlike pyogenic and tuberculous abscesses, aspergillus abscesses did not have central restricted diffusion, which could be a differentiating factor, leading to a timely diagnosis. Antifungals are the main treatment option for aspergillus, although prognosis is often poor with an 88% fatality rate [20].

13.2.4.2 *Candida*

Candida is a diploid fungus and type of yeast that is also endemic and opportunistic. In low birth weight neonates, it has been shown to cause disseminated CNS infection in up to 5% of cases. Similar to *Aspergillus*, *Candida* is also seen in immunocompromised hosts such as patients with HIV or post-surgery, most commonly spreading through hematogenous means. *Candida* has been implicated in superimposed infections after VP shunt or ventriculostomy placement.

Clinical Manifestation

Candida has a variety of presentations and is an infection that often disseminates. Meningitis is the most common presentation of *Candida* presenting with fevers, lethargy, altered mental status, and seizures as frequent signs and symptoms. In immunocompromised hosts, symptoms of increased intracranial pressure can be evident resulting in seizures, focal deficits, and headaches. Similar to *Aspergillus*, *Candida* can also progress to abscess formation.

Imaging

Neurocandidiasis can vary in imaging manifestations and is not well defined in the current literature. CT is normal in most cases. MRI often shows diffuse parenchymal lesions in both the supra- and infratentorial brain parenchyma with possible involvement of the ventricles. In the supratentorial brain, involvement of the basal ganglia and cortex is most characteristic. These lesions often show T1 hyperintensity secondary to microhemorrhage and can also show restriction diffusion. In contrast to *Aspergillus*, neurocandidiasis tends to form micro-abscesses. These can exhibit a similar ring enhancement depending on the patient's immune response. Timely diagnosis and treatment is essential as the mortality for neurocandidiasis ranges between 10% and 30% [21].

13.2.4.3 *Cryptococcus*

Cryptococcus is the most common CNS fungal infection. It is an encapsulated yeast which spreads via inhalation and can be found in bird droppings in the soil. Similar to *Aspergillus*, *Cryptococcus* is more frequently seen in the immunocompromised population, especially those with HIV, diabetes, organ failure, and posttransplantation [1]. *Cryptococcus* still causes significant morbidity and mortality with 1 million new cases and 625,000 deaths yearly [1].

Clinical Manifestation

Cryptococcus spreads through inhalation and eventually through hematogenous means to enter the CNS. Once it disseminates into the CNS, it causes a granulomatous response leading to meningitis, seizures, headaches, blurry vision, and cranial nerve palsies. In more severe cases, it can lead to vasculopathic symptoms and acute infarctions. A distinguishing feature of *Cryptococcus* is the resultant hydrocephalus, which is secondary to the increased intracranial pressure. *Cryptococcus* has a predilection for spreading through the perivascular spaces and into the basal ganglia where it forms cryptococcomas and gelatinous pseudocysts, which have a characteristic soap bubble appearance on pathology.

Imaging

CT and MRI are the mainstays for suspected CNS cryptococcal infection. CT, however, is unreliable as prior studies have shown a normal appearance in up to 43% of cases. The most common CT manifestation of *Cryptococcus* is nonspecific hydrocephalus, which is seen in up to 10% of the cases [22]. MRI is a more reliable modality for diagnosing cryptococcal disease. Leptomeningeal enhancement in the setting of meningitis is a common MRI manifestation of the infection. Cryptococcomas are rare intraparenchymal lesions that typically demonstrate low T1 and high T2 signal with variable enhancement and can been seen in the thalami, basal ganglia, and cerebellum. Corresponding lesions on CT are often hypodense [20] (Fig. 13.10). Gelatinous pseudocysts are most often seen in dilated perivascular spaces and the basal ganglia. They appear intermediate, unlike cryptococcomas, on T1 due to its mucin content and high on T2. Most commonly, dilated perivascular spaces with hydrocephalus in an immunocompromised patient should raise concern for cryptococcal disease. Similar to *Aspergillus*, antifungals are the mainstay of treatment. If left untreated, the infection is often fatal [20].

13.2.5 Human Immunodeficiency Virus

Human immunodeficiency virus (HIV) and its most severe form, acquired immunodeficiency syndrome (AIDS), affect

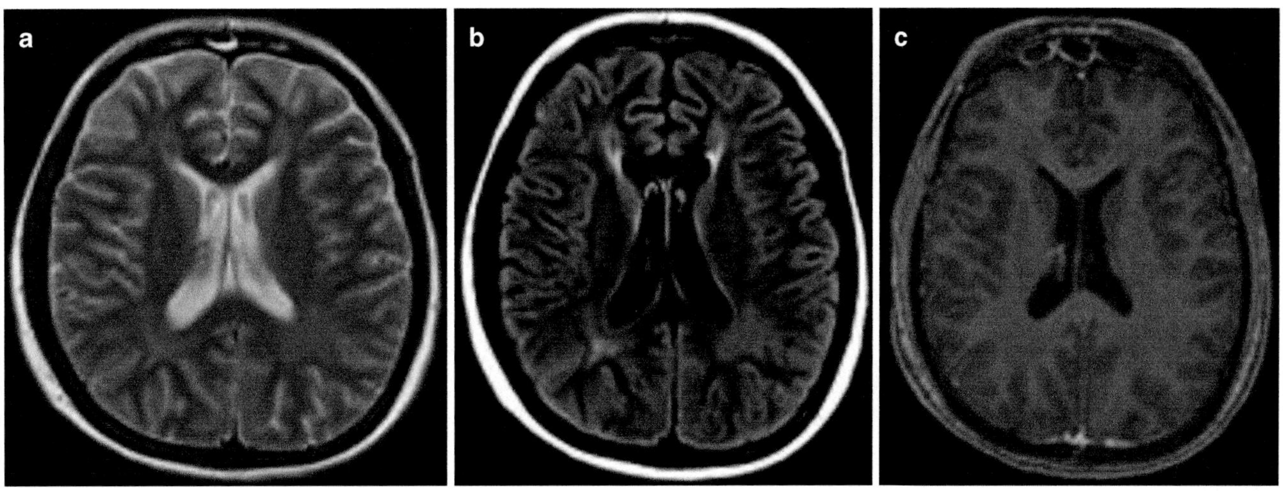

Fig. 13.10 Cryptococcal meningitis. A 16-year-old male with acute lymphocytic leukemia and cryptococcal meningitis showing mild ventricular enlargement with nonspecific increase T2 and FLAIR and mild decrease T1 signal involving the deep white matter of the corona radiate and centrum semiovale of both cerebral hemispheres (**a**, **b**). No enhancing lesion is observed (**c**)

over three million children worldwide and are a significant cause of morbidity and mortality. HIV is a retrovirus that can cross the blood-brain barrier and has a predilection for infecting monocytes, macrophages, oligodendrocytes, and astrocytes leading to impaired function and growth. The progression of HIV differs in children compared to adults where the retrovirus' invasion of the macrophages and astrocytes leads to neuronal loss and eventually brain growth restriction in children [1]. Approximately 60% of children infected with HIV will have neurological manifestations with up to 20% demonstrating CNS symptoms as the first marker of the infection [20]. The virus can lead to impaired immune function directly or indirectly through immunosuppression, leading to a number of potential superimposed infectious processes. CD4 count has been the gold standard for assessing the potential of superinfections in an HIV patient. This review will focus on HIV encephalopathy (HIVE), progressive multifocal leukoencephalopathy (PML), and immune reconstitution inflammatory syndrome (IRIS). More common infections that are intimately associated with HIV are reviewed in other sections of this chapter including TORCH, tuberculosis, and fungal infections. Please refer to those sections for a more detailed review.

13.2.5.1 HIV Encephalopathy

HIV encephalopathy (HIVE) occurs with early CNS infection of the developing pediatric brain caused by the HIV retrovirus. It is the most common primary HIV CNS complication and can be seen in up to 60% of pediatric cases [23]. It is classified based on at least two of the following three criteria as per the Center for Disease Control and Prevention guidelines: failure to achieve normal milestones with loss of intellectual abilities, acquired asymmetric motor deficits, and acquired microcephaly. Multinucleated giant cells, microglial nodules, reactive gliosis, and myelin loss are commonly seen on pathology [24].

Clinical Manifestation

The diagnosis of HIVE includes the loss of intellectual ability specifically impaired early motor and language skills, memory, visual-spatial synthesis, and generalized executive function [23]. Asymmetric motor deficits with loss of muscle tone and deep tendon reflexes as well as impaired coordination are observed.

Imaging

HIVE causes a number of early imaging manifestations. Global cerebral atrophy out of proportion for age in conjunction with basal ganglia calcifications is most characteristic [20] along with symmetric non-enhancing hypodensities within the periventricular and subcortical white matter which do not cause mass effect are commonly seen on CT. Characteristic MRI features include confluent low T1 and high T2 signal within the periventricular and subcortical white matter. These lesions tend to spare the subcortical U-fibers and typically do not enhance, cause mass effect, or restrict (Fig. 13.11). There is a stronger predilection for symmetric frontal lobe atrophy in the setting of global atrophy with possible involvement of the genu of the corpus callosum seen on MRI. Early highly active antiretroviral therapy (HAART) has shown to demonstrate improvement in these areas of MR signal abnormalities up to sevenfold in certain studies [20].

13.2.5.2 Progressive Multifocal Leukoencephalopathy

Progressive multifocal leukoencephalopathy (PML) is a superimposed viral infection seen in HIV that can cause serious neurological complications. It is caused by the JC virus, a papovavirus which infects myelin-producing oligodendrocytes. It is a demyelinating disease of the central nervous system whose only known reservoir is humans. Fewer than 30 cases have been reported in infected and non-infected children and have rarely been reported in immunocompromised pediatric patients infected with HIV. Due to its multifocal nature, it is thought to spread hematogenously with the pathological triad of hyperchromatic oligodendrocytic nuclei, lobulated astrocytes, and multifocal demyelination [25] and will manifest when the CD4 count drops below 100 [20].

Clinical Manifestation

PML has a nonspecific constellation of symptoms. It frequently spares the optic nerves and spinal cord with most signs and symptoms confined to the supratentorial brain. Cognitive abnormalities are seen in at least one third of patients. Nonspecific signs and symptoms such as language impairment, visual deficits, sensory loss, seizures, headaches, and gait abnormalities are possible. In advanced cases, multiple motor deficits have been reported.

Imaging

On CT, multifocal hypodensities scattered throughout the periventricular and subcortical white matter are common. These lesions are asymmetric in contradistinction to HIVE. On MRI, these lesions appear as low T1 and high T2 areas of abnormal signal predominantly centered within the periventricular and subcortical white matter. Unlike HIVE, these are asymmetric, involving the subcortical U-fibers and sometimes even the cortex itself. In contrast to HIVE, there may be mild mass effect with hemorrhage rarely seen. They rarely enhance, do not restrict, and, like HIVE, may also involve the corpus callosum [1, 20]. If enhancement is present, it is often faint and only seen in the periphery of these lesions [20]. Of note, studies have shown that enhancement is associated with improved survival. Although PML lesions

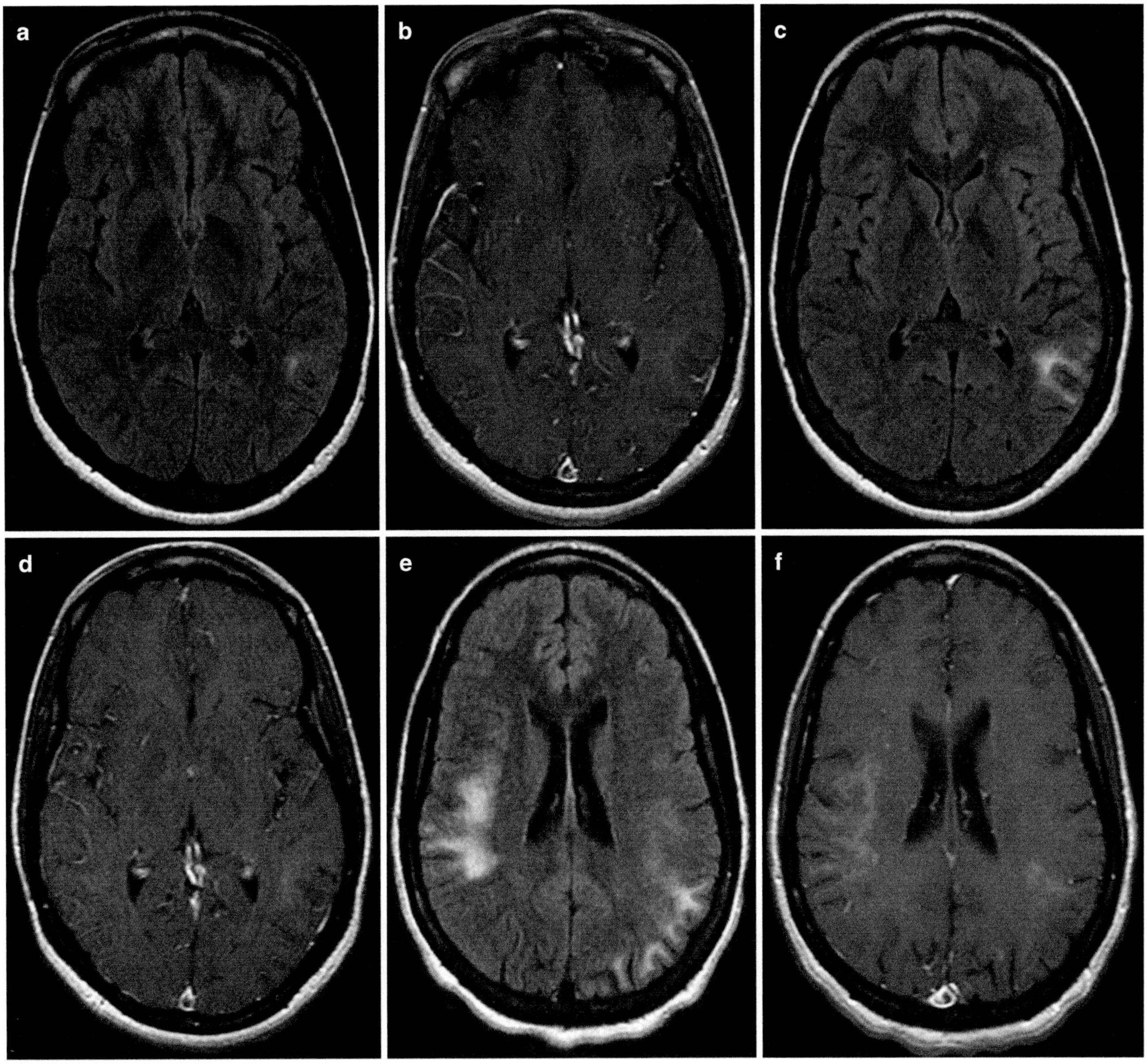

Fig. 13.11 HIV encephalitis. A 17 years youth with initial FLAIR signal abnormality in the left posterior temporal subcortical white matter (**a**) with associated subtle enhancement within the adjacent white matter (**b**). Subsequent mid follow-up images show progressive worsening (**c**, **d**) with further progression and worsening in the left posterior temporal, left occipital, and new involvement in the right temporal regions on late images (**e**) and associated mild progressive enhancement in the later stages (**f**). The findings are consistent with HIV encephalitis with progressive multifocal leukoencephalopathy (PML)

do not restrict, studies have shown that low signal on ADC can be a potential marker of positive treatment response when on HAART therapy. MR spectroscopy can also play a potential role, showing reduced NAA and increased lactate, choline, and lipids as seen in necrosis and neuronal impairment [20].

13.2.5.3 Immune Reconstitution Inflammatory Syndrome (IRIS)

With the advancements in the utilization of the HAART therapy, HIV has become a manageable disease even in the pediatric population by restoring some of the patient's intrinsic immunity. Some patients, however, have an abnormal immune response leading to clinical deterioration, referred to as immune reconstitution inflammatory syndrome (IRIS). IRIS is a T-cell-mediated response after antiretroviral therapy (ART) where there is partial recovery of the immune system or an exuberant immunological response to antigenic stimuli. Patients affected will undergo paradoxical clinical deterioration despite an increase in CD4 and decrease viral load after ART [26]. The pathogens most frequently encountered are mycobacterium tuberculosis (TB), varicella zoster, herpes virus, and cytomegalovirus. The incidence of IRIS is about 10–20% with mycobacteria considered the most common offending agent as it is seen in up to 38% of cases in children, where it is then labeled paradoxical (TB-IRIS) TB-IRIS [27]. A subgroup of IRIS that can also be seen where there is a subclinical infection that reactivates after restoration of immunity is referred to as "unmasking" IRIS. Studies by Puthanakit demonstrated an incidence on up to 19% in Thai children who developed unmasking IRIS after undergoing 4 weeks of HAART therapy. The mortality in children is highest during the first 6 months of HAART treatment reaching a fatality rate of up to 90%.

Clinical Manifestation

IRIS can present clinically in a number of ways depending on the cause. TB-IRIS has a number of major and minor criteria for assessment. Some major criteria include enlarging lymph nodes, radiologically worsened TB disease, meningitis, encephalitis or focal deficits, pleural effusions, ascites, conjunctivitis, and erythema. Meningitis is the most common CNS manifestation of TB-IRIS. A few minor criteria include nonspecific symptoms such as night sweats, fevers, cough, and abdominal pain. Additional causes of IRIS include *Cryptococcus*, CMV, Kaposi sarcoma, and PML.

Imaging

CT and MRI findings in IRIS are mostly dependent on the etiology and tend to follow similar nonspecific radiological signs and features that can commonly be seen with other etiologies. Irrespective of the etiologies, generalized IRIS of the CNS has some characteristic features. These include high FLAIR signal within scattered parenchymal lesions, which also show enhancement and restricted diffusion. Additionally, leptomeningeal enhancement is often seen in conjunction with the parenchymal lesions. These are thought to be due to the fulminant inflammatory response from the restored CD4 count [28]. TB-IRIS, the most common form of CNS IRIS, often demonstrates ring-enhancing intraparenchymal lesions with regional edema. There is also associated ependymal enhancement of the ventricular system [28].

13.3 Other Pediatric CNS Infections

13.3.1 Rasmussen Encephalitis

Rasmussen encephalitis is a rare, progressive pediatric disorder characterized by intractable seizures and multifocal neurologic deterioration. Approximately 85% of cases occur in children under the age of 10 years. Its hallmark is chronic progressive inflammation of one of the cerebral hemispheres resulting in unilateral cortical atrophy. The etiology is unclear, although existing data suggests an immune-mediated response. Diagnosis is reliant upon clinical evaluation, EEG findings, and morphologic examination via neuroimaging or histopathology.

Clinical Presentation

Rasmussen encephalitis has been described as a syndrome with prodromal, acute, and residual stages. The prodromal stage is characterized by nonspecific findings which include relatively low seizure occurrence and seldom mild hemiparesis, with a median duration of about 7 months. Subsequently the acute stage, with a median duration of 8 months, is characterized by high-frequency drug-resistant polymorphic seizures and multifocal central nervous system dysfunction including hemiparesis, cognitive impairment, hemianopsia, and possibly aphasia. This is followed by the residual stage with permanent neurologic dysfunction with development of a fixed hemiplegia and persistent, relatively less frequent, seizures. The most common form of seizure is epilepsia partialis continua seen in about 56–92% of cases. Diagnosis is essential in the early stages of the syndrome with hemispherectomy as the preferred treatment preventing progressive neurologic deterioration and inflammatory spread and ultimate death.

Imaging

Magnetic resonance imaging (MRI) findings are vital to the diagnosis of the childhood infection based on formal criteria. The most common finding is unilateral cortical atrophy with a predilection for the insular and peri-insular regions. Additional findings include cortical swelling, increased white and gray matter signal on T2-weighted and fluid-attenuated inversion recovery sequences, and unilateral atrophy of the head of the caudate nucleus. There is associated ex vacuo dilatation of the lateral ventricle on the affected cerebral hemisphere (Fig. 13.12). The various stages of Rasmussen encephalitis can be seen: grade 1 (cortical swelling, increased T2 signal), grade 2 (normal parenchymal volume, increased T2 signal), grade 3 (cortical atrophy, increased T2 signal), and grade 4 (progressive atrophy, normal T2 signal).

Increased restricted diffusion in the corresponding affected regions has also been reported. Interictal MR/FDG-PET fusion imaging can aid in localizing regions of hypometabolic activity not seen on standard MR sequencing. Proton MR spectroscopy can show reduced N-acetylaspartate (NAA) levels and increased choline (Cho) peaks resulting in a decreased NAA/Cho ratio from neurologic loss or dysfunction in the affected regions and can be used as an adjunct in making the diagnosis.

13.3.2 Acute Disseminated Encephalomyelitis

Acute disseminated encephalomyelitis (ADEM) is an acute monophasic autoimmune demyelinating disorder of the cen-

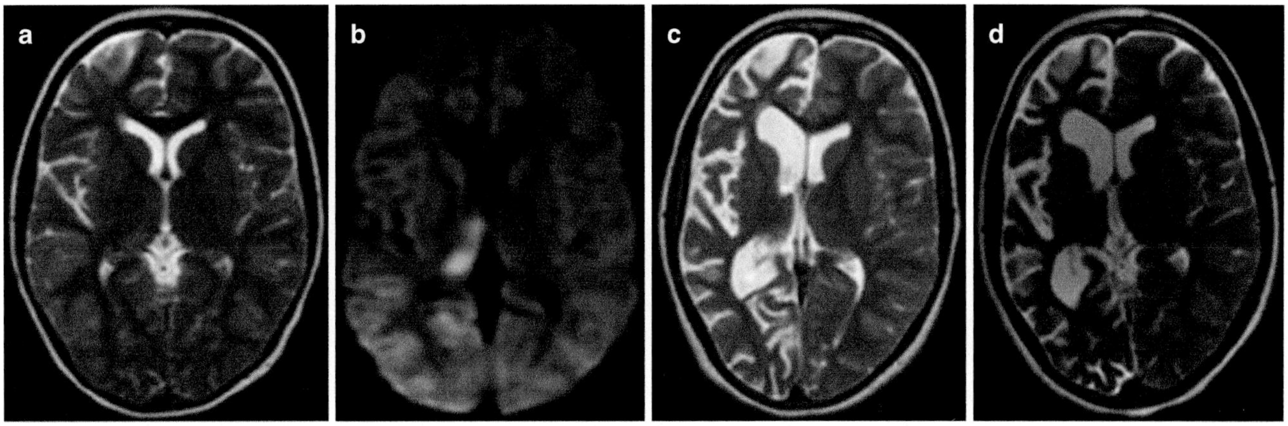

Fig. 13.12 Rasmussen encephalitis. A 7-year-old female initial Ax T2 shows increase signal with cortical swelling involving the right thalamus and right posterior temporal and occipital regions with mild asymmetric prominence of the cortical sulci of the right frontal and anterior temporal regions when compared to the left (**a**). DWI shows corresponding areas of diffusion restriction in the right thalamus and right posterior temporal and occipital regions (**b**). Follow-up imaging axial T2 at 9 years and 10 years shows progressive increase in sulcal prominence of the right cerebral hemisphere (**c**, **d**)

tral nervous system most commonly followed by an infection accounting for patients, less commonly post-vaccination with an incidence of less than 5% with rare incidence of being idiopathic. The disease is thought to be related to an autoimmune reaction to myelin, with peak incidence in children 3–10 years of age. The disorder is characterized by widespread multifocal neurologic signs and imaging findings. Thus, diagnosis is difficult to distinguish initially due to its clinical and imaging manifestations overlapping those of multiple sclerosis. A prior report delineated the two separate disorders if two of the following three criteria are satisfied: (1) clinical symptoms atypical for MS, including one or more of the following: consciousness alteration, hypersomnia, seizures, cognitive impairment, hemiplegia, tetraplegia, aphasia, or bilateral optic neuritis; (2) absence of oligoclonal bands in cerebrospinal fluid analysis; and (3) gray matter involvement such as basal ganglia or cortical lesions. Initial diagnosis is vital due to the favorable outcome seen in ADEM patients.

Clinical Presentation

Fever, headache, vomiting, and meningeal signs are initial prodromal signs and symptoms. Neurologic symptoms of ADEM will be seen approximately 4–13 days following the infection or vaccination, with progression of initial neurologic findings seen within 4–7 days. Acute encephalopathy is a common symptom ranging from lethargy to coma. Additional neurologic features of the disease include pyramidal tract signs, acute hemiparesis, cerebellar ataxia, cranial neuropathies including optic neuritis, and spinal cord dysfunction including transverse myelitis. These neurologic features can last from 2 to 4 weeks, and patients will typically make a complete recovery with no significant long-term sequela. An accurate diagnosis of ADEM is reliant on clinical evaluation and neuroimaging correlation and follow-up.

Imaging

CT plays a limited role as normal findings are generally seen at initial presentation. After 5–14 days following initial presentation, nonspecific multifocal areas of hypoattenuation in the subcortical white matter can be seen. Thus, MRI is the neuroimaging modality of choice for initial diagnosis and subsequent follow-up imaging of ADEM due to its ability to better visualize demyelinating lesions.

The MRI appearance in ADEM is quite variable. A common finding is patchy foci of increased signal on T2-weighted and fluid-attenuated inversion recovery sequences with or without post-contrast enhancement (Fig. 13.13). The most common presentation is multiple large, asymmetric lesions bilaterally although confluent symmetric lesions bilaterally or multiple unilateral lesions have also been visualized. There is a predilection to involve the subcortical and deep white matter in the parieto-occipital, and centrum semiovale with gray matter structures is also affected including the basal ganglia, thalami, and cerebral and cerebellar cortices. Involvement of the brainstem and spinal cord is also commonly seen. Spinal cord lesions are typically intramedullary extending over multiple vertebral segments with an isolated spinal lesion considered rare.

There is a dramatic regression in the number, size, and signal intensity of lesions on subsequent MRI related to treatment (corticosteroids, intravenous immunoglobulins, or plasmapheresis) with resultant improved clinical course. Therefore, prolonged MRI follow-up is considered helpful in separating ADEM from other distinct entities such as multiphasic disseminated encephalomyelitis or multiple sclerosis.

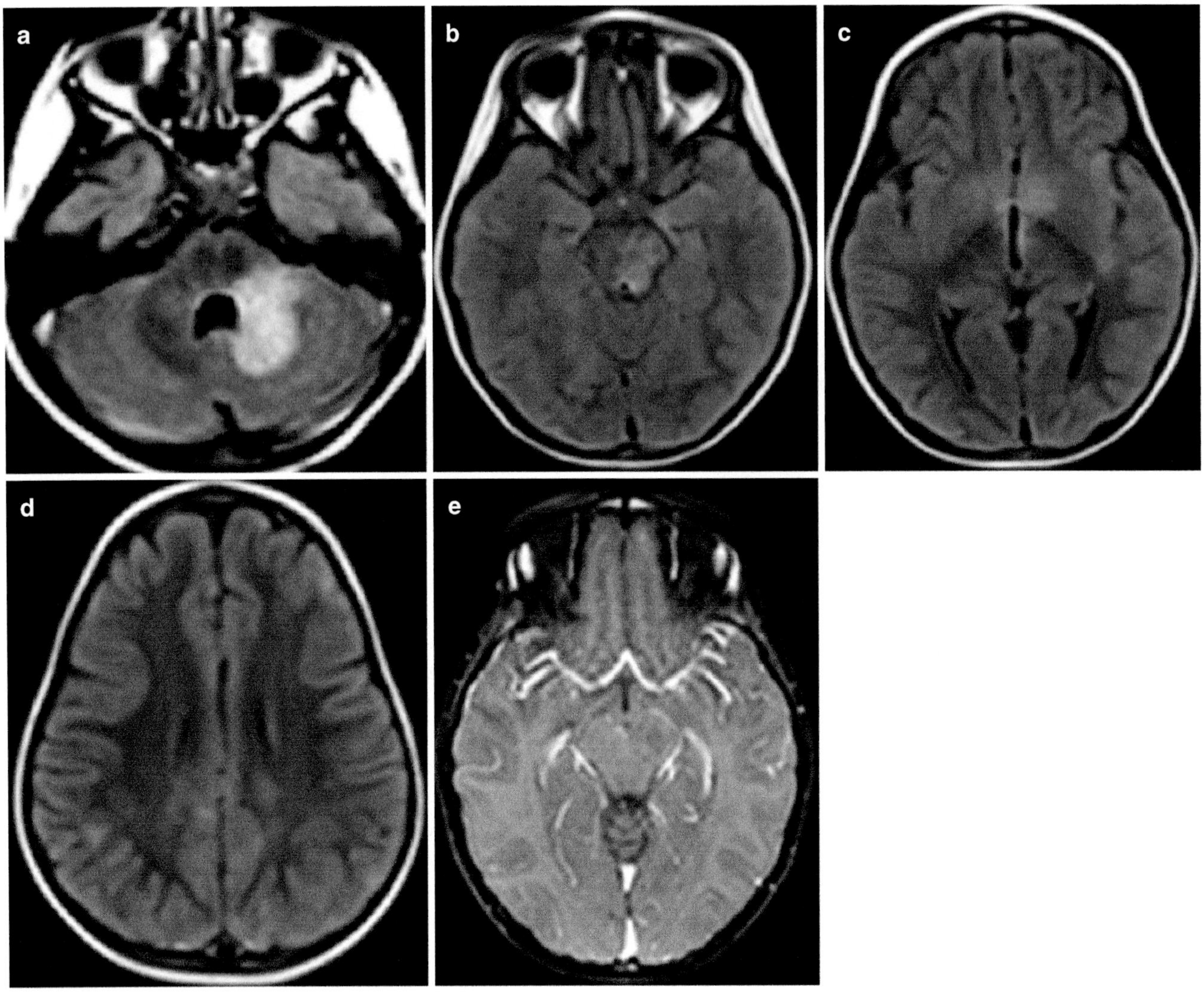

Fig. 13.13 Acute disseminated encephalomyelitis. A 4-year-old child after a 3-week history of viral illness presents with multiple foci of abnormal increase FLAIR signal abnormalities in left dentate nucleus, left middle cerebellar peduncle, and left midbrain with supratentorial lesions in the left anterior commissure and right parietal subcortical white matter and left posterior parietal centrum semiovale (**a**–**d**) with no associated enhancement noted on axial T1 post-contrast images (**e**)

13.4 Neonatal Infections

13.4.1 Cytomegalovirus

Cytomegalovirus (CMV) infection is the most common intrauterine infection in the United States and is the leading cause of congenital infections. CMV is a member of the herpes virus family and results in congenital infection via transplacental transmission in pregnant women experiencing primary or recurrent infections, with roughly 40% of mothers transmitting the virus to the fetus after acquiring primary infection during pregnancy [29–31]. Maternal risk factors for delivery of an infected neonate include close contact with young children, young maternal age, and having multiple sexual partners. Infections can also occur postnatally via transmission through breast milk or blood products; however, these patients typically have a benign clinical course. The incidence of infection is estimated to be approximately 1% of all neonates [29, 31], and 5–10% of these patients will exhibit signs or symptoms indicative of congenital CMV infection [1]. Diagnosis is made via polymerase chain reaction analysis of the newborn's urine, saliva, or blood for the presence of CMV DNA [29].

Clinical Presentation

Most infants who are infected with CMV are asymptomatic. Approximately 5–10% of neonates with congenital CMV infection demonstrate systemic and CNS involvement, with signs and symptoms including microcephaly, hepatosplenomegaly, jaundice, petechiae, chorioretinitis, seizures, neurodevelopmental delay, and sensorineural hearing loss [1, 10, 32]. Sensorineural hearing loss is the most common nongenetic cause of childhood hearing loss seen in 10–15% of patients following congenital infection, and prompt diagnosis is vital to minimize this incidence of loss of hearing. Prognosis is variable depending on the extent of CNS and systemic manifestations.

Imaging

Cranial ultrasonography (US), computed tomography (CT), and magnetic resonance imaging (MRI) are common imaging modalities utilized to help confirm and characterize neonatal CMV infection. Intracranial calcifications are the most common imaging finding reportedly occurring in 34–70% of patients [33]. Calcifications are typically coarse and bulky along the periventricular regions on CT and are seen as hyperechoic foci with or without posterior acoustic shadowing on US. MRI will demonstrate decreased periventricular signal on T2-weighted gradient echo sequences compatible with abnormal susceptibility due to calcifications. Although common, calcifications are not always present and should not exclude a diagnosis of CMV infection.

The most common imaging finding following intracranial calcifications is ventriculomegaly, a nonspecific finding that has been implicated with CMV infection in up to 45% of patients [34, 35]. Ventricular septations or adhesions may be seen in patients as thin strands of tissues crossing ventricles on all modalities.

MRI is the imaging modality of choice and the most common modality in assessing the abnormalities of the brain. White matter disease is seen in up to 22% of patients [34] typically involving the posterior white matter, parietal region, and frontal region or in a random distribution [33]. This will be characterized as focal, patchy, or confluent hypoattenuating areas on CT and hyperintense areas on MR T2-weighted FLAIR sequences relative to the adjacent normal myelinated white matter (Fig. 13.14). Periventricular cysts can be demonstrated in infected patients, with anterior temporal cysts and associated white matter disease somewhat indicative for CMV [34]. Cerebral and cerebellar atrophy can be evident as generalized parenchymal volume loss, ventriculomegaly, and microcephaly, with microcephaly seen in as many as 27% of patients, correlating with poorer outcomes [33, 36].

The gestational age at the time of CMV infection tends to manifest with certain pattern of CNS imaging findings. Fetuses with early CMV infection, occurring before 18 weeks of gestation, generally have a more severe clinical course than those infected at a later gestational age. A variety of migrational abnormalities have been demonstrated in up to 10% of patients with CMV infections [34]. These include most commonly lissencephaly, pachygyria, cerebellar atrophy, and ventriculomegaly with delayed myelination and intracranial calcifications sometimes seen [33] primarily affected early in gestation. Infants infected at a gestational age of 18–24 weeks are associated with more focal migrational abnormalities, including polymicrogyria and schizencephalic clefts as well as cerebellar atrophy [33]. Ventriculomegaly can be seen, although to a lesser degree compared to early CMV infections. Fetuses affected in the third trimester result in delayed or disturbed myelination, white matter disease, intracranial calcifications, and periventricular cysts [33].

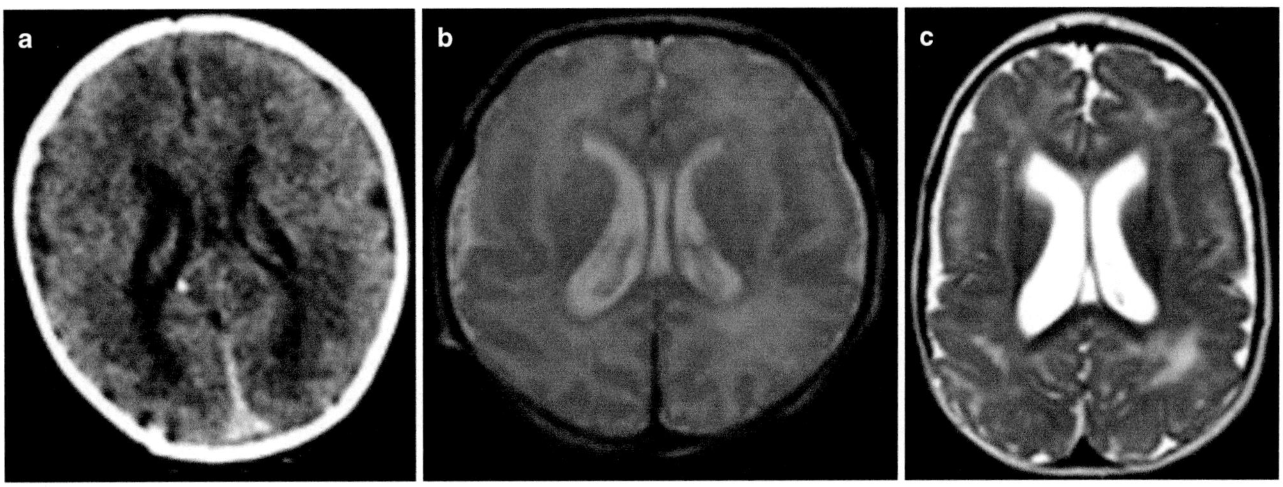

Fig. 13.14 CMV. A 4-day-old newborn axial CT image with focus of calcification along the splenium of the corpus callosum on the right (**a**). MRI at 7 days shows prominent gyral pattern with areas of cortical thickening throughout the frontal and temporal regions bilaterally (**b**). Axial T2 at 7 months of age better defines these areas of cortical thickening in the bilateral frontal and temporal regions with some areas showing poorly defined gray-white differentiation (**c**). Note, the prominent gyral pattern is not as well defined at 7 days compared to 7 months due to incomplete myelination

13.4.2 Toxoplasmosis

Congenital toxoplasmosis is the second most common intrauterine infection following cytomegalovirus infection [1]. *Toxoplasma gondii* is an intracellular protozoan parasite transmitted via transplacental transmission in pregnant women who have been exposed to viable *Toxoplasma gondii* or its infectious oocytes predominantly by ingestion of inadequately cooked meat or feline exposure resulting in a congenital infection. It has therefore been hypothesized that cases of congenital toxoplasmosis can be limited by avoidance of cats and undercooked food during pregnancy. The overall risk of transmission in treated pregnant women is approximately 30% [37]. The incidence of infection varies, with rates ranging from less than 0.1 per 1000 live births in many regions to 1 per 1000 live births in highly endemic regions [1]. Diagnosis can be achieved prenatally or postnatally, with diagnostic tests including polymerase chain reaction analysis of amniotic fluid for the presence of toxoplasmosis DNA prenatally and the presence of toxoplasma-specific humoral antibodies in patient's bodily fluids postnatally [37].

Clinical Presentation

The clinical spectrum of congenital toxoplasmosis infection ranges from asymptomatic patients to neurologic and ocular sequelae to more systemic involvement and possibly even death. Many cases of neonatal congenital toxoplasmosis demonstrate no obvious abnormalities, initially with symptoms presenting 2–3 months following birth [38, 39]. Symptomatic infants can exhibit generalized findings of anemia or lymphadenopathy to a more severe clinical course including mental retardation, blindness, hearing loss, and epilepsy [40, 41]. Jaundice and hepatosplenomegaly has been reported in up to 70% of patients with toxoplasmosis [42] and purpuric or petechial rash in approximately 20–25% of patients [1]. Scarring from chorioretinitis occurs in 75% of patients and sensorineural hearing loss and can develop in untreated cases [1]. Similar to congenital cytomegalovirus, the timing of infection during gestation correlates with severity of disease as earlier infections are associated with poorer outcomes in comparison to later infections [43].

Imaging

Cranial ultrasonography (US), computed tomography (CT), and magnetic resonance imaging (MRI) are the useful modalities to evaluate congenital toxoplasmosis. Findings overall are nonspecific, however are suggestive but not diagnostic for toxoplasmosis infection. US can demonstrate diffuse periventricular hyperechogenicities, subtle intracranial calcifications with or without shadowing, and ventriculomegaly [1 44]. CT and MR images can confirm the presence of intracranial calcifications with CT revealing hyperattenuating structures in a periventricular or scattered intraparenchymal distribution and MR showing decreased signal on T2-weighted gradient echo sequences in a similar distribution. CT and MRI can also demonstrate the presence of passive ventriculomegaly or macrocephaly possibly due to hydrocephalus [1] (Fig. 13.15).

13.4.3 Herpes Simplex Virus

Herpes simplex virus (HSV) is a common cause of devastating encephalitis with significant morbidity and mortality in the United States and other developed regions. The

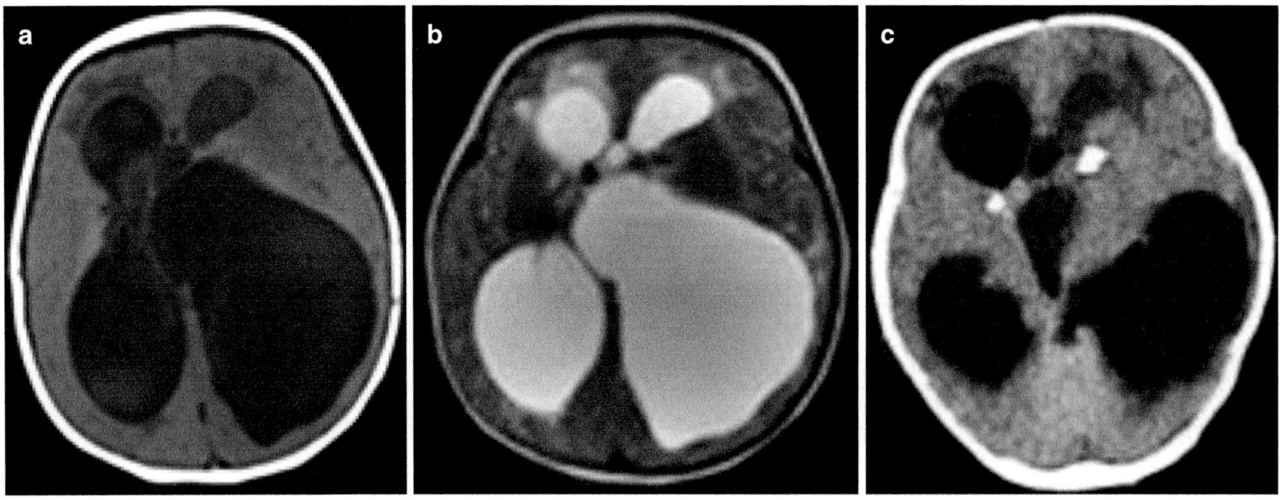

Fig. 13.15 A 4-month-old infant with congenital toxoplasmosis. Images show hydrocephalus with abnormal signal in frontal white matter surrounding the enlarged right frontal horn seen on axial T1 and T2 images despite immature myelinated brain parenchyma (**a**, **b**). Axial CT shows prominent coarse calcifications along the foramen of Monroe and medial basal ganglia (**c**)

age of presentation divides herpes encephalitis into two separate groups, neonatal and children and adults [45], with HSV type 2 typically linked with neonatal infection and HSV type 1 associated with sporadic encephalitis in children and adults. The non-neonatal form of HSV encephalitis caused by HSV type 1 is discussed in the viral encephalitis section of this chapter. Infected mothers with HSV type 2, either thru primary infection or secondary reactivation of latent virus, will typically vertically transmit the infection to neonates during vaginal delivery via asymptomatic cervical shedding of the virus although in utero or postnatal infection can occur [46]. The incidence of infection has been reported to be approximately 1 per 3000–20,000 live births, although only 5–10% of these represent congenital infection. Rapid diagnosis by HSV culture or PCR of CSF/vesicle fluids is essential to prevent significant associated morbidity and mortality, with 15% mortality rate in patients with HSV encephalitis and 57% in patients with disseminated disease [46].

Clinical Presentation

In utero infection results in prematurity and low birth weight, while infants with peripartum infection typically present in the first to third weeks of life [47, 48]. A variety of clinical presentations have been implicated with neonatal HSV infection, ranging from nonspecific signs and symptoms such as irritability, lethargy, fever, and poor feeding to disseminated infection involving multiple sites including the skin, eye, mouth, and central nervous system [46]. Delayed diagnosis results in significant morbidity and mortality and should be suspected in any patient with irritability, lethargy, fever, and poor feeding at 1 week of age. Patients who survive herpes encephalitis or disseminated disease have long-term sequelae which include seizures, psychomotor retardation, blindness, and learning disabilities [46].

Imaging

Computed tomography (CT) and magnetic resonance imaging (MRI) are the imaging modalities of choice for evaluating neonatal HSV encephalitis. In contrast to sporadic encephalitis seen in children and adults having a predilection for temporal lobe involvement, neonatal HSV presents with more widespread abnormalities [49]. CT can demonstrate normal findings or variable distribution of hypoattenuating areas [50]. Calcifications, if present, have a distinct penchant for the basal ganglia and thalamus in congenital HSV encephalitis [51].

MRI is the preferred modality to evaluate the extent of disease. Spectrum of disease can be visualized, ranging from normal appearance to extensive signal abnormalities with diffuse scattered regions of decreased T1 signal and increased T2 signal although particular involvement of the periventricular white matter with sparing of the medial temporal lobes and inferior frontal lobes has been described [52]. Post-contrast sequences can demonstrate heterogeneous enhancement in the involved regions with occasional leptomeningeal enhancement. DWI will reveal restricted diffusion in affected regions that may not been seen on conventional sequences, especially in early infection [53], reinforcing the value of obtaining DWI sequences for assessing HSV encephalitis (Fig. 13.16).

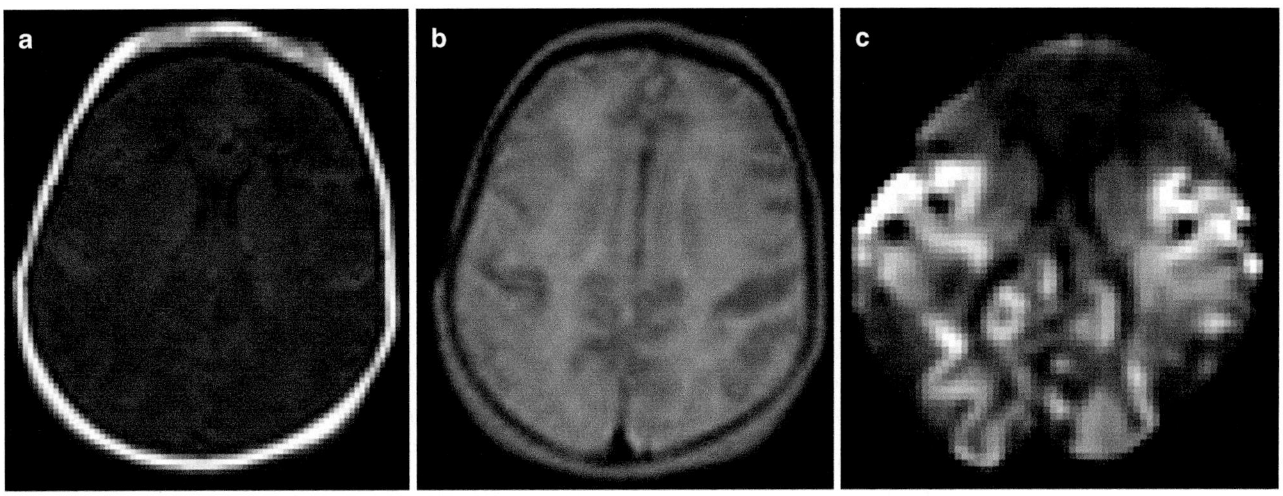

Fig. 13.16 Neonatal form of HSV encephalitis. A 23-day-old infant with diffuse cerebral edema and loss of gray-white differentiation of both cerebral hemispheres on axial T1 and T2 images (**a**, **b**) with areas of diffusion restriction (**c**) consistent with ischemia. Follow-up imaging at 4 weeks shows diffuse heterogeneous signal throughout both cerebral hemispheres consistent with evolving encephalomalacia on axial T1 and T2 images (**d**, **e**) with a focus T1 shortening and abnormal susceptibility in the right thalamus (**d**, **f**) consistent with parenchymal hemorrhage

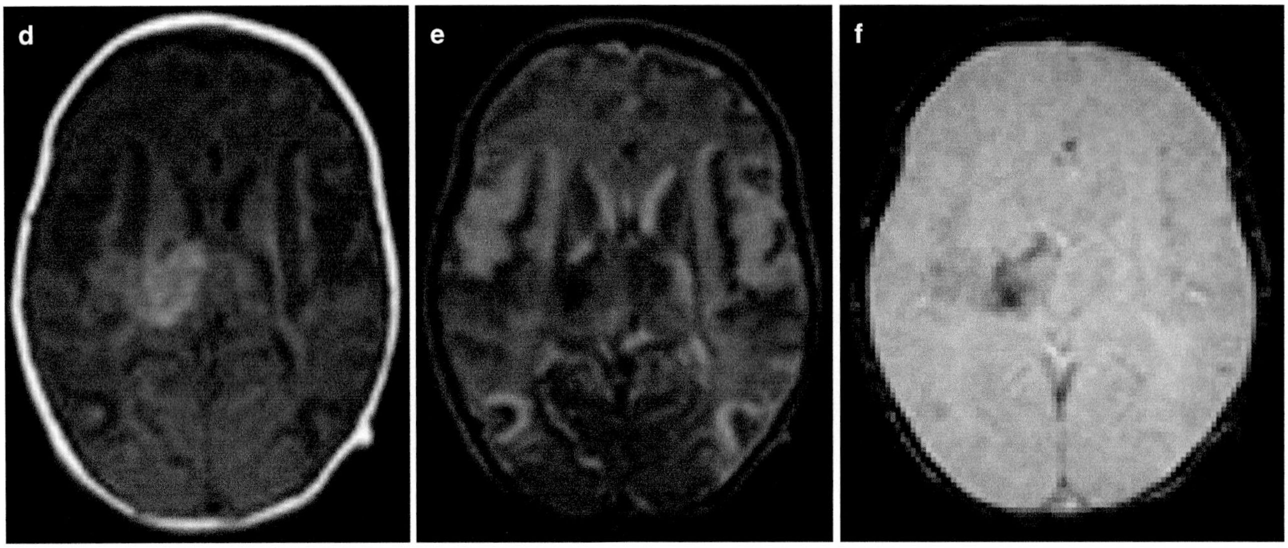

Fig. 13.16 (continued)

13.4.4 Syphilis

Congenital syphilis is caused by the spirochete *Treponema pallidum* and is a potential cause of multisystem infection. The fetus is infected via the placenta typically during the second and third trimester, with the overall transplacental infection risk reported to range from 25% to 80% in untreated mothers. Untreated mothers are also at increased risk for a stillborn fetus or neonatal death [47, 48]. Those infected neonates that survive will display signs and symptoms of congenital syphilis 2–16% of the time. Diagnosis is typically clinical and confirmed with VDRL serology testing.

Clinical Presentation

Many infants will be asymptomatic and remain clinically silent for their life with signs and symptoms of infection divided into early congenital manifestations and late congenital manifestations. Early manifestations, occurring less than 2 years of age, include rash, hepatosplenomegaly, jaundice, and generalized lymphadenopathy [1]. Late manifestations, occurring older than 2 years of age, include saber shins, saddlenose deformity, mulberry molars, frontal bossing, rhagades (perioral fissures), and the Hutchinson triad of sensorineural deafness, interstitial keratitis, and Hutchinson teeth [1]. Neurosyphilis may be asymptomatic, however may result in seizures, stroke, paresis, tabes dorsalis, or meningitis [47, 48, 54].

Imaging

Cross-sectional CT and MR neuroimaging is utilized to evaluate the meningovascular and intracranial parenchymal forms of neurosyphilis. In the meningovascular form, leptomeningeal enhancement is a common finding seen on post-contrast imaging [54]. The enhancement can be associated with perivascular inflammatory infiltrates sometimes extending to the parenchyma, thus almost appearing as an enhancing parenchymal mass [55]. Inflammatory vasculitis can lead to regions of arterial infarctions which would be best demonstrated on DWI MR sequences [55]. Parenchymal disease includes diffuse cerebral and cerebellar atrophy with periventricular calcifications, hydrocephalus, and microcephaly, common features seen in other congenital infections associated with the TORCH (toxoplasmosis, other, rubella, cytomegalovirus, and HSV) complex [54, 56, 57]. As previously described in this section, CT and MR images can confirm the presence of intracranial calcifications with CT showing foci of increased attenuation in a periventricular distribution and MR showing decreased signal on T2-weighted gradient echo sequences in a similar distribution.

13.5 Infections of the Spine

There are three primary sources where pathogens originate as an etiology of spine infections. One is by hematogenous spread through the Batson's plexus, another by direct external inoculation, and lastly by contiguous spread to the bone from the adjacent tissues. The vascularized intervertebral disc in children is made up of vessels in a ringlike fashion across the cartilaginous vertebral plate which disappears after 8 years of age leaving a rich anastomotic network of vessels at the periphery of the disc. The highly vascularized nature of the intervertebral disc of the spine in children therefore explains the higher incidence of disc infection in children compared with adults. In contrary, the intervertebral disc in adults is avascular with intraosseous anastomoses occurring around 30 years of age. Children also have a rich blood network in the metaphysis of the vertebral body, forming an incomplete ring at the base of the pedicle. The metaphyseal rings above and below two adjacent vertebrae communicate through anastomoses of the posterior-lateral region of the disc. This is a common area affected by tuberculosis where destruction of the vertebral body and spread to the adjacent vertebrae through ligaments.

13.5.1 Spondylodiscitis

Childhood spondylodiscitis (SD) is a term thought to encompass a clinical spectrum of rare spinal infections, ranging from discitis (infection of the disc space) to vertebral osteomyelitis (infection of the vertebrae) to spondylodiscitis (concurrent infection of the disc space and adjacent vertebrae). There is increased incidence in children compared to adults due to the vascularized nature of the intervertebral disc at a younger age. A trimodal age distribution in the pediatric population has been described, with groups including the neonate, 6 months to preschool period, and older school-aged children.

Infection can occur at any level of the spine, most commonly involving the lumbar/lumbosacral region (75% of cases), followed by the thoracic and cervical regions. SD can be subdivided into groups including pyogenic (most common), unspecific granulomatous, specific (such as tuberculosis, brucellosis, or fungal), and parasitic. Infection can occur by hematogenous spread from distant infection (most common) or via direct inoculation (via surgery, punctures, or trauma). Different manifestations of SD will occur via two mechanisms essentially representing the same pathologic process: (1) initial discitis with subsequent spread to the adjacent vertebral end plates and bodies and (2) initial vertebral osteomyelitis with subsequent spread to the adjacent intervertebral disc. Implicated pathogens include *S. aureus* (80% of cases in neonates and older children), *K. kingae* (commonly seen between 6 months and 4 years of age), *M. tuberculosis* (commonly seen in nonindustrialized countries), *Brucella* spp. (history of goat cheese consumption), and fungal agents including *Aspergillus* spp., *Candida* spp., and *Cryptococcus neoformans* (commonly seen in immunocompromised patients). Treatment regimen includes bedrest, spinal immobilization, and antimicrobial therapy based on the causative agent.

Clinical Presentation

Clinical presentation of SD is variable with nonspecific signs and symptoms often resulting in delayed diagnosis. Clinical manifestations include difficulty walking, unexplained irritability, back pain, abdominal pain, inability to flex the lower back, loss of lumbar lordosis, dysphagia and stiff neck (if cervical region involved), and low-grade fever or sepsis. Neurologic complications have been reported in approximately 12% of cases, including medullary or spinal nerve compression, meningitis, and progressive weakness/paralysis. Diagnosis is based on imaging findings in correlation with clinical and laboratory evaluation. Most patients make a full recovery following conservative treatment although surgery is indicated in more rare severe cases related to neurologic deficits, spinal deformities and instability, or failure from conservative treatment. Morality rate has been reduced to less than 5% since the advent of antimicrobials.

Imaging

Magnetic resonance imaging (MRI) is the imaging study of choice for the diagnosis of SD due to its relatively high sensitivity (96%) and specificity (93–94%) relative to other imaging modalities. Typical findings include disc space reduction of intervertebral disc height and disc space, decreased signal intensity on T1-weighted sequences, increased signal intensity on T2-weighted sequences, and enhancement of the affected disc on post-contrast sequences. Typical findings of the adjacent vertebrae include end plate irregularity, decreased bone marrow signal intensity on T1-weighted sequences, increased bone marrow signal intensity on T2-weighted and inversion recovery (STIR) sequences, and enhancement on post-contrast sequences. Post-contrast sequences are beneficial in evaluating for an associated paravertebral/spinal inflammatory mass or abscess (Fig. 13.17). MRI is also helpful in evaluating patients with neurologic complications indicative of compressive myelopathy with findings typical of nerve entrapment. It has been suggested that diffusion-weighted images (DWI) can differentiate between acute and chronic SD, with hyperintense disc and vertebral signal in the acute stage of the disease and hypointense disc and vertebral signal in chronic stages. MRI following initial presentation demonstrates a varied appearance, with changes in the disc space resolving after 34 months and changes in the vertebrae resolving after 24 months (Fig. 13.18).

13.5.2 Spinal Abscess

Spinal abscesses are rare entities in the pediatric population. Involvement can be epidural, subdural, or intramedullary; however many are epidural and intramedullary in location. Subdural abscesses, however, are considered rare.

13.5.2.1 Epidural Abscess

Spinal epidural abscesses (SEAs) are medical emergencies requiring urgent intervention rarely seen in children, with an incidence of less than 0.2 to 1.2–1.5 per 10,000 hospital

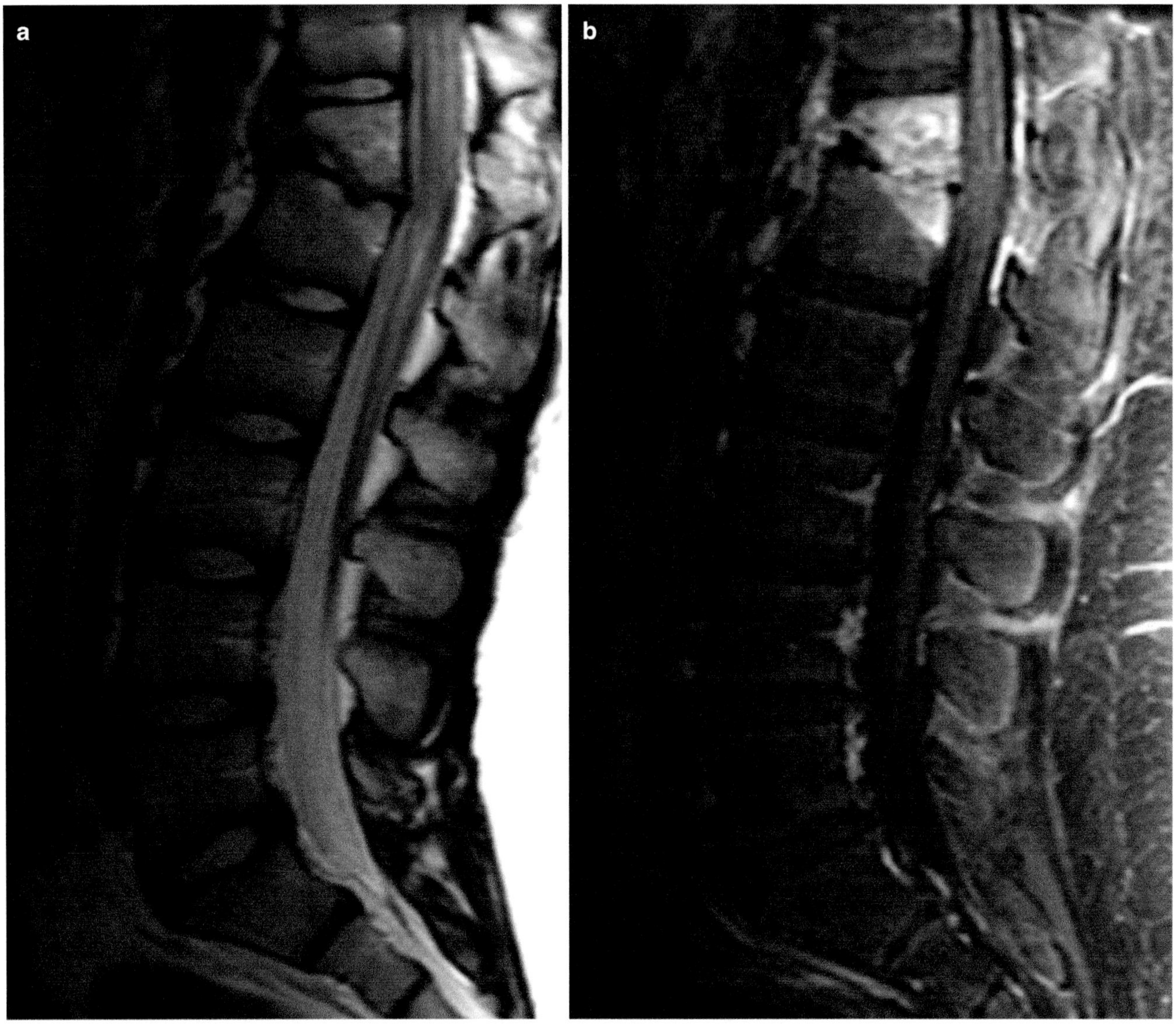

Fig. 13.17 Chronic spondylodiscitis. A 13-year-old male with anterior wedge deformity of T12 with abnormal bone marrow signal and joint space destruction of T12 and L1 on sagittal T2 (**a**). Post-contrast sagittal T1 shows associated enhancement (**b**) consistent with chronic spondylodiscitis. Also of note is enhancement along the dorsal aspect of the canal from T11 through L1 suspicious for a small epidural abscess collection (**b**) with inflammatory changes noted along the dorsal paraspinal soft tissues shown as increased T2 signal (**a**) and mild enhancement on post-contrast T1(**b**)

admissions. Hematogenous spread from distant infection is the most common cause, with additional sources by direct inoculation via prior interventions or trauma and direct spread from adjacent spondylodiscitis. The most common causative agent is *S. aureus*. Clinical presentation is variable and nonspecific, with signs and symptoms including fever, malaise, spinal and hip tenderness, refusal to bear weight, pain with movement, and back pain. SEAs may variably narrow the spinal canal and neural foramen resulting in neurologic symptoms which tend to occur more commonly at the thoracic and lumbar levels posteriorly. Magnetic resonance imaging (MRI) is considered the neuroimaging modality of choice. Typical findings include a focal, loculated epidural collection of increased T2/STIR signal intensity with restricted diffusion and peripheral rim enhancement. Treatment is controversial involving surgical drainage and/or antibiotic therapy.

13.5.2.2 Intramedullary Spinal Cord Abscess

Intramedullary spinal cord abscess is a rare pediatric entity requiring immediate therapy. It is more frequently seen in males with a peak incidence in the first and third decades of life. Commonly located at the thoracic level, they can be classified as acute (<1 week), subacute (1–6 weeks), and chronic (>6 weeks). In up to 85% of cases, the abscesses are secondary to another infection site from a distant focus either

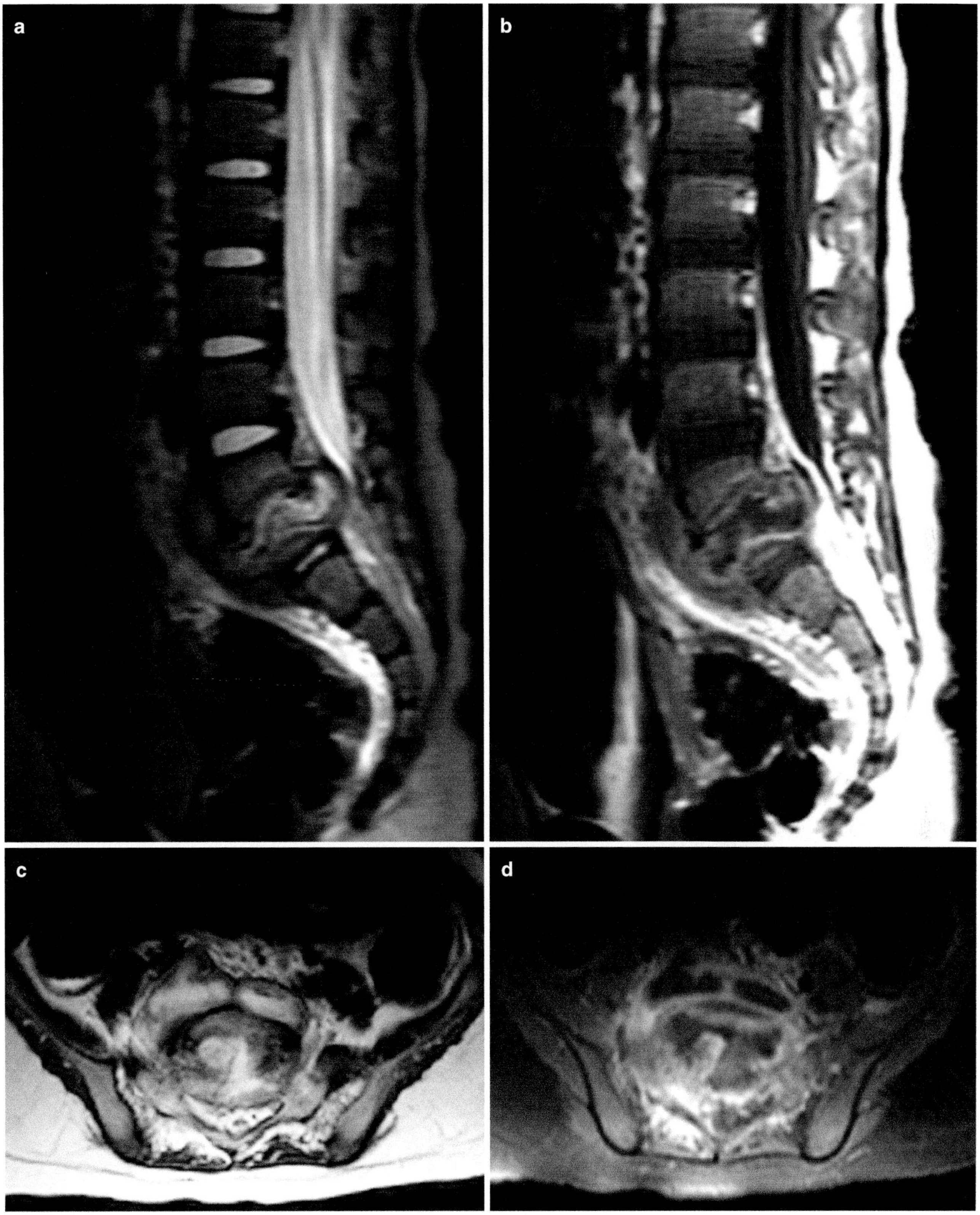

Fig. 13.18 Tuberculous spondylodiscitis. Soft tissue mass of the S1 vertebrae with destruction of the L5-S1 joint space on sagittal and axial T2 (**a**, **b**) with corresponding heterogeneous enhancement (**c**, **d**) in this 2-year-old patient with tuberculous spondylodiscitis

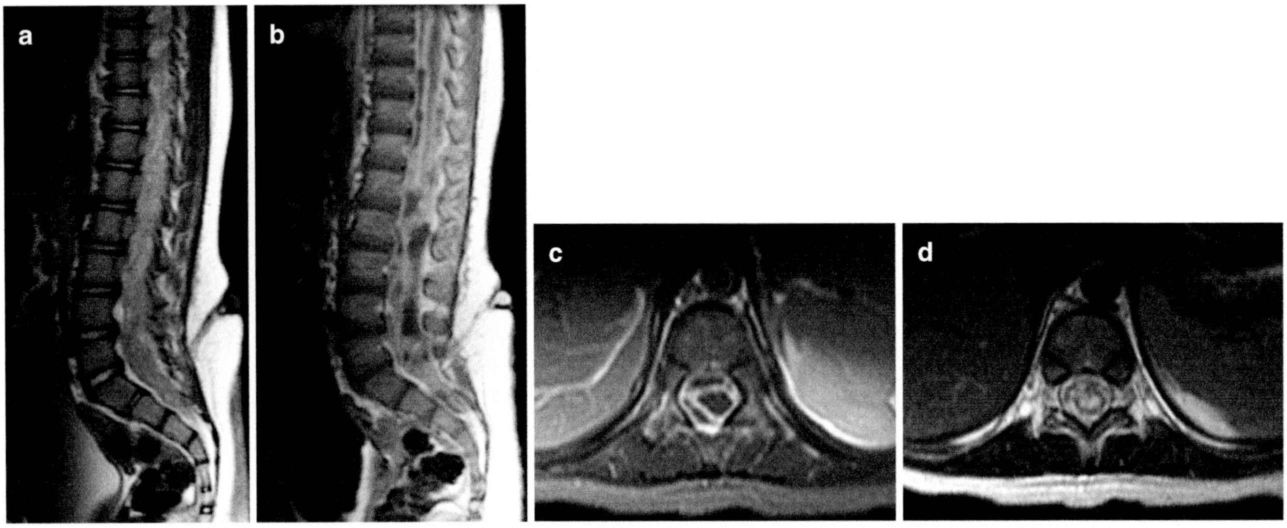

Fig. 13.19 Spinal abscess. A 13-month-old male presents to the emergency room with pus draining from a dermal sinus tract. MR of the lumbar spine shows extensive diffuse heterogeneous abnormal signal and enhancement on throughout the lower thoracic, lumbar, and sacral spinal canal on sagittal T2 (**a**) and sagittal and axial T1 post (**b**, **c**) consistent with and intraspinal abscess. A vitamin E capsule was placed on the dorsal soft tissues marking the sacral dimple on sagittal T2 and T1 post (**a**, **b**). Axial T2 shows increase signal within the spinal cord consistent with edema (**d**)

hematogenous spread or from contiguous spread to the cord via a dermal sinus or neural tube defect. It has been reported that the most common cause of intramedullary spinal cord abscess is a congenital dermal sinus. Clinical presentation can vary based on the age of the abscess, with an acute abscess presenting as a cord syndrome with back pain, fever, malaise, and chronic abscess being less symptomatic with mixed neurologic deficits and features mimicking intramedullary tumor. Approximately 70% of patients will have residual neurologic deficits following treatment. MRI is the modality of choice although imaging findings may overlap with those of spinal tumors. Findings typically include a solitary intramedullary expanded cord region of decreased T1 signal intensity, increased T2 signal intensity centrally with a low T2 signal intense capsule, surrounding increased cord signal intensity on PD/STIR sequences, and peripheral rim enhancement which are all related to the abscess and surrounding spinal cord edema (Fig. 13.19). Restricted diffusion may be present. Treatment involves surgical drainage with antibiotic therapy and steroids for spinal cord swelling and edema.

13.5.2.3 Subdural Abscess

The spinal subdural region is the least common infected area in the CNS. A review of 73 cases of subdural spinal infections in patients under 21 years of age showed a mean age of incidence of 6.5 years, males more frequently affected by a ratio of 2:1, and approximately half of patients (53%) were associated with spinal dysraphism or other spinal abnormalities. Subdural spinal abscesses are secondary to hematogenous spread from a distant focus or iatrogenic. The most common causative agent is *S. aureus* and most common affected regions are the thoracolumbar levels. Clinical presentation can be staged based on the manifestations demonstrated: stage 1 includes fever with or without spinal or nerve root pain; stage 2 includes stage 1 findings with mild neurological deficits; and stage 3 includes paralysis and complete sensory loss occurring below the level of the lesion. MRI is considered the modality of choice in evaluating the extent and location of the abscess which aids emergent neurosurgical planning. Findings typical of spinal abscess will be seen, typically including a subdural collection with decreased T1 signal intensity, increased T2/STIR/PD signal intensity, and peripheral rim enhancement of the collection with heterogeneous subdural enhancement. The collection will efface cerebrospinal fluid which will outline the collection on axial imaging, and there may be impingement and edema of the spinal cord with alteration of intramedullary signal. Treatment is surgical drainage in conjunction with systemic antibiotics.

References

1. Singhi P, Griffin DE, Newton CR. Central nervous system infections in childhood. London: Mac Keith Press; 2014.
2. Ball WS. Pediatric neuroradiology. Philadelphia: Lippencott Raven; 1997.
3. Acosta JH, Rantes CI, Arbelaez A, et al. Noncongenital central nervous system infections in children: radiology review. Top Magn Reson Imaging. 2014;23(3):153–64.
4. Chang LY, Huang LM, Gau SS, et al. Neurodevelopment and cognition in children after enterovirus 71 infection. N Engl J Med. 2007;356(12):1226–34.

5. Idro R, Ndiritu M, Ogutu B, et al. Burden, features, and outcome of neurological involvement in acute falciparum malaria in Kenyan children. JAMA. 2007;297(20):2232–40.
6. Modlin JF. Enterovirus deja vu. N Engl J Med. 2007;356(12):1204–5.
7. Berkley JA, Mwangi I, Ngetsa CJ, et al. Diagnosis of acute bacterial meningitis in children at a district hospital in sub-Saharan Africa. Lancet. 2001;357(9270):1753–7.
8. Hui A, Cheung KF, Lui C, et al. Herpes simplex encephalitis in Hong Kong: a retrospective review. Neurology Asia. 2005;10(Jun):35–8.
9. Singh S, Alexander M, Korah IP. Acute disseminated encephalomyelitis: MR imaging features. AJR Am J Roentgenol. 1999;173(4):1101–7.
10. Baskin HJ, Hedlund G. Neuroimaging of herpesvirus infections in children. Pediatr Radiol. 2007;37(10):949–63.
11. Solomon T. Flavivirus encephalitis. N Engl J Med. 2004;351(4):370–8.
12. Handique SK, Barkataky N. MR imaging in biphasic Japanese encephalitis. AJNR Am J Neuroradiol. 2008;29(3):E3.
13. Lo CP, Chen CY. Neuroimaging of viral infections in infants and young children. Neuroimaging Clin N Am. 2008;18(1):119–32. viii.
14. Maloney JA, Mirsky DM, Messacar K, et al. MRI findings in children with acute flaccid paralysis and cranial nerve dysfunction occurring during the 2014 enterovirus D68 outbreak. AJNR Am J Neuroradiol. 2015;36(2):245–50.
15. Awasthi M, Parmar H, Patankar T, et al. Imaging findings in rabies encephalitis. AJNR Am J Neuroradiol. 2001;22(4):677–80.
16. Burrill J, Williams CJ, Bain G, et al. Tuberculosis: a radiologic review. Radiographics. 2007;27(5):1255–73.
17. Trivedi R, Saksena S, Gupta RK. Magnetic resonance imaging in central nervous system tuberculosis. Indian J Radiol Imaging. 2009;19(4):256–65.
18. Gupta RK, Vatsal DK, Husain N, et al. Differentiation of tuberculous from pyogenic brain abscesses with in vivo proton MR spectroscopy and magnetization transfer MR imaging. AJNR Am J Neuroradiol. 2001;22(8):1503–9.
19. DeLone DR, Goldstein RA, Petermann G, et al. Disseminated aspergillosis involving the brain: distribution and imaging characteristics. AJNR Am J Neuroradiol. 1999;20(9):1597–604.
20. Smith AB, Smirniotopoulos JG, Rushing EJ. From the archives of the AFIP: central nervous System infections associated with human immunodeficiency virus infection: radiologic-pathologic correlation. Radiographics. 2008;28(7):2033–58.
21. Lin DJ, Sacks A, Shen J, et al. Neurocandidiasis: a case report and consideration of the causes of restricted diffusion. J Radiol Case Rep. 2013;7(5):1–5.
22. Popovich MJ, Arthur RH, Helmer E. CT of intracranial cryptococcosis. AJR Am J Roentgenol. 1990;154(3):603–6.
23. Donald KA, Walker KG, Kilborn T, et al. HIV Encephalopathy: pediatric case series description and insights from the clinic coalface. AIDS Res Ther. 2015;12(1):2.
24. Bell JE, Brettle RP, Chiswick A, et al. HIV encephalitis, proviral load and dementia in drug users and homosexuals with AIDS. Effect of neocortical involvement. Brain. 1998;121(Pt 11):2043–52.
25. Berger JR, Aksamit AJ, Clifford DB, et al. PML diagnostic criteria: consensus statement from the AAN neuroinfectious disease section. Neurology. 2013;80(15):1430–8.
26. Murdoch DM, Venter WD, Feldman C, et al. Incidence and risk factors for the immune reconstitution inflammatory syndrome in HIV patients in South Africa: a prospective study. AIDS. 2008;22(5):601–10.
27. Orikiiriza J, Bakeera-Kitaka S, Musiime V, et al. The clinical pattern, prevalence, and factors associated with immune reconstitution inflammatory syndrome in Ugandan children. AIDS. 2010;24(13):2009–17.
28. Post MJ, Thurnher MM, Clifford DB, et al. CNS-immune reconstitution inflammatory syndrome in the setting of HIV infection, part 2: discussion of neuro-immune reconstitution inflammatory syndrome with and without other pathogens. AJNR Am J Neuroradiol. 2013;34(7):1308–18.
29. Dollard SC, Grosse SD, Ross DS. New estimates of the prevalence of neurological and sensory sequelae and mortality associated with congenital cytomegalovirus infection. Rev Med Virol. 2007;17(5):355–63.
30. Demmler GJ. Infectious Diseases Society of America and Centers for Disease Control. Summary of a workshop on surveillance for congenital cytomegalovirus disease. Rev Infect Dis. 1991;13(2):315–29.
31. Kenneson A, Cannon MJ. Review and meta-analysis of the epidemiology of congenital cytomegalovirus (CMV) infection. Rev Med Virol. 2007;17(4):253–76.
32. Griffiths PD, Walter S. Cytomegalovirus. Curr Opin Infect Dis. 2005;18(3):241–5.
33. Fink KR, Thapa MM, Ishak GE, et al. Neuroimaging of pediatric central nervous system cytomegalovirus infection. Radiographics. 2010;30(7):1779–96.
34. van der Knaap MS, Vermeulen G, Barkhof F, et al. Pattern of white matter abnormalities at MR imaging: use of polymerase chain reaction testing of Guthrie cards to link pattern with congenital cytomegalovirus infection. Radiology. 2004;230(2):529–36.
35. de Vries LS, Gunardi H, Barth PG, et al. The spectrum of cranial ultrasound and magnetic resonance imaging abnormalities in congenital cytomegalovirus infection. Neuropediatrics. 2004;35(2):113–9.
36. Noyola DE, Demmler GJ, Nelson CT, et al. Early predictors of neurodevelopmental outcome in symptomatic congenital cytomegalovirus infection. J Pediatr. 2001;138(3):325–31.
37. Pomares C, Montoya JG. Laboratory diagnosis of congenital toxoplasmosis. J Clin Microbiol. 2016;54(10):2448–54.
38. Carter AO, Frank JW. Congenital toxoplasmosis: epidemiologic features and control. CMAJ. 1986;135(6):618–23.
39. Wilson CB, Remington JS, Stagno S, Reynolds DW. Development of adverse sequelae in children born with subclinical congenital Toxoplasma infection. Pediatrics. 1980;66(5):767–74.
40. Stamos JK, Rowley AH. Timely diagnosis of congenital infections. Pediatr Clin North Am. 1994;41(5):1017–33.
41. Lynfield R, Guerina N. Toxoplasmosis. Pediatr Rev. 1997;18(3):75–83.
42. Boppana SB, Pass RF, Britt WJ, et al. Symptomatic congenital cytomegalovirus infection: neonatal morbidity and mortality. Pediatr Infect Dis J. 1992;11(2):93–9.
43. Holliman RE. Congenital toxoplasmosis: prevention, screening and treatment. J Hosp Infect. 1995;30(suppl):179–90.
44. Malinger G, Werner H, Rodriguez Leonel JC, et al. Prenatal brain imaging in congenital toxoplasmosis. Prenat Diagn. 2011;31(9):881–6.
45. Becker LE. Infections of the developing brain. AJNR Am J Neuroradiol. 1992;13(2):537–49.
46. Rudnick C, Hoekzema G. Neonatal herpes simplex virus infections. Am Fam Physician. 2002;65(6):1138–42.
47. Caserta M, et al. Neonatal Herpes Simplex Virus (HSV) infection. Merck Manual Prof Version; 2015.
48. Caserta M, et al. Congenital syphilis. Merck Manual Prof Version; 2015.
49. Tyler KL. Update on herpes simplex encephalitis. Rev Neurol Dis. 2004;1(4):169–78.
50. Vossough A, Zimmerman RA, Bilaniuk LT, et al. Imaging findings of neonatal herpes simplex virus type 2 encephalitis. Neuroradiology. 2008;50(4):355–66.

51. Hutto C, Arvin A, Jacobs R, et al. Intrauterine herpes simplex virus infections. J Pediatr. 1987;110(1):97–101.
52. Leonard J, Moran C, Cross D, Wippold F, et al. MR imaging of herpes simplex type i encephalitis in infants and young children: a separate pattern of findings. AJR Am J Roentgenol. 2000;174(6):1651–5.
53. Bajaj M, Mody S, Natarajan G. Clinical and neuroimaging findings in neonatal herpes simplex virus infection. J Pediatr. 2014;165(2):404–7.
54. Barkovich AJ, Raybaud C, et al. Pediatric neuroimaging. 5th ed. Philadelphia: Lippincott Williams and Wilkens; 2012.
55. Shah G, et al. Central nervous system infections. Elsevier Health Sciences; 2012.
56. Blaser S, Jay V, Becker L, Ford-Jones EL. Neonatal brain infection. In: Ruthford M, editor. MRI of the neonatal brain. London: WB Saunders; 2002. Imaging; Part 4 Chapter 10.
57. de Fatima Vasco Aragao M, van der Linden V, Brainer-Lima AM, et al. Clinical features and neuroimaging (CT and MRI) findings in presumed Zika virus related congenital infection and microcephaly: retrospective case series study. BMJ. 2016;353:i1901.

Part III

Immunological Diseases of CNS

Overview of Neuroimmunology

14

Heng Liu, Li Li, and Hongjun Li

14.1 Introduction

Patients with neuroimmunological syndromes have presented many clinical challenges for the attending physician. Even experienced clinicians occasionally reach the point where diagnostic, identification, treatment, or prognostic thinking becomes blocked.

The field of classical neuroimmunology includes the immune response in infectious, ischemic, degenerative, traumatic, autoimmune-mediated, and especially neoplastic diseases of the nervous system, which focus on immune-mediated demyelination [1]. Immune responses of the nervous system are the subject of classical neuroimmunology, which has also been named "immunoneurology" [2].

Classical neuroimmunology, (1) autoimmune diseases: acute demyelinating encephalomyelitis (ADEM), multiple sclerosis, chronic immune-related demyelinating polyradiculoneuropathy (CIDP), Guillain-Barré-Strohl syndrome, Lambert-Eaton myasthenic syndrome, myasthenia gravis pseudoparalytica, dermatomyositis, polymyositis, inclusion body myositis, vasculitides, and collagenoses. (2) Neuroinfections: encephalomyelitis, encephalitis, meningitis, polyradiculitis, or polyneuritis caused by bacteria such as *burgdorferi*, *Clostridium botulinum*, *Clostridium tetani*, and viruses such as rabies, herpes, HIV, JC, Coxsackie, measles, mumps, RS, and polio virus. (3) Other diseases: cerebrovascular diseases (stroke, intracerebral hemorrhage), neurodegenerative diseases (Alzheimer's disease, Huntington's disease, Parkinson's disease, and amyotrophic lateral sclerosis), psychic diseases (schizophrenia, epilepsy, major depressive disorder, and narcolepsy), neoplastic diseases (leukemias, primary brain tumor, lymphomas, and paraneoplastic syndromes), traumata (spinal cord injury), and so on.

Recently more evidence suggests that a broader interaction between the immune and nervous systems through morphological connections shared common mechanisms of signal transduction and signal molecules. The nervous and immune systems establish functional and structural networks of their cellular components, which communicate through cell-cell contact and soluble factors, respectively [3]. Therefore, immune processes impact nervous functions and vice versa under pathologic/physiologic conditions. This includes vegetative and neuroendocrine influences on the immune response, including immunosuppression and conditioned immunostimulation as well as effects of immune mediators on psychic and neuronal functions (Fig. 14.1).

The essential structure of the cell-cell contact complies with the same principles in these systems (Dustin and Colman) [4]. Both types of synapses even share the same matrix molecule agrin [2]. The other structures that enable direct cell-to-cell communication between the immune and nervous system are gap junctions [5] and tunnelling nanotubules [6]. These findings have a significant impact on strategies for the treatment of somatic and psychiatric diseases in the future.

Here we will introduce neuroimmunological syndromes from the following six types of diseases (Fig. 14.2).

H. Liu (✉)
Department of Radiology, Affiliated Hospital of Zunyi Medical University, Zunyi, China

L. Li · H. Li
Department of Radiology, Beijing You'an Hospital, Capital Medical University, Beijing, China

B. Gao et al. (eds.), *Imaging of CNS Infections and Neuroimmunology*, https://doi.org/10.1007/978-981-13-6904-9_14

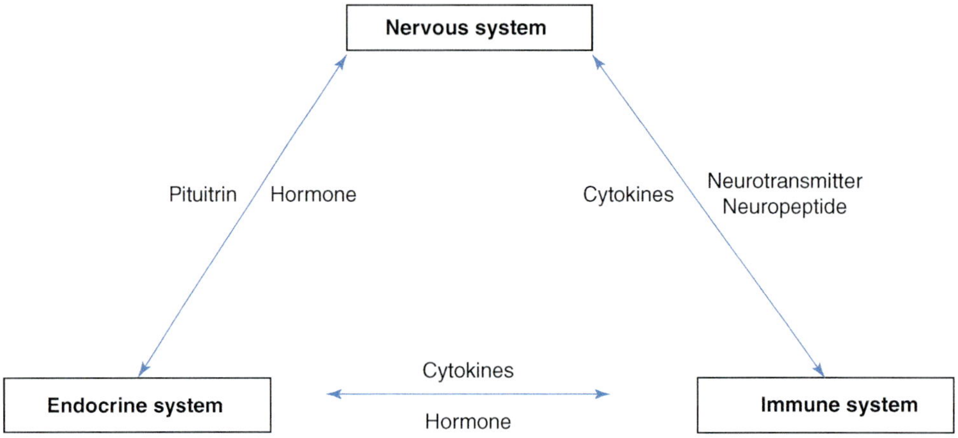

Fig. 14.1 Interaction between the immune and nervous systems

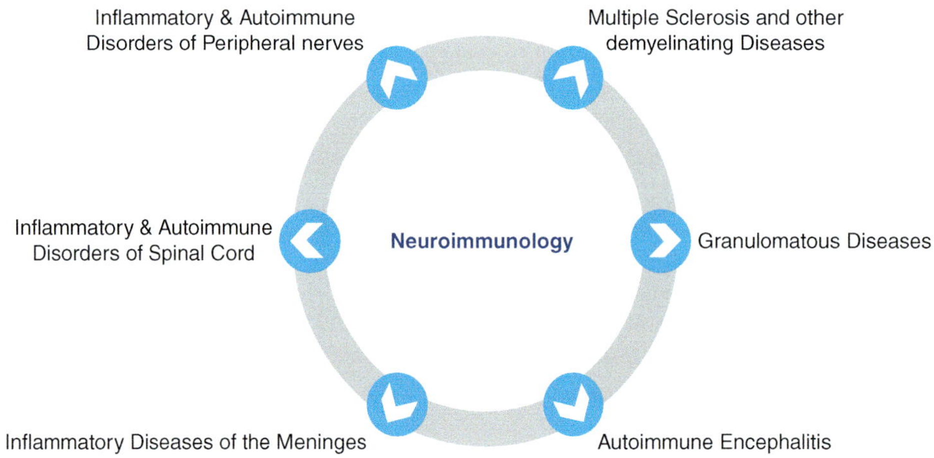

Fig. 14.2 Six types of diseases included in neuroimmunological syndromes

14.2 Multiple Sclerosis and Other Demyelinating Diseases

Multiple sclerosis (MS) is the most common idiopathic demyelinating disease of the central nervous system (CNS). MS is thought to be an example of development of autoimmunity to self-antigens within the CNS through multiple initiating events, which include infections and other environmental factors [7]. Moreover, MS lesions are growing and changing in space as time passes by.

MS usually occurs in young adults, with a peak between 20 and 40 years. The ratio of women to men is about 2–3:1. There is evidence for the first manifestations of MS at childhood and older ages as well. According to the area involved, MS patients have different symptoms. The classical patient triad (of Charcot) is intention tremor, scanning speech, and nystagmus (Jerky, back-and-forth movements of the eyes). The diagnosis of MS requires evidence for at least two anatomically distinct lesions. The lesions are consistent with white matter damage in an individual who has a history of at least two distinct episodes of focal neurological dysfunction (symptom dissemination in space and time). They are not difficult to prove in accepted MS. But in the stages of the disease, MS presents with a clinically isolated symptom of MS. In recent years, application and new progress of image technology may contribute to the diagnosis and prognosis of MS.

CT as a preliminary investigation method of MS discovers the rate of hardened plaque which is 42–47%. Magnetic resonance imaging (MRI) is the preferred imaging modality. MRI can find the rate of hardened plaque up to 95%. Lesion conspicuity is related to the field strength of the MR scanner; therefore, priority should be given to the high-magnetic-field scanners [8]. Lower field-strength magnets with an open configuration, however, may be the only option to check extremely claustrophobic or obese patients [9]. Its symbol signs: Multiple hyperintense T2 signal plaques in the white matter are seen classically at the periventricular area along the lateral ventricles and the occipital horns, the internal capsule, the pons, the corpus callosum, and the middle cerebral peduncles. Ring enhancement occurs in acute stage of the disease only. Contrast study is not recommended after therapy with intravenous steroid administration as active plaques will usually not enhance [10]. DTI is used to monitor the therapy and disease progression of white matter tracts lesions, which mainly affects the corticospinal tract. DTI may be a sensitive marker for early detection of inflammatory disease activity in MS [11].

14.3 Granulomatous Diseases

Granulomatous diseases (GD) are a group of rare primary phagocytic function defects. It is caused by mutations in gene-encoding protein subunits of the nicotinamide adenine dinucleotide phosphate (NADPH) oxidase complex [12]. Granulomatous diseases have a varied etiology, including autoimmune, idiopathic, infectious, and hereditary causes [13]. Infective granulomas may be due to fungal agents or bacterial [14]. Non-infective granulomas are sarcoidosis, amyloidosis, Wegener's granulomatosis, chemical granuloma, and reparative giant cell granuloma.

GD has systemic manifestations, affecting the whole body, especially the natural barriers of the human body, such as the lymph nodes, skin, and the respiratory tract [15]. The liver, spleen, bones, and brain can also be affected by infections. These diseases mostly involve the small vessels, which can lead to a good pathological condition in the central nervous system. And inflammation can be the first clinical manifestation.

Chronic granulomatous disease (CGD) is an essential immunodeficiency caused by the deficiency of phagocyte nicotinamide adenine dinucleotide phosphate (NADPH) oxidase, which leads to the dysregulation of inflammation and increases the susceptibility to infections. The prevalence of CGD at birth is 1 per 120,000–250,000 people [13, 16]. The ratio of women to men affected is about 1:9, usually within 6 months of birth. The classical clinical manifestations of CGD are recurrent severe infection as well as the formation of recurrent infection pigmentation characterized by granulomas.

It's a difficult diagnostic challenge for radiologists. According to the disease, different anatomical structures are affected. Imaging findings of GD can appear nonspecific, with considerable overlap with imaging findings of other conditions, including malignancy [15]. Lymphadenopathy is a common manifestation. It often shows that granuloma formation may lead to osseous erosion and progressive destruction of cartilage; to granuloma location, scope, and influence on surrounding structures, with central necrosis; to fibro calcification on CT. MR imaging shows the exact location, elongation, and influence on surrounding structures [15]. FDG-PET/CT is deemed as a useful diagnostic tool to evaluate the accuracy and activity of disseminated GD. In addition, PET/CT is advantageous to assess the therapeutic response and time course of the disease [17].

14.4 Autoimmune Encephalitis

Autoimmune encephalitis (AIE) is a common cause of encephalitis and increasingly regarded as the cause of a variety of neuropsychiatric syndromes that can be severe and prolonged. However, its incidence is still difficult to estimate. AIE is more frequent in immunocompetent [18] and also tend to occur in young adults, adolescents, and children [19].

The classic manifestations of AIE include behavior and cognition, memory, seizures, speech, dyskinesia, autonomic dysfunction, loss of consciousness, and central hypoventilation [20, 21]. The symptoms occur rapidly in a few days or weeks [22]. There is substantial overlap of symptoms among the different types of autoimmune encephalitis, making it difficult for us to diagnose.

The diagnosis of AIE often relies on clinical manifestations and various laboratory tests, including antibody testing, biopsy, cancer screening, imaging, and so on [23]. Many imaging applications can be used to assist the diagnosis of AIE.

Brain MRI can be used for the differential diagnosis, particularly in limbic encephalitis. Patients with autoimmune or paraneoplastic limbic encephalitis often have increased T2/FLAIR signal in the medial temporal lobes; patients with paraneoplastic encephalitis often show contrast enhancement [18, 22, 24]. Post-contrast MRI can show the situation of dural invasion [25].

As one of exclusion examinations, the imaging of the brain vessels, looking for other evidence of vasculitis, may be useful [26].

PET/SPECT shows diverse regions of regional hyper- or hypometabolism in patients, providing evidence of cerebral functional changes underlying the clinical manifestation [26, 27].

14.5 Inflammatory Diseases of the Meninges

Inflammatory diseases of the meninges that surround the brain and the spinal cord is the most common infection of the CNS [28, 29]. And it contains meningitis. Many factors can be lead to the diseases, such as viruses, bacteria, fungi, parasites, radiation, or tumors, and so on. Infection can be due to hematogenous spread during systemic infection and brain injury with disruption of the dura mater [28, 30]. It often occurs in immunocompromised patients, like infant nursing [31].

Different etiologies may lead to various clinical symptoms and different onset times. In most cases, meningitis begins with unspecific prodromes, such as abnormal fatigue growing pains, which may last for several hours before the onset of meningeal symptoms. The features are usually associated with nervous system and the cause itself. For example, bacterial meningitis often presents with at least two of the following symptoms: neck stiffness; fever; changes in mental status-the classical triad and headache. TBM begins with unusual symptoms such as ill humor, diminished appetite, fatigue, elevated temperature, and headache [28].

It's hard to diagnose the disease. Mostly, clinical manifestations, history, and analysis of the CSF will provide the differential diagnosis clues. Imaging is important in cases of suspected infectious meningitis to show the extent of the disease, the typical lesion patterns, and the potential involvement of brain structures. In addition, neuroimaging may identify sources of infection, such as infection of the temporal bone or mastoid, fractures of the skull base, and to rule out other, noninfectious causes of inflammatory disease of the meninges [28]. At the initial stage of the disease, imaging might be normal appearance of the meninges and the brain.

In infectious or inflammatory conditions, meninges can be involved in the process. Bacterial and viral meningitis is usually associated with leptomeningeal enhancement. Fungal meningitis may cause nodular, thicker enhancement of the meninges. However, nodular enhancement is much more specific for leptomeningeal carcinomatosis. In granulomatous infections, intracranial contrast enhancement is often confined to the basal cistern and may be related to other findings such as hydrocephalus, ischemia/infarct, subdural fluid collection, or brain parenchymal lesions. Sarcoidosis may be associated with the meninges. Usually the leptomeninges are involved, and contrast enhancement usually extends along the contour of the brain into sulci [28].

In the following, we will review the main signs of the diseases in imaging. Plain radiography can hardly provide us with direct information. CT as a fast, simple, and basic tool can clearly display cerebral structures and provide primary information for probable pathologies of the skull base, the nasal sinus, and the temporal bone. In the cases of bacterial meningitis, CT may reveal slight enlargement of the ventricles and the subarachnoid space (SAS) and demonstrate linear leptomeningeal enhancement. To neurosarcoidosis, CT might show osteolytic skull lesions.

MRI can provide more valid information. In bacterial meningitis, enhanced T1-weighted images are more effective in demonstrating meningeal enhancement than contrast-enhanced CT. In addition, MRI might reveal an increase in the SAS signals on T2-weighted and FLAIR images. DWI is highly sensitive in displaying of small cortical or deep white matter infarctions. Vascular changes can be visualized directly with MRA [32]. Conventional MRI can hardly see the infarcts. fMRI is useful to obtain functional information which is useful for deciding the use of high-dose steroid therapy [28].

The neuroimaging findings of tuberculous meningitis (TBM) are enhancement of the basal cisterns and the corresponding leptomeninges caused by dense fibrinous exudate [33]. Moreover, findings of MRI are little effect on hydrocephalus and basal enhancement [28, 34]. There are four most characteristics of tuberculous meningitis: hydrocephalus, infarcts, the presence of basal exudates, and tuberculoma. These neuroimaging features can give confidence in the clinical diagnosis without bacteriological confirmation. Some imaging findings are quite characteristic for tuberculous meningitis. Surgical intervention requires a repetitive imaging. Neuroimaging is essential in the evaluation of subjects suffering from tuberculous meningitis [34].

Viral meningitis is most of MRI scans are normal. T2 images in the caudate nucleus, thalami, brain stem, or the cerebellum may indicate the presence of meningitis.

Cryptococcal meningoencephalitis is mainly characterized by diffuse meningeal enhancement and ventriculitis, accompanied by characteristic cystic and punctuated lesions in the basal ganglia due to cryptococcal invasion of the perivascular spaces, namely, the "soap-bubble lesions."

Imaging findings of aspergillus meningeal infection include dural enhancement near the affected paranasal sinus or the orbit; typically, bony structures are involved. More than 50% of the patients develop vasculitis of the perforating arteries of the basal ganglia caused by hemorrhagic infarctions.

Small-vessel arteritis is the typical direct change of meningitis. Approximately one-third of the patients have normal findings. There is little systematic data about neuroradiological findings in neurosyphilis.

To neurosarcoidosis, enhanced CT and MRI have an extensive spectrum of leptomeningeal enhancement (basal SAS and cranial nerve involvement). Neurosarcoid infiltration impacts the chiasma, infundibulum, and hypothalamus. The changes of the pachymeninges and in the SAS display low signal intensity on T2 images and isointense on T1 images.

14.6 Inflammatory and Autoimmune Disorders of the Spinal Cord

Spinal cord disease can be caused by a variety of pathologic processes, including inflammatory and demyelinating diseases [35]. Inflammatory is caused by viruses, bacteria, spirochetes, Rickettsia, parasites, protozoa, mycoplasma, and other biological infection or white matter that infect gray matter or/and inflammatory lesions of the spinal cord, and the lesions is lower than the level of limb paralysis, sensory, autonomic dysfunction, and its clinical features. It has been reported to occur occasionally (1–3%) in a large amount of autoimmune disorders, e.g., SLE, antiphospholipid syndrome, Sjögren's syndrome, Behçet's disease, mixed connective tissue disease, rheumatoid arthritis, ankylosing spondylitis, etc. [36]. The clinical symptoms can be carried out according to the lesion site and range. Lesions in the spinal cord often affect the pyramidal and spinothalamic tract and the dorsal column system. They lead to more severe physical disability [36]. Inflammatory and infectious disorders of the spine are less common in children than in adults [37].

The diagnosis and treatment relay on a clinical and physical examination. Hemogram and CSF analysis show signs of spinal cord inflammation. Electrophysiological study is helpful in diagnosing and judging prognosis. Imaging findings often provide a basis for clinical diagnosis:

Spinal X-ray plain display normal. MRI showed the swelling of the spinal cord. The plaques or patchy lesions show significantly homogeneous low signal intensity on T1-weighted MR imaging, and high signal intensity on T2-weighted MR imaging. These lesions are generally, but they are not necessarily. Some cases can always be normal. CT reveals that the spinal cord is slightly thickened and the density is uneven. Myelography: diffuse swelling of the spinal cord or may be normal. Mainly used for clinical manifestations of atypical cases and other diseases.

14.7 Inflammatory and Autoimmune Disorders of Peripheral Nerves

Peripheral neuritis, also known as multiple neuritis, results from a variety of reasons of peripheral neuritis (including cranial nerve and spinal nerve) symmetry or asymmetry damage. The cause of the illness is not clear, including infection, autoimmune disorders, genetic factors, and so on. It occurs at any ages and is not contagious. The clinical manifestations are different for the various causes.

At present, the assessment of peripheral nerve disorders mainly relays on clinical examination supported by electroneurography and electromyography [38]. And imaging technology can be beneficial to diagnose it. Since 1895, Roentgen has discovered X-ray and medical imaging techniques such as X-ray films, CT, and ultrasound images, which can be applied to the clinic when visualizing the anatomy and disease of peripheral nerve, but there are still many limitations and shortcomings. While MRI is an effective technique for nerve injury detecting on T2 images, it lacks specificity. MRI of the peripheral nervous system was mainly manifested by the compression of neural bundles that exclude the surrounding structures [39]. MRI can show axonal injury and be used to evaluate plexus lesions and nerve regeneration, monitor the invasion of hematogenous macrophages and secondary nerve injury in skeletal muscle, identify focal mass lesions in the peripheral nerve: inflammation or tumor [38]? MR neuroimaging can be helpful for the differential diagnosis of pure motor syndromes, multifocal motor neuronopathy, lower motor neuron syndrome, pure motor CIDP, and amyotrophic lateral sclerosis [38]. What's more, the increase of MRI function brings more information. For instance, in CIDP MRI of the sciatic and tibial nerves, FA, and ADC can find the obvious abnormalities of the peripheral nerves associated with the severity of neuropathy [40].

References

1. Mix E, Goertsches R, Zettl UK. Immunology and neurology. J Neurol. 2007;254(2):II2–7.
2. Gao B, Zee CS. Neuroinfection & neuroimmunology: new opportunities, new challenges. Radiol Infect Dis. 2016;3:51–3.
3. Watkins SC, Salter RD. Functional connectivity between immune cells mediated by tunneling nanotubules. Immunity. 2005;23(3):309–18.
4. Dustin ML, Colman DR. Neural and immunological synaptic relations. Science. 2002;298(5594):785–9.
5. Hoftberger R. Neuroimmunology: an expanding frontier in autoimmunity. Front Immunol. 2015;6:206.
6. Rustom A, Saffrich R, Markovic I, et al. Nanotubular highways for intercellular organelle transport. Science. 2004;303(5660):1007–10.
7. Goldenberg MM. Multiple sclerosis review. Pharm Ther. 2012;37(3):175.
8. Hagens M, van Berckel B, Barkhof F. Novel MRI and PET markers of neuroinflammation in multiple sclerosis. Curr Opin Neurol. 2016;29(3):229–36.
9. Tomassini V, d'Ambrosio A, Petsas N, et al. The effect of inflammation and its reduction on brain plasticity in multiple sclerosis: MRI evidence. Hum Brain Mapp. 2016;37(7):2431–45.
10. Barkhof F, Filippi M, Miller DH, et al. Comparison of MRI criteria at first presentation to predict conversion to clinically definite multiple sclerosis. Brain. 1997;120(11):2059–69.
11. Werring D, Clark C, Barker G, et al. Diffusion tensor imaging of lesions and normal-appearing white matter in multiple sclerosis. Neurology. 1999;52(8):1626–32.
12. Rawat A, Bhattad S, Singh S. Chronic granulomatous disease. Indian J Pediatr. 2016;83(4):345–53.
13. Roxo-Junior P, Simão HML. Chronic granulomatous disease: why an inflammatory disease? Braz J Med Biol Res. 2014;47(11):924–8.
14. Wu U-I, Holland SM. A genetic perspective on granulomatous diseases with an emphasis on mycobacterial infections. Semin Immunopathol. 2016;38:199–212. Springer.
15. Razeka AAKA. Imaging appearance of granulomatous lesions of head and neck. Eur J Radiol. 2010;76(1):52–60.
16. Roos D. Chronic granulomatous disease. Br Med Bull. 2016;118:50.
17. Isaac NM. In: Henderson RW, editor. Granulomatous diseases. PET-CT. New York: Springer; 2016. p. 289–306.
18. Armangue T, Leypoldt F, Dalmau J. Auto-immune encephalitis as differential diagnosis of infectious encephalitis. Curr Opin Neurol. 2014;27(3):361–8.
19. Dalmau J, Rosenfeld MR. Autoimmune encephalitis update. Neuro-Oncology. 2014;16(6):771–8.
20. Armangue T, Petitpedrol M, Dalmau J. Autoimmune encephalitis in children. J Child Neurol. 2012;27(11):1417–21.
21. Guan HZ, Ren HT, Cui LY. Autoimmune encephalitis: an expanding frontier of neuroimmunology. Chin Med J. 2016;129(9):1122–7.
22. Leypoldt F, Armangue T, Dalmau J. Autoimmune encephalopathies. Ann N Y Acad Sci. 2010;85(10):94–114.
23. Graus F, Titulaer MJ, Balu R, et al. A clinical approach to diagnosis of autoimmune encephalitis. Lancet Neurol. 2016;15(4):391–404.
24. Deramecourt V, Bombois S, Debette S, et al. Bilateral temporal glioma presenting as a paraneoplastic limbic encephalitis with pure cognitive impairment. Neurologist. 2009;15(4):208–11.

25. Aupy J, Collongues N, Blanc F, et al. [Autoimmune encephalitis, clinical, radiological and immunological data]. Rev Neurol. 2013;169(2):142–53.
26. Lancaster E. The diagnosis and treatment of autoimmune encephalitis. J Clin Neurol. 2016;12(1):1–13.
27. Baumgartner A, Rauer S, Mader I, et al. Cerebral FDG-PET and MRI findings in autoimmune limbic encephalitis: correlation with autoantibody types. J Neurol. 2013;260(11):2744–53.
28. Rohde S. Inflammatory diseases of the meninges. Berlin: Springer; 2012.
29. Dalmau J, Graus F, Villarejo A, et al. Clinical analysis of anti-Ma2-associated encephalitis. Brain. 2004;127(Pt 8):1831–44.
30. Schär M, Wiesmann E. [Inflammatory diseases of the meninges. Epidemiology and examination methods]. Bibl Tuberc. 1967;23:1–11.
31. Fowler MI, Weller RO, Heckels JE, et al. Different meningitis-causing bacteria induce distinct inflammatory responses on interaction with cells of the human meninges. Cell Microbiol. 2004;6(6):555–67.
32. Jan W, Zimmerman RA, Bilaniuk LT, et al. Diffusion-weighted imaging in acute bacterial meningitis in infancy. Neuroradiology. 2003;45(9):634–9.
33. Andronikou S, Smith B, Hatherhill M, et al. Definitive neuroradiological diagnostic features of tuberculous meningitis in children. Pediatr Radiol. 2004;34(11):876–85.
34. Garg RK, Malhotra HS, Jain A. Neuroimaging in tuberculous meningitis. Neurol India. 2016;64(2):219–27.
35. Manelfe C, Sarrazin JL. Spinal cord inflammatory and demyelinating diseases. In: Diseases of the brain head & neck spine. Milan Berlin Heidelberg, New York: Springer; p. 195–9.
36. Demaerel P, Ross JS. Spinal cord inflammatory and demyelinating diseases. Cham: Springer; 2016.
37. Castillo M, Tortori-Donati P. Infectious and inflammatory disorders of the spine. Berlin: Springer; 2005.
38. Stoll G, Bendszus M, Perez J, et al. Magnetic resonance imaging of the peripheral nervous system. Phys Med Rehabil Clin N Am. 2001;12(2):399–432.
39. Judmaier W. Introduction to magnetic resonance imaging of the peripheral nervous system: general considerations and examination technique. Berlin: Springer; 2013.
40. Markvardsen LH, Vaeggemose M, Ringgaard S, et al. Diffusion tensor imaging can be used to detect lesions in peripheral nerves in patients with chronic inflammatory demyelinating polyneuropathy treated with subcutaneous immunoglobulin. Neuroradiology. 2016;58(8):745–52.

Multiple Sclerosis and Other Demyelinating Diseases

15

Yongmei Li

15.1 Introduction

Multiple sclerosis (MS) is characterized by localized areas of demyelination, axonal loss, and glial scar formation in the brain [1, 2]. The disease usually begins in young adults with onset at the age of 20–50 years old [3, 4]. It is the most common cause of non-traumatic disability in young adults [5]. The estimated populations affected are about 2.5 million globally, which are unevenly occurring throughout the world. The prevalence of MS increases with the distance from the equator rising [6]. The exact etiology involved in the disease remains uncertain. Genetic, environmental, and immunological factors may contribute to the pathogenesis.

The pathologic features of MS are consisting of focal areas of demyelination characterized by variable gliosis, inflammation, and relative axonal preservation. The location, size, number, and shape of these plaques vary greatly among MS patients. Lesions have a predilection of involving optic nerves, periventricular white matter regions, spinal cord, brainstem, and cerebellum. Acute active plaques are characterized by relative axonal preservation by myelin-laden macrophages evenly distributed in the lesion. Chronic active plaques have relative axonal preservation and sharply defined margins.

The last 10 years have witnessed major advancements in the ability to diagnose MS and other demyelinating diseases with the aid of MRI and other instrumental and laboratory tools. Conventional MRI plays an important role in diagnosing and in monitoring the disease course. Advanced MRI techniques provide higher specificity and sensitivity to both lesions and normal-appearing gray/white matter contributing in better understanding of MS pathophysiology.

Y. Li (✉)
Department of Radiology, First Hospital of Chongqing Medical University, Chongqing, China

15.2 Clinical Presentations

Based on its highly variable clinical course, MS could be divided into four main clinical types [7]: relapsing-remitting MS (RRMS), primary progressive MS (PPMS), secondary progressive MS (SPMS), and progressive relapsing MS (PRMS). The additional subtypes include clinically isolated syndrome (CIS) and radiologically isolated syndrome (RIS) [8, 9].

Visual symptoms include diplopia, blurred vision, diminution, or loss of visual acuity and visual field defects [6]. Limb weakness is the most common sign of corticospinal tract involvement, almost always present in advanced cases. The cerebellum and brainstem are usually involved with the symptoms of dysarthria, gait ataxia, tremor, and incoordination of the trunk or limbs. Paresthesias and sensory impairment are common when spinothalamic tract is involved. The patients would frequently feel tingling or numbness in the limbs, trunk, or face [6]. Other manifestations, such as fatigue, urinary symptoms, sexual dysfunction, psychiatric disorder, and cognitive, judgment, and memory disorders, may also present sometimes.

15.3 Diagnosis of Multiple Sclerosis

The diagnosis of MS is depending on the complete clinical history, neurological examination, cerebrospinal fluid (CSF) test, neuroimaging, as well as electrophysiology. MRI, oligoclonal IgG bands (OCBs) in CSF test, and visual-evoked potentials (VEPs) are of greatest value for confirming the diagnosis [10]. Up to 90% of MS patients have two or more immunoglobulin G (IgG). Conventional MRI is currently regarded as the most sensitive noninvasive tool for supporting MS diagnosis and evaluating treatment response after anti-inflammatory agents.

Conventional MRI protocols include T1WI, T2WI, FLAIR, and contrast enhancement T1WI (Fig. 15.1).

B. Gao et al. (eds.), *Imaging of CNS Infections and Neuroimmunology*, https://doi.org/10.1007/978-981-13-6904-9_15

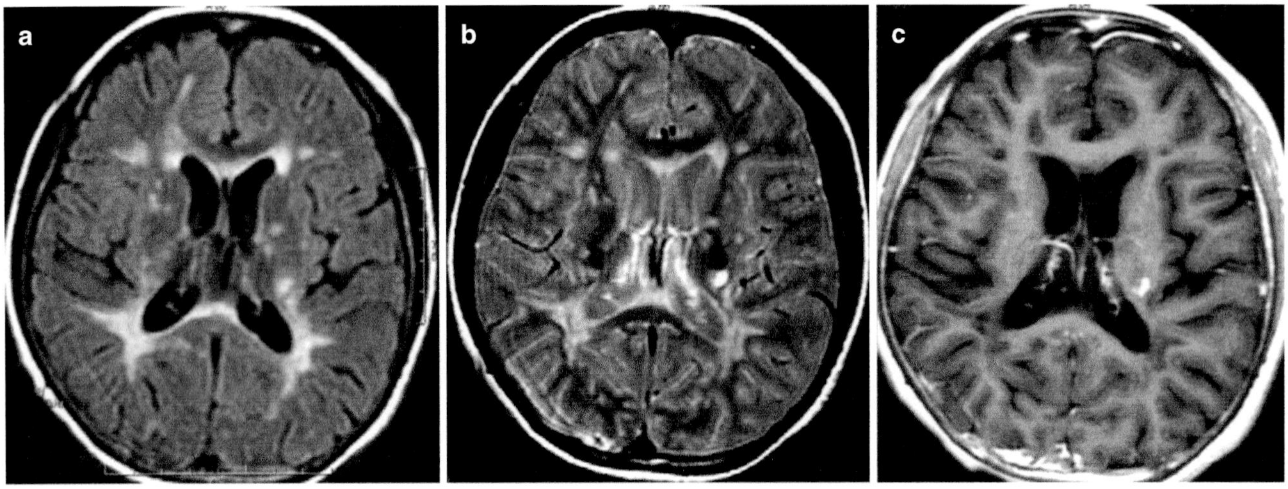

Fig. 15.1 A 40-year-old man with RRMS. (**a**) Axial T2-FLAIR shows several patchy and punctiform hyperintense (arrow) in the periventricular areas; (**b**) PD image shows the multiple hyperintense plaque (arrow) located in the same areas; (**c**) axial contrast-enhanced T1WI shows a small nodular enhancement in the left periventricular area (with permission from the patient)

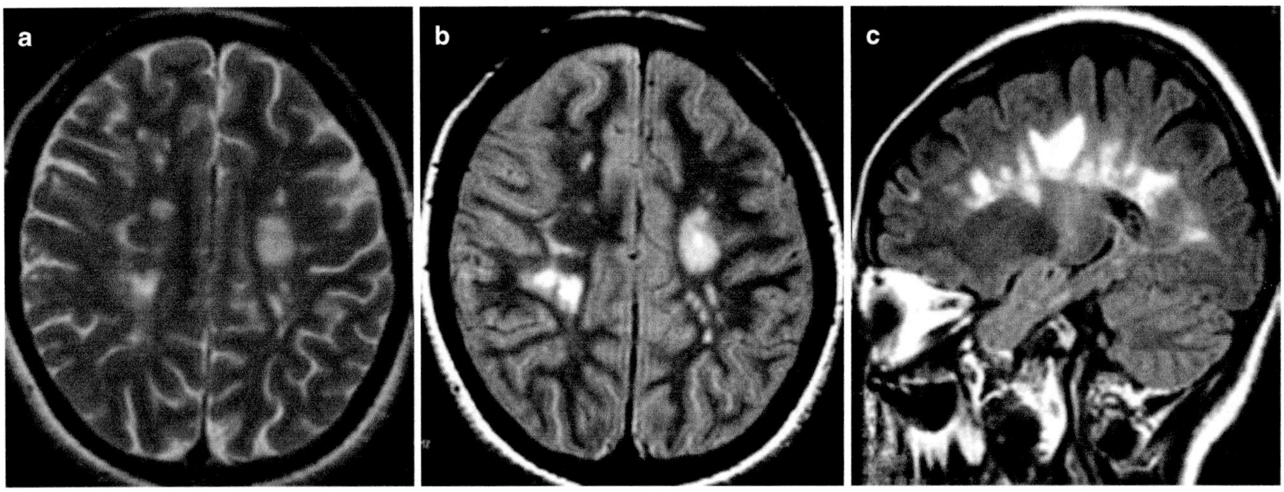

Fig. 15.2 A 26-year-old female with SRMS. (**a**) Axial T2WI shows multiple patchy and nodular lesions in the bilateral centrum semiovale areas. (**b**) Axial PDWI shows the hyperintense were more obviously in the same areas. (**c**) Sagittal T2-FLAIR shows the confluent plaques perpendicular to the body of the lateral ventricles, also called "Dawson's fingers"

1. T1WI: Lesions are typically hypointense; chronic plaques are distinctly demarcated, firm, slightly retracted, and also called T1 black holes, which are the result of demyelination, thinned matrix, and loss of axons.
2. T2WI: Lesions are typically hyperintense. Acute lesions often present marked hyperintense in the center with peripheral edema.
3. Fluid-attenuated inversion recovery (FLAIR): Lesions are typically hyperintense and may occur in the juxtacortical, brainstem, cerebellum, or spinal cord. Periventricular ovoid lesions arranged perpendicular to lateral ventricles as fingerlike projections, best visualized on sagittal images, are called "Dawson's fingers" [11]. FLAIR is more sensitive than T2WI in detection of juxtacortical and periventricular lesions, while T2WI is more sensitive of infratentorial lesions (Fig. 15.2).
4. T1 C+: Gadolinium is useful in defining active inflammation. The enhancement pattern is variable and may appear homogeneous, curvilinear, or nodular. Active lesions often show incomplete peripheral enhancement as "open-ring sign"; the enhancing part of the ring represents advanced front of demyelination and indicates the white matter side of the lesion, whereas the open part of the ring usually point toward the side of gray matter.

The spinal cord is another suffering site of predilection of MS. The cord abnormalities are detected on MRI scans in up to 89% of patients with established disease. So the spinal

Table 15.1 Updates of McDonald's criteria of MS

McDonald's criteria	2001	2005	2010
MRI DIS	≥3 of the following; • ≥1 Gadolinium enhancing lession or ≥9 T2 hyper intense lesions • ≥3 periventricular lesions • ≥1 juxtacortical lesion • ≥1 infratentorial lesion 1 cord lesion can substitute 1 brain lesion	≥3 of the following; • ≥1 Gadolinium enhancing lession or ≥9 T2 hyper intense lesions • ≥3 periventricular lesions • ≥1 juxtacortical lesion • ≥1 infratentorial lesion Any number of cord lesions can be included	≥1 T2 bright lesions in ≥2 of the following locations: • Periventricular • Juxtacortical • Infratentorial • Spinal cord
MRI DIT	≥l new gadolinium enhancing lesions on a scan performed at least 3 months after CIS onset ≥l new- hyperintense T2 lesions on a scan performed at least 3 months after CIS onset	≥1 new gadolinium enhancing lesions on a scan performed at least 3 months after CIS onset ≥l new- hyperintense T2 lesions on a scan performed at least 1 months after CIS onset	A new T2 and/or gadolinium enhancing lesion(s) on follow-up MRI at any time Simultaneous presence of asymptomatic enhancing and non-enhancing lesions at any time
CSF	+	+	–

MRI magnetic resonance imaging, *DIS* dissemination in space, *DIT* dissemination in time, *CIS* clinically isolated syndrome, *CSF* cerebrospinal fluid

cord abnormalities play a major role in the development of clinical disability. 86% of patients with MS at postmortem examination have spinal cord lesions. The cervical portion lesions are more frequent, are located more peripherally and, in less than half the cross-sectional area of the cord, are limited to two vertebral segments in length, and are not visible as T1 hypointensities. Acute cord lesions can cause swelling of the cord and enhance after Gd-DTPA administration.

Although MS has long been regarded as a WM disease, during the last decade, the extensive involvement of gray matter (GM) pathology has become evident. On histopathologic examination, GM pathology is characterized by focal demyelination, activation of microglia with little inflammatory infiltration, lymphocyte in filtration, and disruption of the blood-brain barrier. GM damage is present from the earliest stage of the disease and accumulates with disease progression. Due to the cortical GM lesion size, relaxation characteristics, and partial volume effect with CSF, focal and widespread demyelinating lesions in GM are rather inconspicuous by conventional MRI. They are often missed on conventional T2-weighted images. More recently, new MRI techniques have been developed to improve the displaying of cortical GM lesions. Recent studies have shown that both double inversion recovery (DIR) and phase-sensitive inversion recovery (PSIR) increase cortical lesion detection sensitivity and accuracy. GM atrophy is more strongly associated with neurologic disability and cognitive impairment than other imaging metrics (T2 and T1 lesion volumes and WM atrophy). Although GM atrophy has emerged as a promising marker for neural degeneration, the underlying pathologic substrates and mechanisms are not completely understood.

The diagnosis of MS is established on the base of disseminated in both space (i.e., multiple lesions) and time (i.e., lesions in different age). McDonald criteria is a guidelines of the diagnostic criteria of MS in 2001, revised in 2005 and 2010. This latest revision has improved sensitivity from 46% to 77% with specificity from 94% to 92% and accuracy of 86% in the definite diagnosis of MS after the first CIS [12]. The updates of McDonald's criteria are summarized (Table 15.1).

The revised McDonald's criteria in 2005 modified the definition of dissemination in time (DIT) to a new hyperintense T2 lesion scanning at least 1 month (instead of 3 months) after CIS onset [13]. The lesion in spinal cord was defined as multiple spinal cord lesions may be as a substitute for the brain and infratentorial lesion criteria, as long as they are >3 mm in size, the length <2 vertebral body heights, and the lesion occupies only a portion of the cord cross section (Fig. 15.3). An enhancing lesion in spinal cord may be replaced by an enhancing brain lesion.

Modifications of McDonald's criteria in each successive revision have resulted in earlier and easier diagnosis of MS. The 2010 revised McDonald's criteria simplified the definition of dissemination in space (DIS), including at least one T2 bright lesions in two or more typical sites (periventricular, juxtacortical, infratentorial, or spinal cord) [14]. Gadolinium-enhancing lesion was no more required for DIS. The criteria for DIT were also modified to include a new T2 and/or gadolinium-enhancing lesion(s) on follow-up at any time or asymptomatic-enhancing and non-enhancing lesions simultaneously existing anytime [15]. These revised DIT can be identified on a single baseline MRI scan and be made early diagnosis of MS. CSF examination for oligoclonal IgG bands was no longer needed for the diagnosis of RRMS.

MS diagnosis depends on the "DIS and DIT" evidence of the disease, which leads to the over diagnosis of MS. Therefore, Filippi et al. developed a more practical diagnostic criteria in 2016 [16]. The new guidelines remain

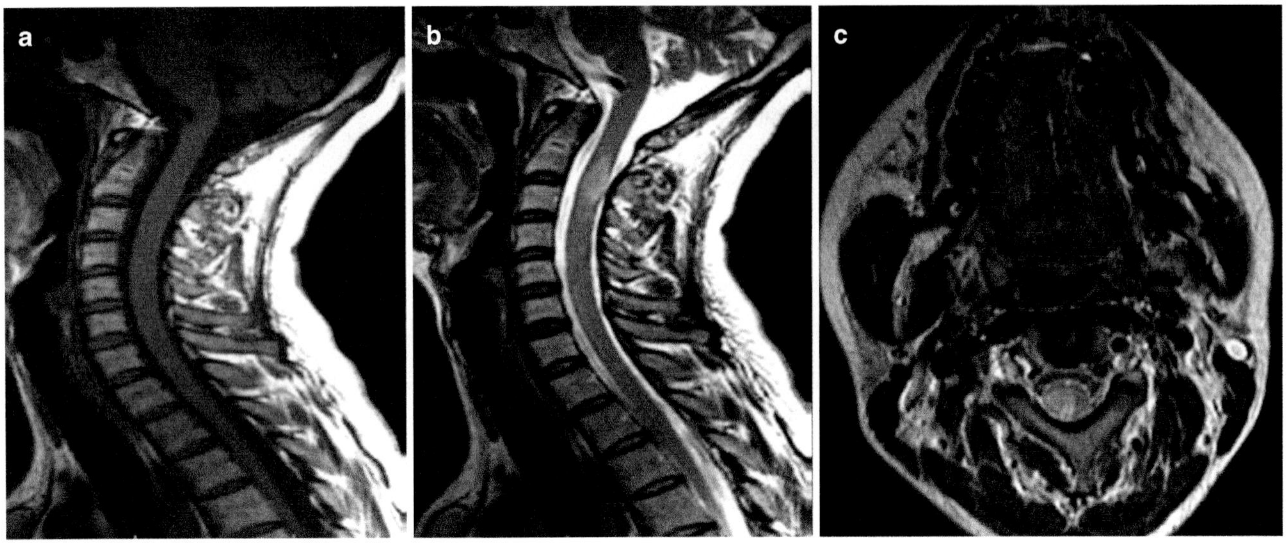

Fig. 15.3 A 20-year-old female with MS lesion in spinal cord. (**a**, **b**) Sagittal T1WI and T2WI show a strip lesion at the C2–C3 level in the cervical cord. (**c**) Axial T2WI shows the plaque in the lateral cord

the DIT requirements; however, there are four different key points compared to the criteria in 2010. Firstly, DIS requirements have a litter change, they propose an increase in the number of lesions necessary to confirm involvement of the periventricular area from one to three, then expand the concept of juxtacortical lesion including all cortical lesion types and white matter next to the cortex, and the lesion in the optic nerve should be added to the criteria [16]. Secondly, symptomatic and asymptomatic MRI lesions are included in the diagnostic criteria [17]. Thirdly, imaging of the whole spinal cord is recommended to define dissemination in space [18]. Fourthly, new criteria can be used both in primary progressive multiple sclerosis and relapse-onset multiple sclerosis [19].

Recommended 2016 MAGNIMS modifications to the 2010 McDonald criteria in the diagnosis of MS (proposed revisions): Three or more lesions are characterized to define the involvement of the periventricular WM and to establish dissemination of lesions in space. The presence of lesion in the optic nerve should be added into the criteria for dissemination in space as an additional site. The combined term cortical/juxtacortical is recommended to expand the concept of juxtacortical lesion in the criteria for dissemination in space. Imaging of the whole spinal cord is recommended to define the dissemination in space. 2016 MAGNIMS MRI criteria are recommended to establish disease dissemination in space in multiple sclerosis. Dissemination in space can be shown by involvement of at least two of five areas of the CNS as follows: three or more periventricular lesions, one or more infratentorial lesion, one or more spinal cord lesion, one or more optic nerve lesion, and one or more cortical or juxtacortical lesion.

15.4 Clinical Variants

Benign MS It accounts for about 20% of all MS patients. The patients remain fully functional in all neurological systems for 15 years after initial onset. Serial follow-up brain MRI shows few new or enlarging lesions with lower incidence of enhancement [20].

Malignant (Fulminant) MS or Marburg Disease It has a rapid deteriorating course with severe relapses, leading to disability or death within weeks to months after onset. The lesions are characterized by massive macrophage infiltration with diffuse demyelination, severe axonal injury, and destruction. MRI shows defined rings and incomplete ring enhancement lesions. Compared with prototypical MS, the Marburg variant has the most impressive feature of marked destruction of the lesions.

Schilder's Disease (SD) It is rare and usually affects children and young adults. The clinical symptoms include aphasia, dementia, personality changes, balance instability, seizures, headache, and visual disturbances. A single or two symmetrically lesions with size of at least 2–3 cm arranged in the centrum semiovale with the symptoms unusual for MS. MRI shows large ring-enhancing lesions in each brain hemisphere [21].

Baló's Concentric Sclerosis (BCS) It is a rare and aggressive demyelination leading to death within weeks to months after the onset. Pathologically, it is characterized by alternating

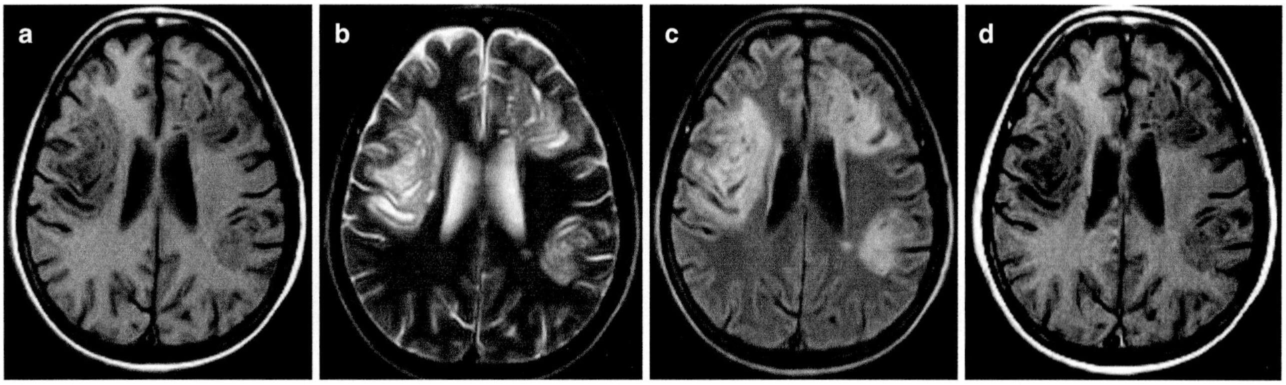

Fig. 15.4 A 48-year-old woman with left limbs paralyzed for 2 months. (**a–c**) Axial T1WI reveals multiple concentric rings with hypo-/isointense in bilateral frontoparietal cerebral white matter, on axial T2WI showing whirlpool hyperintense concentric rings, as well as on FLAIR image. (**d**) Axial T1WI after administration of gadolinium-DTPA shows minor enhancement (Courtesy of Hui Yu MD., Department of Radiology, Affiliated Hospital of Guizhou Medical University, Guiyang, China)

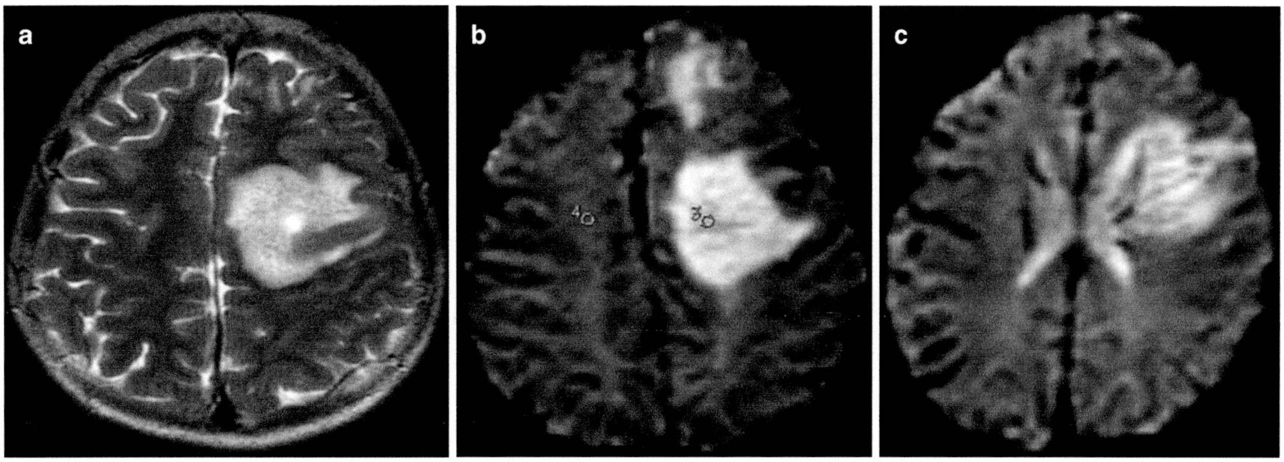

Fig. 15.5 An 18-year-old male with a diagnosis of tumefactive demyelinating MS. (**a**) Axial T2WI shows a hyperintense mass with ill-defined borders and edema in the left frontal lobe; a small lesion is located in the front of the frontal lobe. (**b**) Axial DWI shows the hyperintensity. (**c**) Axial PWI shows some linear vessels dilation in the lesion

layers of preserved and destroyed myelin [22]. These alternating bands result in the characteristic imaging appearance of T2WI concentric hypointense bands corresponding to areas of demyelination, alternating with isointense bands corresponding to normal myelinated white matter (Fig. 15.4). Gadolinium-enhanced T1WI show concentric rings of enhancement that depict active demyelination.

Tumefactive MS It presents with at least one large (>2 cm) lesion with edema, mass effect, and single or multiple focal lesions that may mimic brain tumor clinically and radiologically. Clinical presentations often include headache, confusion, aphasia, apraxia, and seizures. T1WI shows lesion hypointense and T2WI hyperintense with open-ring enhancement [23, 24]. Tumefactive demyelination is differentiated from brain tumor in the presence of multiple lesions and decrease of size or detection of new lesions on serial MRI. Marked enhancement of dilated veins running through the outside and inside of the lesion is specific for confirming the diagnosis (Fig. 15.5).

15.5 Advanced MRI Technique

Conventional MRI lacks pathological specificity and sensitivity to the presence of gray matter (GM) lesions and to the microscopic injury occurring in normal-appearing WM and GM. In the last few years, new MRI techniques, which provide better correlation with pathological features such as de- and remyelination, neuroaxonal injury, and astrogliosis, have been developed. More advanced neuroimaging techniques have been used to study of MS and other demyelination disease.

Proton Magnetic Resonance Spectroscopy (^{1}H-MRS) ^{1}H-MRS allows to measure metabolites within the lesions and normal-appearing white matter (NAWM). In active enhancing MS lesions, increased Cho, Cr, myoinositol, and glutamate and a decrease of NAA are usually observed. A similar pattern of abnormal metabolites can be detected in NAWM. In chronic lesions, NAA is markedly decreased, myoinositol is increased, and glutamate is normal [25]. Decreased ratio of NAA/Cr within MS lesions and NAWM correlates well with physical and cognitive impairment in MS patients [26]. For the low pathological specificity of ^{1}H-MRS, it is not routinely used in assessing and monitoring MS patients (Fig. 15.6).

Magnetization Transfer Imaging (MTI) The base of MTI is the interactions between protons in free water and protons bound to macromolecules. Magnetization transfer is quantified by magnetization transfer ratio (MTR), whereas a reduced MTR indicating the damage to myelin and axonal membranes [27]. And, reduced MTR has been documented in normal-appearing gray/white matter and more pronounced in progressive forms of MS [28–30]. Due to lack of standardization in acquisition protocols, it is not widely used in routine.

Diffusion-Weighted Imaging (DWI) and Diffusion Tensor Imaging (DTI) Diffusion MRI allows to asses microscopic properties. Cellular structures in the CNS restrict water molecular random motion; therefore, pathologic processes that interrupt tissue integrity would result in increased diffusion coefficient. The diffusivity in brain tissue is lower than that of free water, called the apparent diffusion coefficient (ADC). Active plaques of MS may demonstrate restricted diffusion on DWI/ADC. Mean diffusivity (MD) reflects cellular integrity, fractional anisotropy (FA) reflects fibers integrity and directionality, radial diffusivity (RD) provides a specific measure of myelin integrity, and axial diffusivity (AD) correlates with axons injury. DTI allows the segmentation and visualization of the major WM tracts. Analogous to MTI, DTI is sensitive to tissue injury and is abnormal in MS lesions and normal-appearing brain tissues [31]. DTI abnormalities have confirmed that damage to the brain in MS patients is not limited to focal and macroscopic lesions. This damage is also present in the normal-appearing gray matter, even at early stages of the disease. Abnormal gray matter diffusivity correlates with disease progression and cognitive impairment [32].

Perfusion MRI Perfusion MRI is used to analyze brain tissue perfusion with either bolus tracking of exogenous tracers or endogenous arterial water (arterial spin labeling). Active MS lesions are characterized by increased perfusion, whereas normal-appearing brain tissues have relatively decreased perfusion [33]. Utilizing perfusion MRI, we may characterize the stage of MS lesion and optimize disease management.

Susceptibility-Weighted Imaging (SWI) SWI uses the paramagnetic susceptibility effect of iron to demonstrate susceptibility differences between tissues [34]. Veins associated with MS plaques and iron-laden tissues can be visualized on SWI. Haacke et al. [35] demonstrated nearly 50% more lesions can be visualized when combining conventional imaging and SWI. Unfortunately, SWI could not provide enough specificity to differentiate MS from small vessel disease involving white matter lesions (Fig. 15.7).

Functional MRI (fMRI) fMRI measures the level of blood oxygenation, by detecting the signal generated by changes in the local magnetic field secondary to the increased amount of oxygenated hemoglobin in the venous system. fMRI is a

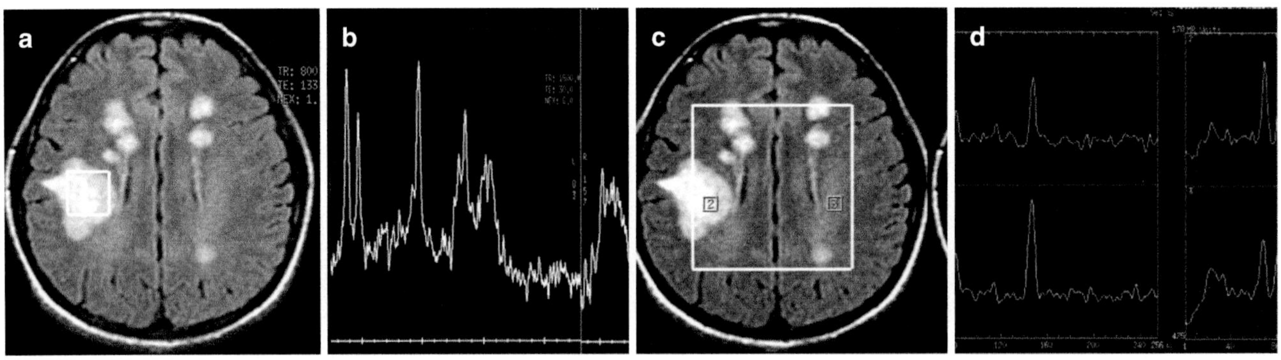

Fig. 15.6 MRS in a female patient with RRMS. (**a**, **c**) are the locations of the MR spectroscopy, (**a**) is the single volume spectroscopy, and (**c**) is the multi-voxel spectroscopy, respectively. Image (**b**) shows the increase of the lactate peak within the active lesion. Image (**d**) shows the decreased NAA within the same lesion

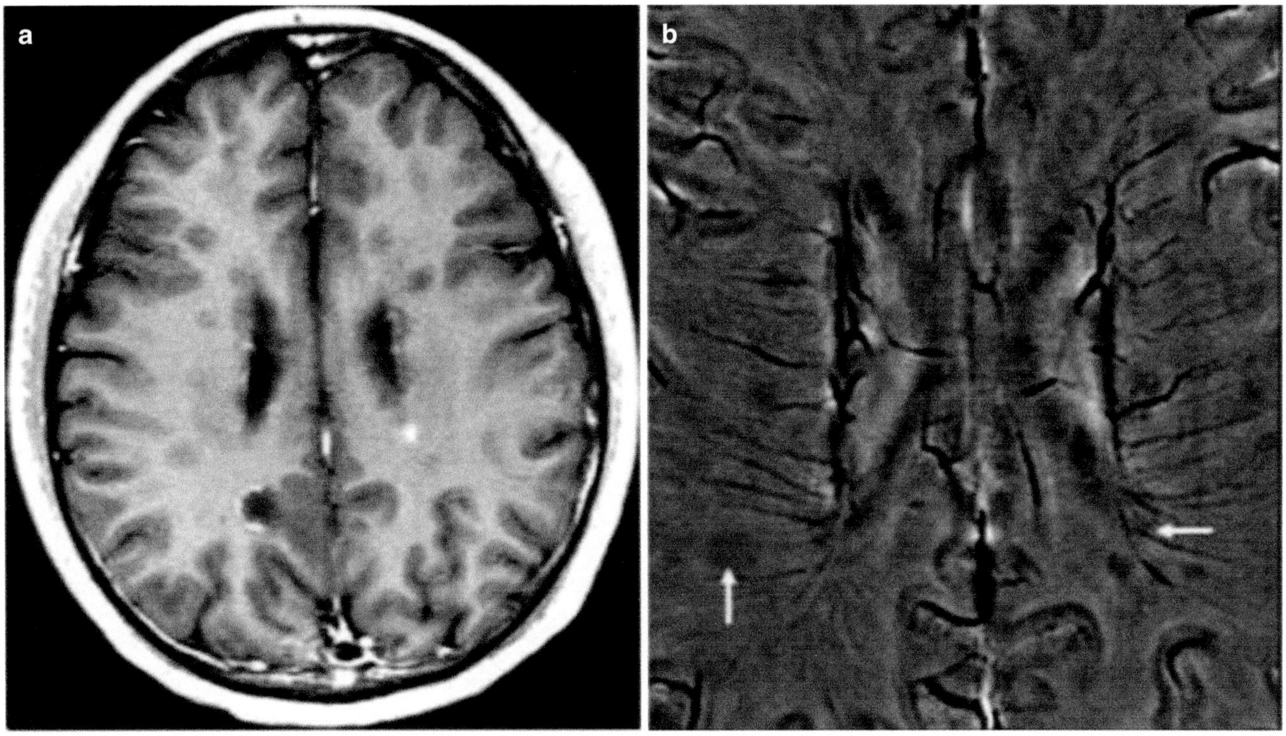

Fig. 15.7 Images in a male patient with active MS lesion. (**a**) T1WI with contrast shows some active lesions in the white matter (arrowhead). (**b**) Phase image of the SWI shows some medullary vein dilated (arrowhead)

technique used to obtain functional information by visualization of cortical activity. It detects subtle alteration in blood flow in response to stimuli or actions. It has been used in research settings to examine the neural correlates of known motor, visual, sensory, and neuropsychological deficits. The combination of measures of functional connectivity with measures of structural damage within specific white matter fiber bundles is likely to improve our understanding of the relation between structural and functional abnormalities in RRMS patients [36]. An abnormal pattern of brain activation is also correlated with fatigue [36].

Higher-Field Imaging High-field (3 T) and ultrahigh-field (>7 T) MRI equipments are more sensitive to detect T2 and gadolinium-enhancing lesions than that of 1.5 T MRI scanner [37, 38]. Higher-field-based imaging can improve the early diagnosis of MS [39]. Some specific scanning sequences such as double inversion recovery (DIR) imaging can further improve the detection of cortical MS lesions in vivo [39, 40].

15.6 Differential Diagnosis

MS must be differentiated from the following clinical entities:

Non-specific White Matter T2 Hyperintensities Old age, hypertension, diabetes, smoking, vasculitis, and migraine, all are high risk factors of non-specific T2 hyperintensities in white matter. Leukoaraiosis or small vessel disease usually shows white matter T2 hyperintensities in elderly. Location, size, clinical history, and laboratory test may help to differentiate it from MS plaques.

Acute Disseminated Encephalomyelitis (ADEM) ADEM usually precedes viral or bacterial infections or vaccinations [41]. It typically occurs within 2–4 weeks of viral infection or vaccination, with up to 90% of patients reporting a preceding infection. It can occur at any ages but more common in children and adolescents [42]. The pathology of ADEM consists of "sleeves" of demyelination with indistinct margins surrounding small, engorged venules and is associated with significant inflammatory infiltrates. It is typically monophasic. The clinical course is rapidly progressive, leading to focal or multifocal neurologic deficits that are often associated with encephalopathy (Fig. 15.8). It predominantly involves the subcortical white matter in up to 90% of cases and can also be seen in the deep nuclei, cerebellum, brainstem, and spinal cord. The spinal cord is usually affected with large, tumefactive lesions [43]. ADEM lesions are usually larger, more edematous, and symmetric or asymmetric distribution compared

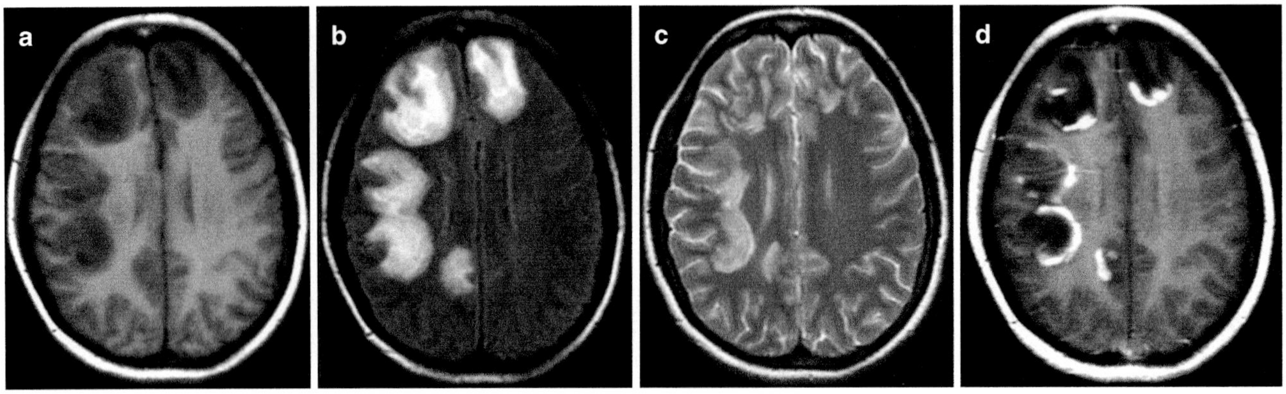

Fig. 15.8 A female with ADEM. (**a**) Axial T1WI shows multiple hypointense lesions involving the subcortical white matter. (**b**) Axial T2-FLAIR shows the hyperintensity. (**c**) Axial TIWI with contrast shows multiple open-ring enhancement lesions. (**d**) Axial PD image shows the marked improvement after therapy with steroid

to MS [44]. It is estimated that 21% of ADEM convert to MS after a mean period of 2.36 years and 27% after 5.64 years [45].

Neuromyelitis Optica (NMO) *Neuromyelitis optica (NMO)*, also known as Devic's disease, is characterized by severe relapsing attacks that usually target the optic nerves and central spinal cord. NMO is an acute, severe demyelination. It usually presents with bilateral optic neuritis and myelitis. Spinal cord imaging is characterized by longitudinally extensive myelitis and cord lesions involving more than three vertebral segments [14] (Fig. 15.9). NMO-IgG is a serum autoantibody marker that binds at or near the blood-brain barrier (BBB) which distinguishes NMO from MS. The water channel aquaporin-4 (AQP4) proved to be the target of NMO-IgG. It is highly concentrated in the astrocytic foot processes, particularly in the subpial, subependymal areas and in the hypothalamus. Demyelination and necrosis in NMO also involve the gray matter of the spinal cord and the deep gray matter. Brain MR imaging usually shows bilateral swollen optic nerve with T2 hyperintensity and contrast enhancement. Unlike MS, white matter lesions are absent or few and non-specific [46]. The term NMO spectrum disorders (NMOSDs) was introduced in 2007 to include AQP4 IgG-seropositive patients. In 2015, the Panel for NMO Diagnosis proposed new diagnostic criteria for NMOSD, which stratified further by serologic anti-AQP4 status. Immunosuppressive therapy reduces the frequency of NMO relapses, and interferon-β, commonly used for the treatment of MS [47].

Neoplastic Disease Primary CNS tumors or systemic metastases usually show gadolinium enhancement. Lymphoma can create multifocal lesions and should be included in the differential diagnosis of MS. The response to corticosteroid treatment may be helpful, as well as advanced MRI such as PWI [48].

Rheumatologic Diseases Rheumatologic diseases such as systemic lupus erythematosus (SLE), Wegener granulomatosis, polyarteritis nodosa, etc. may sometimes mimic MS. These can present with subcortical T2 hyperintensities; however, the T2 lesion burden is far lower than those in MS [48].

Sarcoidosis The characteristic MRI findings of meningeal thickening with gadolinium enhancement, hypothalamus involvement, and persistent enhancement on follow-up imaging despite treatment with corticosteroids are helpful to differentiate sarcoidosis from MS [49].

CNS Infectious Diseases Toxoplasmosis and Lyme disease may show similar imaging findings to MS; exposure histories and serology may differ from MS [50]. Progressive multifocal leukoencephalopathy (PML) usually presents as subcortical, T2 hyperintensities, which do not enhance on post-contrast T1WI.

Cerebral Autosomal Dominant Arteriopathy with Subcortical Infarcts and Leukoencephalopathy (CADASIL) CADASIL is an inherited arterial disease caused by mutations of the Notch gene on chromosome. It is characterized by recurrent transient ischemic attacks, followed by recurrent strokes, dementia, depression, pseudobulbar palsy, and hemiplegia or quadriplegia. It usually presents as confluent subcortical or periventricular areas of T2 hyperintensities and does not enhance after gadolinium administration. It mainly affects the subcortical U-fibers, anterior-inferior temporal lobes, and inferior frontal lobes [50]. Family history, cognitive features, and the absence of oligoclonal bands in the CSF may help the differentiation.

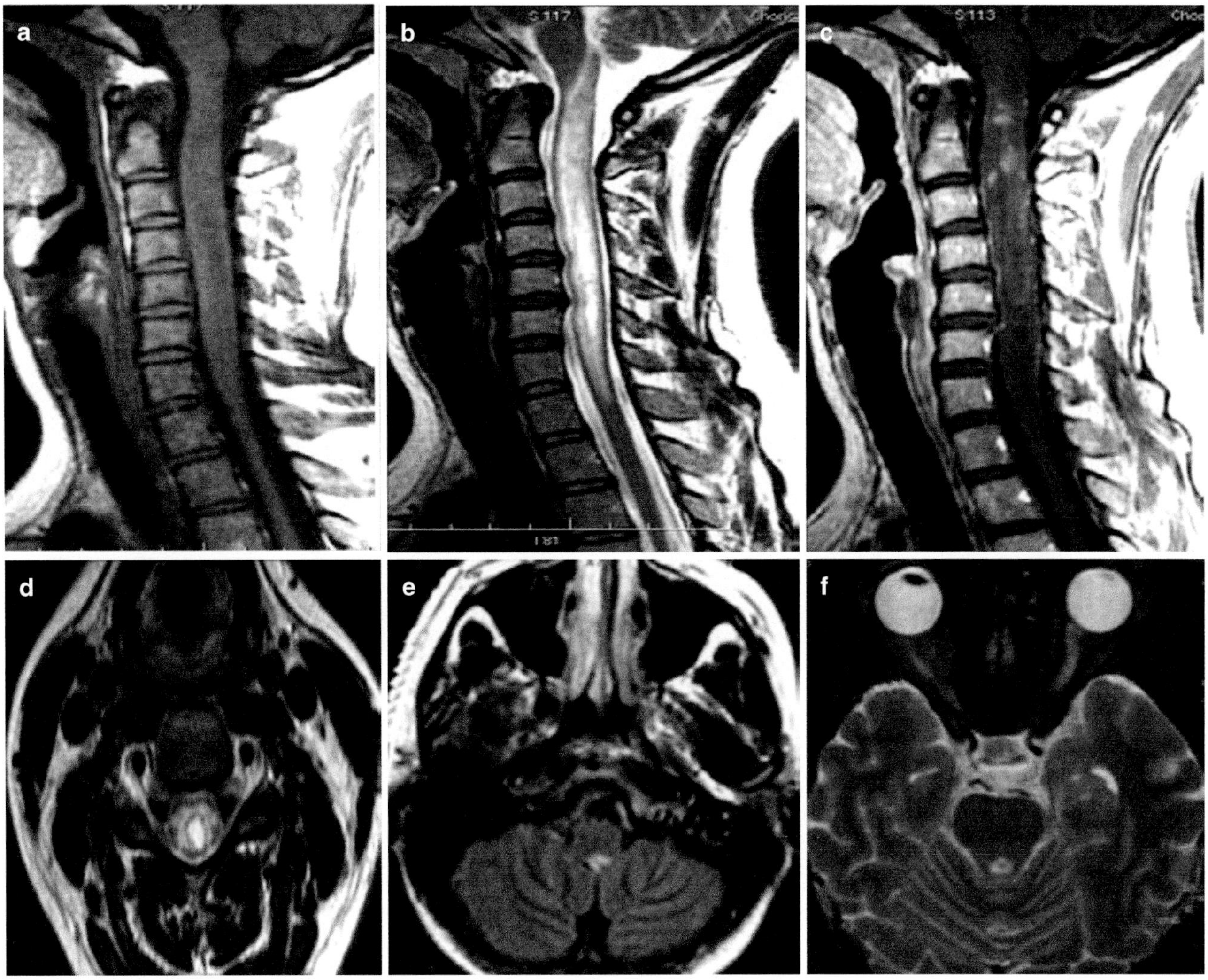

Fig. 15.9 A 22-year-old man with NMO. (**a**) Sagittal T1WI and (**b**) sagittal T2WI show hypointensity and hyperintensity signal (arrow) was extended from C1 to T1. And marked swelling of the cervical cord lesion could be noticed on T2WI. (**c**) Sagittal T1WI with contrast shows the patchy enhancements (arrow). (**d**) Axial T2WI shows lesion located in the center of the spinal cord. (**e**) Axial T2-FLAIR shows a small patchy hyperintense signal in the medulla. (**f**) Axial fat-suppressed T2WI demonstrates marked swelling of the optic nerves. The optic nerves and optic nerve sheaths cannot be identified

References

1. Berer K, Krishnamoorthy G. Microbial view of central nervous system autoimmunity. FEBS Lett. 2014;588(22):4207–13.
2. Frohman EM, Racke MK, Raine CS. Multiple sclerosis—the plaque and its pathogenesis. N Engl J Med. 2006;354(9):942–55.
3. Milo R, Miller A. Revised diagnostic criteria of multiple sclerosis. Autoimmun Rev. 2014;13(4-5):518–24.
4. Krupp LB, Banwell B, Tenembaum S. Consensus definitions proposed for pediatric multiple sclerosis and related disorders. Neurology. 2007;68(16 Suppl 2):S7–12.
5. Milo R, Kahana E. Multiple sclerosis: geoepidemiology, genetics and the environment. Autoimmun Rev. 2010;9(5):A387–94.
6. Compston A, Coles A. Multiple sclerosis. Lancet. 2008;372(9648):1502–17.
7. Lublin FD, Reingold SC. National Multiple Sclerosis Society Advisory Committee on Clinical Trials of New Agents in Multiple Sclerosis. Defining the clinical course of multiple sclerosis: results of an international survey. Neurology. 1996;46(4):907–11.
8. Miller D, Barkhof F, Montalban X, et al. Clinically isolated syndromes suggestive of multiple sclerosis, part I: natural history, pathogenesis, diagnosis, and prognosis. Lancet Neurol. 2005;4(5):281–8.
9. Okuda DT, Mowry EM, Beheshtian A, et al. Incidental MRI anomalies suggestive of multiple sclerosis: the radiologically isolated syndrome. Neurology. 2009;72(9):800–5.
10. Tsang BK, Macdonell R. Multiple sclerosis-diagnosis, management and prognosis. Aust Fam Physician. 2011;40(12):948–55.
11. Dawson JW. XVIII.-the histology of disseminated sclerosis. Trans R Soc Edinb. 1914;50:517–740.
12. Swanton JK, Fernando K, Dalton CM, et al. Modification of MRI criteria for multiple sclerosis in patients with clinically isolated syndromes. J Neurol Neurosurg Psychiatry. 2006;77(7):830–3.
13. Polman CH, Reingold SC, Edan G, et al. Diagnostic criteria for multiple sclerosis: 2005 revisions to the "McDonald criteria". Ann Neurol. 2005;58(6):840–6.

14. Polman CH, Reingold SC, Banwell B, et al. Diagnostic criteria for multiple sclerosis: 2010 revisions to the McDonald criteria. Ann Neurol. 2011;69(2):292–302.
15. Montalban X, Tintoré M, Swanton J, et al. MRI criteria for MS in patients with clinically isolated syndromes. Neurology. 2010;74(5):427–34.
16. Filippi M, Rocca MA, Ciccarelli O, et al. MRI criteria for the diagnosis of multiple sclerosis: MAGNIMS consensus guidelines. Lancet Neurol. 2016;15(3):292–303.
17. Caucheteux N, Maarouf A, Genevray M, et al. Criteria improving multiple sclerosis diagnosis at the first MRI. J Neurol. 2015;262(4):979–87.
18. Sombekke MH, Wattjes MP, Balk LJ, et al. Spinal cord lesions in patients with clinically isolated syndrome: a powerful tool in diagnosis and prognosis. Neurology. 2013;80(1):69–75.
19. Kelly SB, Kinsella K, Duggan M, et al. A proposed modification to the McDonald 2010 criteria for the diagnosis of primary progressive multiple sclerosis. Mult Scler. 2013;19(8):1095–100.
20. Cañellas AR, Gols AR, Izquierdo JR, et al. Idiopathic inflammatory-demyelinating diseases of the central nervous system. Neuroradiology. 2007;49(5):393–409.
21. Sastregarriga J, Rovira A, Río J, et al. Clinically definite multiple sclerosis after radiological Schilder-like onset. J Neurol. 2003;250(7):871.
22. Gharagozloo AM, Poe LB, Collins GH. Antemortem diagnosis of Balo concentric sclerosis: correlative MR imaging and pathologic features. Radiology. 1994;191(3):817–9.
23. Jeong IH, Kim SH, Hyun JW, et al. Tumefactive demyelinating lesions as a first clinical event: clinical, imaging, and follow-up observations. J Neurol Sci. 2015;358(1-2):118–24.
24. Mabray MC, Cohen BA, Villanueva-Meyer JE, et al. Performance of apparent diffusion coefficient values and conventional MRI features in differentiating tumefactive demyelinating lesions from primary brain neoplasms. AJR Am J Roentgenol. 2015;205(5):1075–85.
25. Srinivasan R, Sailasuta N, Hurd R, et al. Evidence of elevated glutamate in multiple sclerosis using magnetic resonance spectroscopy at 3 T. Brain. 2005;128(Pt 5):1016–25.
26. Khan O, Shen Y, Caon C, et al. Axonal metabolic recovery and potential neuroprotective effect of glatiramer acetate in relapsing-remitting multiple sclerosis. Mult Scler. 2005;11(6):646–51.
27. Wolff SD, Balaban RS. Magnetization transfer imaging: practical aspects and clinical applications. Radiology. 1994;192(3):593–9.
28. Filippi M, Iannucci G, Tortorella C, et al. Comparison of MS clinical phenotypes using conventional and magnetization transfer MRI. Neurology. 1999;52(3):588–94.
29. Filippi M, Rocca MA. Magnetization transfer magnetic resonance imaging of the brain, spinal cord, and optic nerve. Neurotherapeutics. 2007;4(3):401–13.
30. Filippi M, Agosta F. Magnetization transfer MRI in multiple sclerosis. J Neuroimaging. 2007;17(S1):22S–6S.
31. Henry RG, Joonmi O, Nelson SJ, et al. Directional diffusion in relapsing-remitting multiple sclerosis: a possible in vivo signature of Wallerian degeneration. J Magn Reson Imaging. 2003;18(4):420–6.
32. Yu HJ, Christodoulou C, Bhise V, et al. Multiple white matter tract abnormalities underlie cognitive impairment in RRMS. NeuroImage. 2012;59(4):3713–22.
33. Bakshi R, Thompson AJ, Rocca MA, et al. MRI in multiple sclerosis: current status and future prospects. Lancet Neurol. 2008;7(7):615–25.
34. Haacke EM, Xu Y, Cheng YC, Reichenbach JR. Susceptibility weighted imaging in MRI. Magn Reson Med. 2004;52(3):612–8.
35. Haacke EM, Makki MY. Characterizing iron deposition in multiple sclerosis lesions using susceptibility weighted imaging. J Magn Reson Imaging. 2009;29(3):537–44.
36. Rocca MA, Pagani E, Absinta M, et al. Altered functional and structural connectivities in patients with MS: a 3-T study. Neurology. 2007;69(23):2136–45.
37. Sicotte NL, Voskuhl RR, Bouvier S, et al. Comparison of multiple sclerosis lesions at 1.5 and 3.0 Tesla. Investig Radiol. 2003;38(7):423–7.
38. Kollia K, Maderwald S, Putzki N, et al. First clinical study on ultra-high-field MR imaging in patients with multiple sclerosis: comparison of 1.5T and 7T. AJNR Am J Neuroradiol. 2009;30(4):699–702.
39. Wattjes MP, Harzheim M, Kuhl CK, et al. Does high-field MR imaging have an influence on the classification of patients with clinically isolated syndromes according to current diagnostic mr imaging criteria for multiple sclerosis? AJNR Am J Neuroradiol. 2006;27(8):1794–8.
40. Calabrese M, Battaglini M, Giorgio A, et al. Imaging distribution and frequency of cortical lesions in patients with multiple sclerosis. Neurology. 2010;75(14):1234–40.
41. Menge T, Hemmer B, Nessler S, et al. Acute disseminated encephalomyelitis: an update. JAMA Neurol. 2005;62(11):1673–80.
42. Tenembaum S, Chitnis T, Ness J, et al. Acute disseminated encephalomyelitis. Neurology. 2007;68(16 Suppl 2):S23–36.
43. Dale RC, Branson JA. Acute disseminated encephalomyelitis or multiple sclerosis: can the initial presentation help in establishing a correct diagnosis? Arch Dis Child. 2005;90(6):636–9.
44. Bennetto L, Scolding N. Inflammatory/post-infectious encephalomyelitis. J Neurol Neurosurg Psychiatry. 2004;75(Suppl 1):i22–8.
45. Hartung HP. ADEM: distinct disease or part of the MS spectrum? Neurology. 2001;56(10):1257–60.
46. Ghezzi A, Bergamaschi R, Martinelli V, et al. Clinical characteristics, course and prognosis of relapsing Devic's Neuromyelitis Optica. J Neurol. 2004;251(1):47–52.
47. Pittock SJ, Weinshenker BG, Lucchinetti CF, et al. Neuromyelitis optica brain lesions localized at sites of high aquaporin 4 expression. Arch Neurol. 2006;63(7):964–8.
48. Rovaris M, Viti B, Ciboddo G, et al. Brain involvement in systemic immune mediated diseases: magnetic resonance and magnetisation transfer imaging study. J Neurol Neurosurg Psychiatry. 2000;68(2):170–7.
49. Joseph FG, Scolding NJ. Sarcoidosis of the nervous system. Pract Neurol. 2007;7(4):234–44.
50. Karussis D, Weiner HL, Abramsky O. Multiple sclerosis vs Lyme disease: a case presentation to a discussant and a review of the literature. Mult Scler. 1999;5(6):395–402.

16 Granulomatous Diseases of the Central Nervous System

Mei Wang and Zhongxiang Ding

16.1 Introduction

Granulomatous diseases of the central nervous system (CNS) are divided into two subgroups, specific and nonspecific. Specific types comprise the following: (1) tuberculosis (TB), (2) neurosyphilis, (3) Lyme disease, (4) nocardiosis, (5) fungal granulomas (*Cryptococcus neoformans* meningitis, *Aspergillus* meningitis, and candidosis), (6) cerebral parasitosis (cerebral cysticercosis, schistosomiasis, cerebral paragonimiasis, amoebiasis, toxoplasmosis, cerebral echinococcosis, and cerebral malaria), (7) fatal bacterial granuloma after trauma (FBGT), and (8) primary central lymphomatoid granulomatosis (LyG) [1]. Nonspecific types are also known as cryptogenic granulomas. In immunocompetent individuals, the most common granulomatous diseases are tuberculosis, sarcoidosis, idiopathic chronic scleroderma, granulomatous vasculitis, and herpes zoster (VZV) [2].

In developing countries, CNS infection is not uncommon. Infective substances enter the central nervous system through the bloodstream and cause tissue destruction. Some lesions form similar to tumors. Although enhancement can be found in the tumor on enhanced CT and MR examinations and have peripheral edema, infectious lesions may also have similar characteristics [3]. As knowledge deepens, the types of pathogens we know became more and more, which increases the difficulty of diagnosis. Mostly infectious disease will be treated conservatively, if the diagnosis is established by a noninvasive method [4].

CNS infection threatens human life. The diagnosis of infectious diseases depends on laboratory tests, but neuroimaging also plays an important role in early diagnosis because laboratory tests take longer time. Magnetic resonance imaging (MRI) is considered a good means of examination. It has high specificity and sensitivity, which is helpful to clarify the disease and assist in the implementation of treatment decisions. In addition, advanced MR techniques (such as DWI, SWI, and MRS) can also assist physicians in the diagnosis and identification of possible complications of neurological infections, thereby reducing morbidity and mortality [5].

When a neurologist is facing an immigrant or traveler who has neurological symptoms, diagnosing a potential central nervous system infection is crucial. The neurologist should think of possible underlying causes and perform appropriate diagnostic tests such as laboratory tests and neuroimaging examinations to aid diagnosis [6]. Similarly, radiologists should also understand the clinical manifestations and complications of the disease and deal with regional specific infections [7].

16.2 Tuberculosis of the CNS

Tuberculosis (TB) of the CNS is divided into two types according to the location of the lesion, including intracranial TB and spinal cord TB. Intracranial TB is usually secondary to hematogenous dissemination of pulmonary TB or TB of other regions, and it often occurs in children and adolescents. There are three different types of TB, including tuberculous meningitis, cerebral tuberculoma, and tuberculous abscess of the brain; these types may occur separately or in combination. TB of the CNS is typically characterized by tuberculous granuloma, also known as a tuberculous nodule. After anti-TB treatment, TB can be reduced, calcified, and even completely absorbed. However, sequelae of CNS TB, including arachnoid adhesion, encephalatrophy, and hydrocephalus, may persist [8].

Spinal cord TB infection with tubercle bacillus usually derives from other organs, such as the lung or kidney, via the blood circulation, or occurs via direct spinal TB infection. Spinal cord TB is also known as tuberculous meningomyelitis because of the frequent involvement of the meninges. Spinal symptoms typically progress slowly, along with other symptoms including low-grade fever, anorexia, loss of body weight, and night sweats.

M. Wang · Z. Ding (✉)
Department of Radiology, Affiliated Hangzhou First People's Hospital, Zhejiang University School of Medicine, Hangzhou, China

B. Gao et al. (eds.), *Imaging of CNS Infections and Neuroimmunology*, https://doi.org/10.1007/978-981-13-6904-9_16

16.2.1 Clinical Presentation and Pathology

The pathology of intracranial TB is described in the following text [9]. Meninges exhibit a large amount of inflammatory exudate with tuberculous nodules. The lesions mainly involve the pia mater, especially the area of the suprasellar cistern. Hydrocephalus may be found due to a blockage of cerebrospinal fluid (CSF). Cerebral parenchyma contains single or multiple small caseous nodules (central necrosis). A few cases present irregular malacic foci.

Cerebral tuberculoma, which is often located in the cortex with a rich blood supply, is nodular or lobulated and ranges in size from 2 to 6 cm. There is a fibrous coat on the periphery and caseous necrosis in the central region, with calcification in a few cases. Pus is formed in very few cases. There are few inflammatory cells, but astrocytosis can be observed. Hydrocephalus is observed.

Cerebral arteritis is characterized by cerebral infarction.

Tuberculous abscess of the brain, which is very rare and often multilocular, has a general pathology similar to purulent abscesses, exhibiting granulation tissue in most peripheral areas.

Cases with mainly intraspinal cord involvement may present single or multiple intramedullary tuberculous granuloma or tuberculoma, and severe cases might exhibit cavity formation. The cases with mainly spinal cord involvement often exhibit a thickening spinal membrane and nerve root, and they might also have tuberculous meningitis or vasculitis. The spinal cord ischemia caused by secondary spinal cord compression or obstruction may result in pathological changes in ischemic injury in the spinal cord [10].

16.2.2 Clinical Presentations

Intracranial TB

Tubercular meningitis: Its symptoms include systemic poisoning, signs of meningeal irritation, intracranial hypertension, epilepsy, nervous disorders, brain stem injury, conscious disturbance, CSF drainage by high lumbar pressure, and moderately elevated protein content in cells.

Cerebral tuberculoma: Similar to the general intracranial space-occupying lesions, this condition presents intracranial hypertension and fixed nervous system signs in the affected location. For supratentorial tuberculoma, headache, epilepsy, hemiplegia, aphasia, and abnormal sensation may occur. Infratentorial tuberculoma is associated with intracranial hypertension and cerebellum malfunction. TB abscess of the brain: This condition mainly manifests as headache, vomiting, fever, and encephalitis.

Spinal Cord TB

This condition is more common in young adults, and the patient may have a history of TB exposure or TB. Onset is usually slow. In addition to showing spinal cord symptoms, patients may also experience low-grade fever, anorexia, loss of body weight, and night sweats. The spinal cord damage is often incomplete, showing below-lesion level symptoms such as limb paralysis, sensory disturbance, and defection dysfunction. Lesions that mainly involve damage in the spinal membrane and spinal arachnoid membrane exhibit radicular pain as a main sign, with dispersed, asymmetric, and segmental sensory disorders.

16.2.3 Imaging Characteristics

X-Rays Tubercular meningitis sometimes shows increased intracranial pressure, with calcification near the top of the sella turcica in the late stage, mainly near the cisterna ambiens and suprasellar cistern. The cerebral angiography mainly shows uniform or irregular narrowing of the basilar artery trunk lumen. A wide range of cerebral veins may also become thinner. The characteristic manifestation of tuberculoma is calcification, but the incidence is not high. The cerebral angiography of the disease is the same as other hypovascular-occupying lesions. The plain film of the tuberculous abscess is similar to that of the purulent abscess, but no gas shadows are observed. A chest X-ray examination shows active or old tuberculous lesions. Complicated spinal TB or tuberculous paravertebral abscesses are shown in some cases. Spine X-rays of these patients reveal the following typical changes in spinal TB: vertebral body destruction, kyphosis, angulation deformity, and paravertebral cold abscess.

Computed Tomography (CT) A plain scan shows an increased density of the subarachnoid, especially in the suprasellar cistern and lateral fissure cistern, with punctate calcification during the late stage. For enhanced scanning, an obvious irregular enhancement is observed in the above areas, with cerebral edema, hydrocephalus, and cerebral infarction, among other symptoms. Plain and enhanced scans provide results similar to pyogenic abscess of the brain without air. The lesions are single or multiple or even widely distributed. For the latter, plain scanning shows multiple small nodules exhibiting iso-density or low density in the intracerebral parenchyma; these nodules are diffusely distributed in the brain and cerebellar areas. The enhanced scanning shows enhancement of the nodules. A plain scan shows nodules exhibiting iso-density, low density, or mixed density, with nodule calcification in some cases. Approximately 80% are single lesions and 20% are multiple lesions, with mild edema in the surrounding area showing a mass effect.

Magnetic Resonance Imaging (MRI) Tubercular meningitis commonly occurs at the base of the brain, manifesting as extensive inflammation, leakage, adhesion, and thickening of the pia mater and subarachnoid at the base of the brain. T1-weighted images show an increased signal in the brain basal cistern, with an even higher signal in the T2-weighted image (Figs. 16.1 and 16.2). Enhanced MRI shows an abnormal signal in the arachnoid space. The following three complications often result from tubercular meningitis: tuberculous meningoencephalitis, cerebral infarction, and communicating hydrocephalus. Tuberculous meningoencephalitis is common in the brain parenchyma near the basis cerebri, thalamus, and basal ganglia. Spot-shaped hyperintensity in the above areas of the brain parenchyma are observed in T2-weighted images. The parenchyma appears scattered or sliced, with the low-signal shadows indicating caseation, with peripheral enhancement in the enhanced image. Cerebral infarction is common in the blood supply area of the middle cerebral artery, with little infarction. T2-weighted image showed small sheets of hyperintensity scattered in the basal ganglia and parietal and occipital lobes. The inflammatory TB exudate in the basal cistern of the brain could easily involve the mesencephalic aqueduct to cause the blockage. MRI shows ventricular dilatation and effusion above the aqueduct. The enhanced image shows a strip-shaped enhancement in the aqueduct. T1-weighted images show a weak signal (capsule exhibiting an iso-signal), and T2-weighted image is uneven (capsule exhibiting a low or slightly elevated signal). Tuberculoma calcification shows a weak signal on both T1- and T2-weighted images.

The MRI of spinal cord TB shows the involvement of swollen spinal cord. The tuberculoma manifests as an equivalent or low-signal lesion in the T1-weighted image and a low and

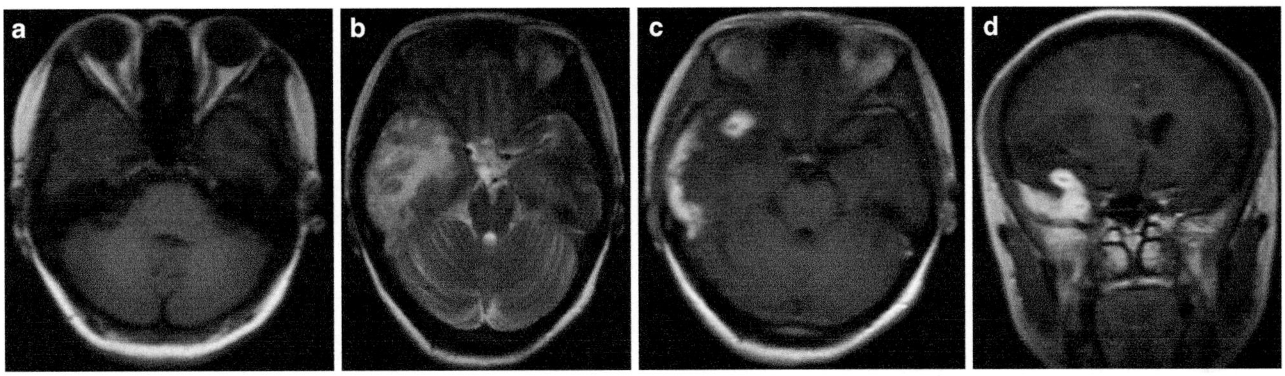

Fig. 16.1 Intracranial tuberculous granuloma; a nodular abnormal signal is observed in the right temporal lobe. The T1-weighted image demonstrates slight hypointensity (**a**) while the T2-weighted image mixed signal intensity (**b**). Significant heterogeneous ring-like enhancement of the lesions with obvious edema around the lesion was noted on post-contrast images, as well as the right temporal meningeal thickening (**c**, **d**)

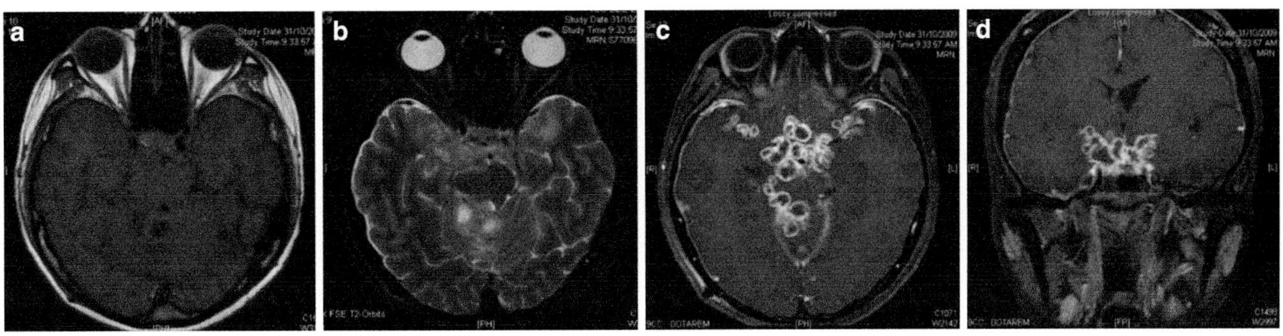

Fig. 16.2 Intracranial tuberculous granuloma; multiple thick-walled capsule-like abnormalities in the bilateral temporal lobe, brain stem, and cerebellar vermis are observed. The T1-weighted image isointensity with slight hypointensity centrally (**a**) and hyperintensity on the T2-weighted image with obvious edema around the lesion (**b**). Clear ring-like enhancement is observed on the post-contrast T1 images (**c**, **d**)

equivalent high-signal lesion in the T2-weighted image. After intravenous administration of the contrast agent, nodular enhancement on the edge of or inside the lesion is observed. The involvement of the spinal membrane and spinal arachnoid membrane manifests as a thickening lumbar nerve root and as the disappearance of the subarachnoid space on MRI. After injecting Gd-DTPA, the posterior nerve root and spinal cord surface show the following types of line-like signal enhancement: dural, arachnoid, and plaque-like signal enhancement (Figs. 16.3, 16.4, and 16.5).

16.2.4 Diagnosis and Differential Diagnosis

Intracranial TB The CT and MRI results for tubercular meningitis are similar to those for meningitis caused by other pathogens. Therefore, the qualitative diagnosis must be performed in combination with clinical information. It is not difficult to make a diagnosis if there is a history of TB with the following clinical findings, based on CT and MRI results: slow onset, toxic systemic symptoms, signs of meningeal irritation, moderately elevated CSF cell numbers and protein

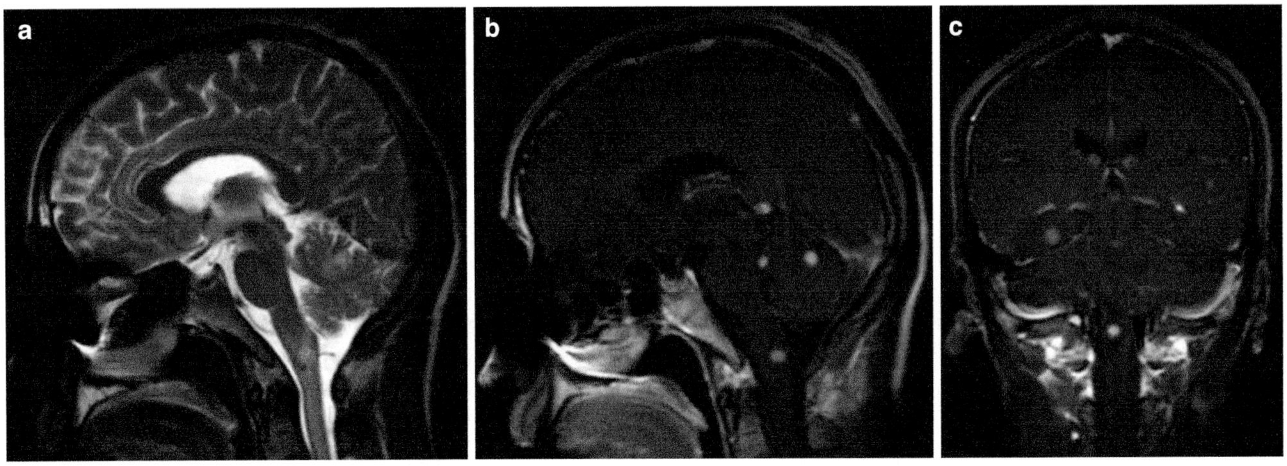

Fig. 16.3 Cervical spinal cord TB; multiple abnormal signal shadows can be observed in the medulla oblongata, cerebellum, right temporal lobe, and upper cervical spinal cord. T2-weighted image demonstrates a slightly increased signal (**a**) and significant homogeneous enhancement on post-contrast T1 images (**b, c**)

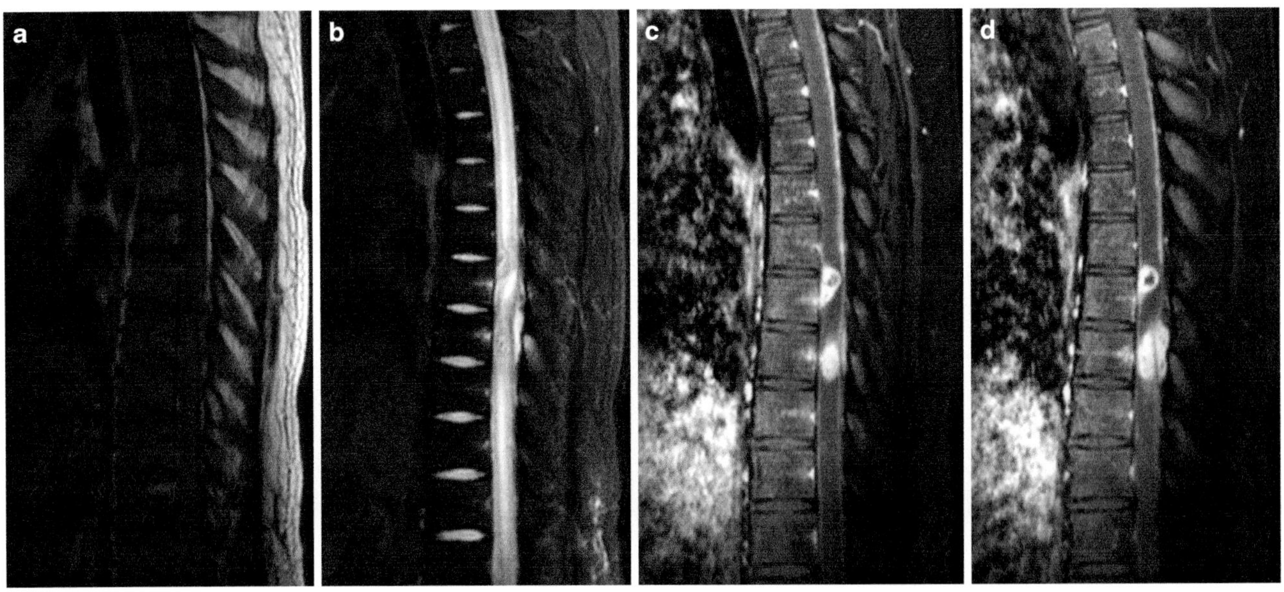

Fig. 16.4 Thoracic spinal cord TB. A thick-walled capsule-like abnormal signal intensity can be observed in the spinal cord at T7–8 vertebral level. On the T1-weighted image, the capsule wall shows an equivalent signal, and the inner capsule shows a weak signal (**a**); on the T2-weighted image, the capsule wall shows an equivalent signal, and the inner capsule shows a weak signal (**b**). The enhanced scan shows ring enhancement with edema around the lesion (**c, d**)

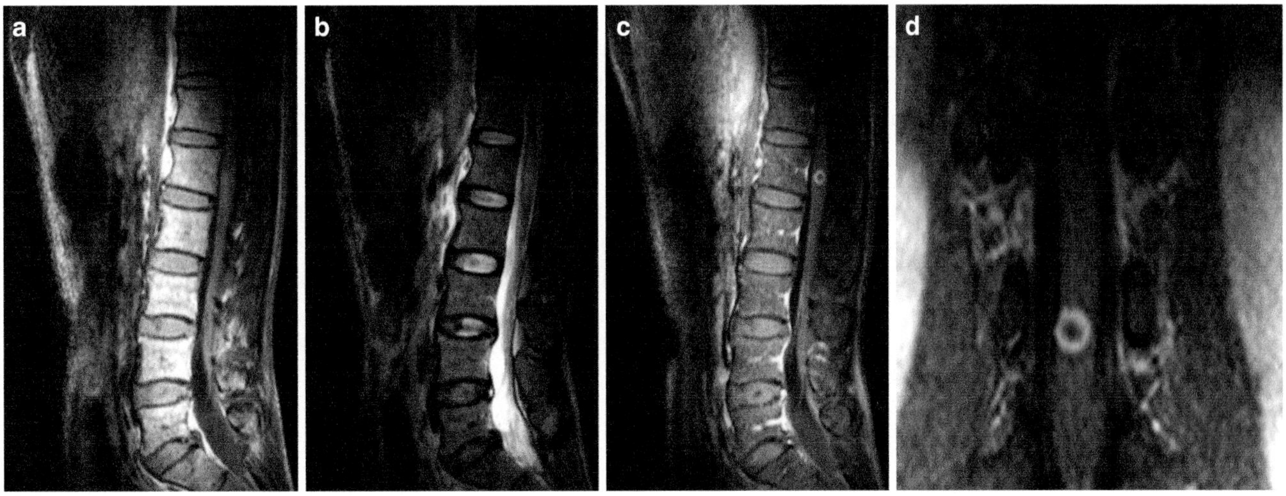

Fig. 16.5 Lumbar cord TB. A thick-walled capsule-like abnormal signal shadow can be observed in the spinal cord at lumbar 1 vertebral level. The capsule wall shows an equivalent signal in the T1- and T2-weighted images (**a, b**). The enhanced scan shows ring enhancement with edema around the spinal cord (**c, d**)

contents, and decreased chloride and glucose levels. The occurrence of calcified plaques in the cerebral-based cistern facilitates the differential diagnosis. The above imaging findings together with the history and clinical manifestations of TB infection allow for the consideration of a diagnosis of TB. Approximately 50% patients may have no history of TB, and CT and MRI manifestations are not typical, for which a differential diagnosis based on primary intracranial tumors and metastatic tumors is difficult. Tuberculous abscess in the brain is rare, and a differential diagnosis based on a pyogenic abscess of the brain and a brain tumor is usually difficult.

Spinal Cord TB Based on a history of TB, impaired symptoms of chronic or subacute onset of the spinal cord and/or the spinal membrane, specific changes in the CSF, and X-ray and MRI images of the spinal cord, diagnosis is generally not difficult. In clinical practice, tuberculous myelitis must still be differentiated from arachnoiditis of the spinal cord and subacute encephalomyelitis due to other causes. The symptoms of spinal arachnoid often fluctuate, and a spinal X-ray is commonly needed. In addition, the protein level can be slightly elevated in the CSF, but the glucose and chloride levels are generally normal. Identification of the CSF changes in chronic and subacute pyogenic encephalomyelitis with tuberculous encephalomyelitis is extremely difficult and should be based on the medical history and observation of the spinal MRI [11].

16.3 Neurosyphilis

Neurosyphilis is a group of clinical syndromes involving damage of the meninges, brain, vessels, or spinal cord of the nervous system by *Spirochaeta pallida*. It can occur during all syphilis stages, often because of an absence of radical testing during early syphilis infection. Neurosyphilis is usually an important manifestation of the systemic damage of terminal syphilis. With the use of penicillin, the incidence of syphilis has been declining, but after the 1970s, the incidence showed an upward trend, particularly among patients with acquired immune deficiency syndrome (AIDS) and poor immunity.

16.3.1 Clinical Presentation and Pathology

The pathological change during the early stage of syphilis is meningitis, which manifests as an infiltrate of meningovascular peripheral lymphocytes and monocytes. Basilar meningitis can invade cranial nerves, leading to a predisposition to the palsy symptoms associated with cranial nerves III, VI, and VII. The inflammation involving meningeal arterioles can cause arteritis obliterans and brain or spinal cord focal ischemic necrosis. After meningitis, the inflammatory corpuscle further migrates to the pallium and small cortical vessels, resulting in cortical neuron loss and gliocyte proliferation, in which the microspironema pallidum can be detected in the cerebral cortex of the patient. Syphilitic tabes dorsalis show inflammation of the spinal membrane and small vessels associated with the dorsal root and funiculi posterior degeneration. Optic nerve injury in syphilis shows optic atrophy and nutrient vessel inflammatory reactions.

16.3.2 Clinical Manifestations

Asymptomatic neurosyphilis refers to CSF abnormalities without neurological signs and symptoms. Syphilis of the meninges can occur during any stage of syphilis infection and is more common at 1 year after syphilis infection, manifesting as syphilitic meningitis. Meningovascular syphilis may involve the blood vessels of the brain, causing cerebral infarction. Cerebral tabes and tabes dorsalis are a group of clinical syndromes characterized by degeneration and necrosis in the nerve cells caused by invasion of the microspironema pallidum to the funiculi posterior of the spinal cord and dorsal root. Gummatous neurosyphilis is rarely observed, including syphilitic gumma of the brain and spinal cord gumma, and manifests characteristics similar to a brain tumor, intracerebral abscess, or TB of the brain, whereas spinal cord gumma is a granuloma of the spinal membrane.

16.3.3 Imaging Characteristics

CT Syphilitic gumma of the brain can occur in any part of the brain tissue. Imaging examination reveals single or multiple lesions. CT shows a low density or iso-density surrounded by an area of edema, potentially with ring enhancement.

MRI Brain MRI of patients with syphilitic gumma is typical. The lesion is similar to a rotundity on a T2-weighted image; it is approximately 2 cm in diameter and is located in the cerebral cortex and subcortex. The caseous necrosis in the center of the lesion shows a low, equivalent, or low mixed signal, with a surrounding hypointensity caused by a relatively large area of edema exhibiting a mass effect. Caseous necrosis in T2-weighted images show hyperintensity or mixed signal intensity, with hyperintensity of the surrounding area of edema. Gd-DTPA contrast-enhanced scanning shows irregular ring enhancement in the lesion because the brain barrier for the new vessel is not mature in the peripheral inflammatory granulation tissue of the necrotic area. The surrounding meningeal enhancement indicates meningeal involvement (Fig. 16.6).

Tabes dorsalis: MRI of the spine reveals atrophy of the cord and intramedullary hyperintensity on T2-weighted images, without any enhancement of the Gd-DTPA, suggesting focal myelitis.

16.3.4 Diagnosis and Differential Diagnosis

Other inflammatory granulomas, metastatic encephaloma, and malignant meningioma can all show similar imaging

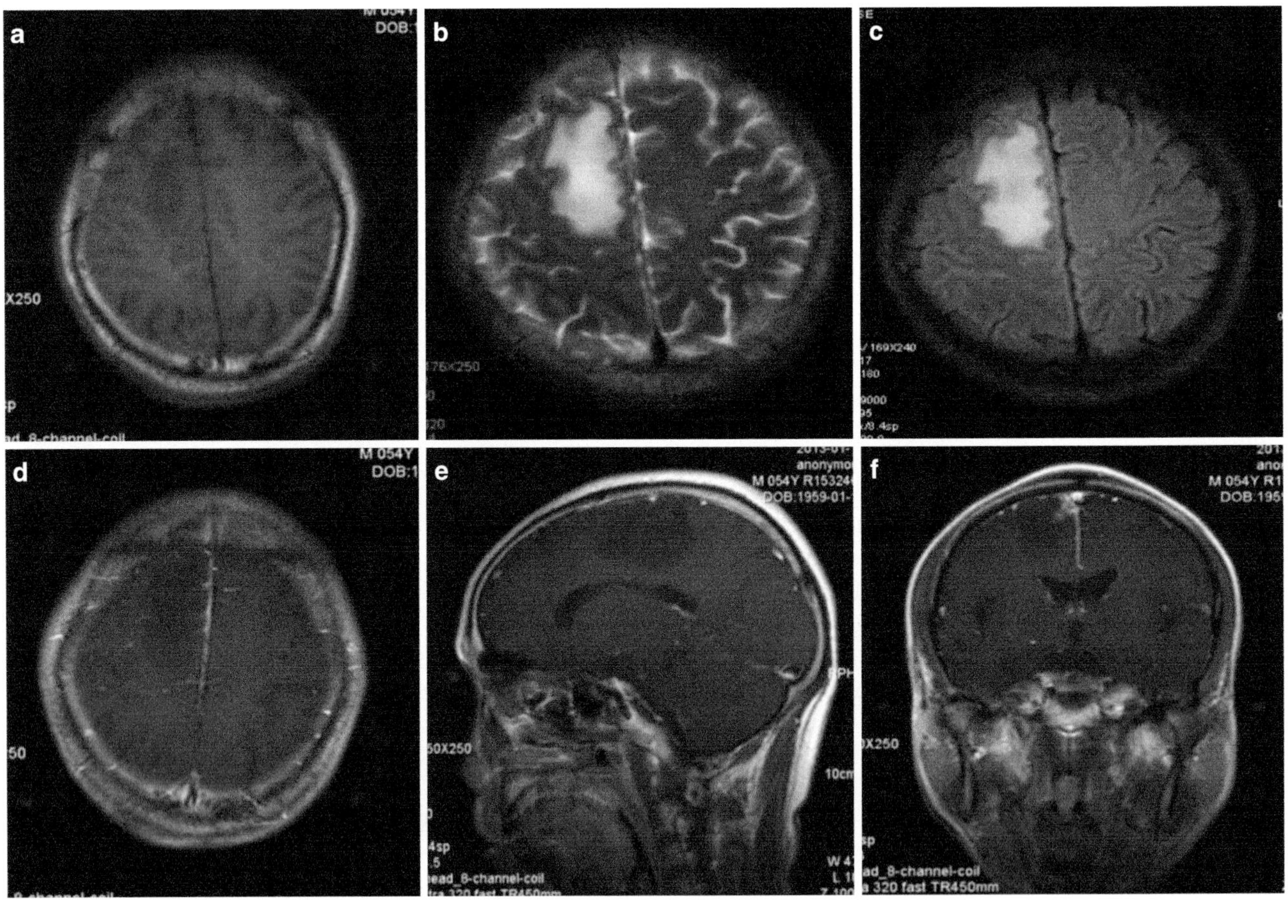

Fig. 16.6 Intracranial syphilitic granuloma; an irregular shadow representing the nodules can be observed near the superior sagittal sinus of the right forehead. The T1-weighted image shows a slightly weak signal (**a**), and the T2-weighted and FLAIR image shows a slightly increased signal (**b, c**). The lesions in the enhanced scan are significantly enhanced, with clear borders and significant edema around the lesion (**d–f**)

manifestations, with markedly enhanced nodules, central necrosis, and a large surrounding area of edema. The key points for identification are as follows: (1) Gummas mostly originate in and thus have a close relationship with the meninges. The maximum lesion level exhibits a focal edge, and peripheral meninges intersect at an obtuse angle. In contrast, other inflammatory granulomas (such as tuberculoma, cryptococcosis, and toxoplasmic granuloma) are mostly located in the brain parenchyma, so the obtuse angle intersection and metastatic meningeal tumors are generally not observed; the extensive meningeal enhancement and small nodules can be easily identified. (2) The lump of the malignant meningioma is generally larger than that of the gumma. If the lesion is small, then the chance of central necrosis is low. Tabes dorsalis must be differentiated from motor neuron disease, cervical spondylosis, MS, and spinal cord tumor, and tabes dorsalis must also be differentiated from the subacute combined degeneration of diabetes mellitus and pseudotabes.

16.4 Lyme Disease

Lyme disease is a natural focal disease caused by *Borrelia burgdorferi*. It is the most popular arthropod infectious disease in the Europe and United States. The most important clinical manifestation of the disease is the damage of the nervous system. The disease is more common in young adults and is closely related to occupations. The infection rate of field workers and forest workers is high [12].

16.4.1 Clinical Presentation and Pathology

The neurological damage of Lyme disease is manifested as *Borrelia burgdorferi* highly neurotropic. The first stage of Lyme disease is characterized by characteristic skin lesions (chronic erythema) and systemic infections (fever, headache, nausea, vomiting, and lymphadenopathy). The second stage is mainly manifested as nervous system damage and heart conduction disorder. The third stage mainly manifested as recurrent arthritis and chronic atrophic limb dermatitis, and some patients had mental abnormalities. About 10–15% of the patients had obvious symptoms of nervous system damage, multiple manifestations, and no specificity. The pathology showed cerebrovascular lymphocytes, plasma cell infiltration, and intimal thickening, and spirochetes can be found (the second stage).

16.4.2 Imaging Characteristics

Cerebral imaging of Lyme disease manifests as non-specific white matter changes. T2-weighted MR images showed that the lesions in the subcortical white matter have normal or slightly higher signal, but no obvious enhancement after enhanced MR scan, and in the brain stem and basal ganglia can have little damage. The meninges are locally thickened and abnormally enhanced. Spinal cord involvement can also be seen, characterized by a number of multiple lesions that are abnormally enhanced along the spinal cord [13].

16.4.3 Diagnosis and Differential Diagnosis

The diagnosis of neural Lyme disease is based on epidemiological, meningitis, radiculitis, encephalopathy, and myelopathy and performance-specific serological diagnostic tests. Biting history and erythema chronicum migrans (ECM) can prompt diagnosis. The disease should be identified with idiopathic facial neuritis, aseptic meningitis, and multiple sclerosis. The lack of specificity of early symptoms makes it very important for physicians to strengthen their understanding of the disease.

16.5 Nocardiosis

Nocardiosis is an infectious disease caused by *Nocardia* that can invade the lungs, skin, soft tissues, central nervous system, and heart, leading to purulent inflammation and abscess formation at the lesion site. The disease mostly occurs in patients with reduced immune function, and the *Nocardia* species that causes human disease is mainly Nocardia asteroides. Its invasive pathways include the respiratory tract and direct contamination of wounds and occasionally the gastrointestinal tract. The incidence of primary central nervous system disease without evidence of epineurium involvement is approximately 5–33%, and the involvement of central nervous system in disseminated disease ranges from 20% to 40% [14].

16.5.1 Clinical Presentation and Pathology

The disease easily occurs in immunosuppressed individuals, but there are also reports of disease in immunocompetent individuals. Unlike the form of propagation of nocardiosis in the lungs, central nervous system infections may be characterized by no fever or leukocytosis, and these manifestations may affect the clinical diagnosis of the origin of the infection.

In cerebral nocardiosis, the CNS is affected in one-third of cases. Most cases of disease derive from the lungs, and a few can also result from primary lesions. Lesions invade the brain to cause meningitis, and they invade the brain parenchyma to form multiple abscesses that can also undergo fusion into a large abscess. Symptoms of meningeal irritation or cerebral space-occupying lesions are observed, with headache, dizziness, nausea, vomiting, irregular fever, fatigue, convulsion, numbness, hemiplegia, stiff neck, visual impairment, confusion, papilledema, blood stasis, and peripheral white blood cell count increased performance.

The central nervous system infection caused by nocardiosis usually presents as an abscess, which is more common in the brain, but cerebellar abscess and spinal abscess can also occur. Nocardia meningitis and endophthalmitis are less common, but the condition is equally severe. Meningitis often causes death, and endophthalmitis usually blinds the affected eye. The main pathological changes were pyogenic granuloma with massive neutrophils, plasma cells, and histiocytic infiltration. Tissue necrosis forms abscesses that tend to fuse, and hyphae can be found within the abscesses.

16.5.2 Imaging Characteristics

Abscesses are usually formed by agglomeration of multiple small lesions and are mostly multilocular. These findings are indistinguishable from other purulent brain abscesses and tumor necrosis. Diffusion-weighted imaging (DWI) and magnetic resonance spectroscopy (MRS) may play an important role in differential diagnosis. The acute abscesses in MRS are mostly manifested as elevated levels of amino acids and bacterial metabolites, including succinate, lactate, and acetate [14].

16.5.3 Diagnosis and Differential Diagnosis

The clinical manifestations of Nocardia encephalitis have no apparent specificity. The T2-weighted MR images showed hypointensity around microcystic lesions, and the multiloculated patterns with relatively small mass effects after administration of gadolinium chelate on the T1-weighted images prove this diagnosis even if the lesion is single and there is no immunosuppression [14]. Patients with suspected disease should be examined in a timely manner using multiple techniques. The differential diagnosis should be performed with related diseases such as actinomycosis, TB, bacterial cerebral abscess, and cerebral tumor, among others.

16.6 Fungal Granulomas of the CNS

Fungal granulomas of the CNS are caused by severe fungal infection. Therefore, any fungus that can cause deep tissue infection can lead to this disease, including *Cryptococcus histolyticus*, *Aspergillus*, actinomycetes, *Histoplasma capsulatum*, *Monilia*, *Allescheria boydii*, and phycomycetes, among which *Cryptococcus histolyticus*, *Aspergillus*, and actinomycetes are the most common [15].

Fungi are widely distributed in nature. When human resistance is reduced, inhaled fungi can form a pulmonary lesion and spread from the lungs to other organs and the brain through the blood. A small number of fungi (such as aspergillus, actinomycetes, and blastomycetes) can directly invade the CNS through lesions in the oral cavity, nasal cavity, paranasal sinus, orbit, and vertebra in the head and face. The patients usually experience low-grade fever and occasionally high-grade fever. The primary symptom is headache associated with signs of meningeal irritation, including nausea, vomiting, and neck rigidity. The course of disease ranges from a few weeks to 6 months, and it can occasionally extend to more than 1 year. Few cases can be alleviated and relapse is common.

Imaging characteristics are non-specific and include enhancing intraparenchymal and extraparenchymal (skull-base) mass lesions with peripheral edema, basal meningeal enhancement, hydrocephalus, and infarcts, with or without hemorrhage. Imaging may also provide evidence of sinus, orbit, and mastoid involvement. The mass lesions may have homogenous (granuloma) or peripheral ring (abscess) enhancement (Fig. 16.7). Common differential diagnoses for fungal mass lesions include pyogenic abscess, tuberculoma, lymphoma, metastasis, glioma, and meningioma if the mass is dural based. A common differential diagnosis of rhinocerebral disease is sinonasal malignancy [16].

16.7 *Cryptococcus Neoformans* Meningitis

Cryptococcus neoformans meningitis is the most common fungal infection of the CNS and is caused by infection with *Cryptococcus histolyticus*, manifesting clinically as fever, headache, and vomiting, in addition to other subacute, chronic meningitis, or meningoencephalitis symptoms. A small number of patients can present intracranial space-occupying lesions.

16.7.1 Clinical Presentation and Pathology

Cryptococcus histolyticus mainly invades the brain parenchyma and meninges, generally showing extensive thickening and vascular engorgement of the meninges, parenchymal edema, narrowed gyri and sulci, and a diffuse opacity of the pia mater, especially at the bottom of the brain. Small granular nodules or a small bladder can be observed in the sulci,

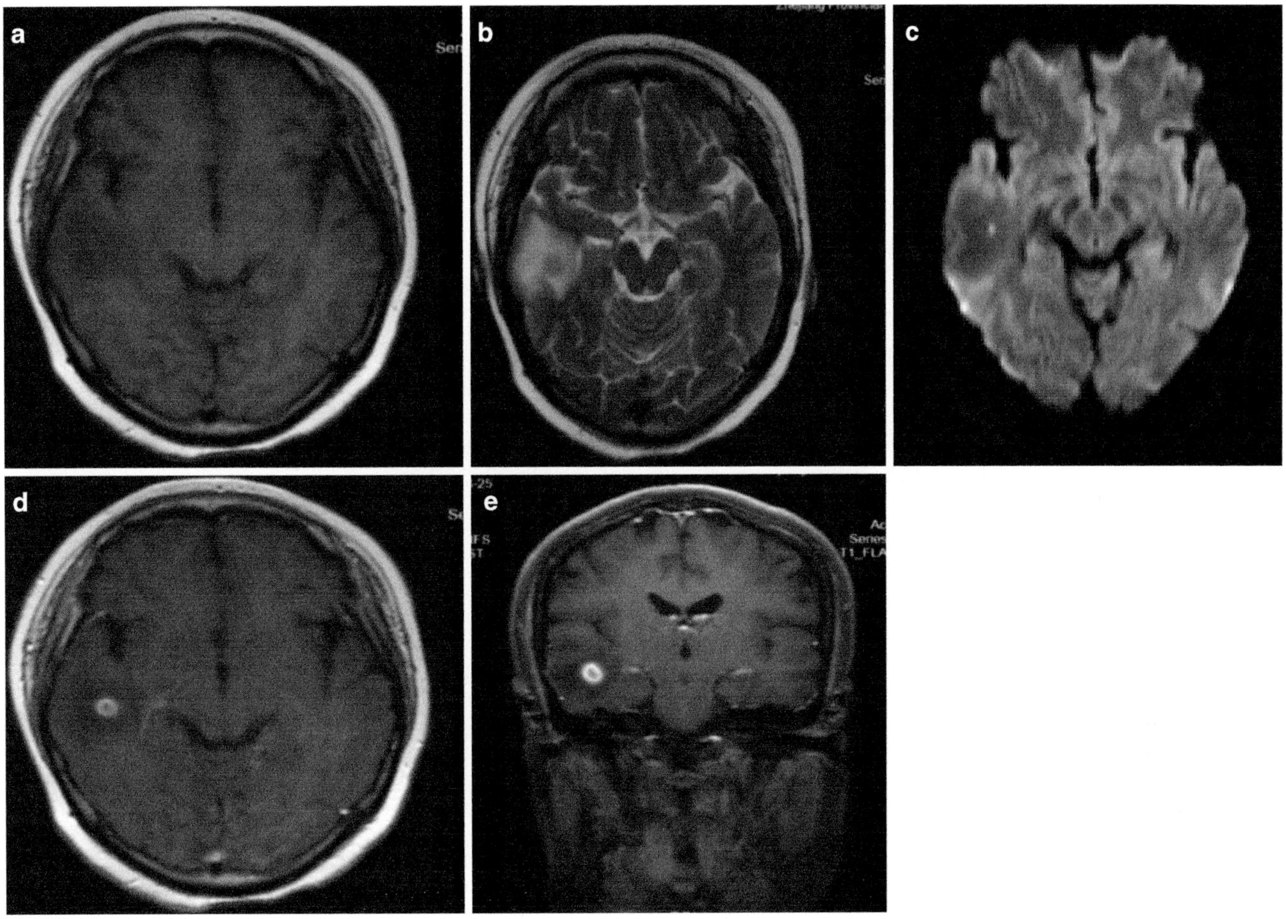

Fig. 16.7 Systemic lupus erythematosus fungal granuloma. An abnormal nodular signal is observed in the right temporal lobe, and the border is clear. The T1-weighted image shows an equivalent signal (**a**), and the T2-weighted image shows a slightly increased signal (**b**). The DWI shows a localized spot-like hyperintense signal in the right temporal lobe (**c**). The enhanced scan shows ring enhancement, with a large area of peripheral edema (**d, e**)

cistern, or parenchyma, with a glue-like exudate and encephalocele expansion. Early pathological changes show lymphocytes, mononuclear cell infiltration, and an abundance of *Cryptococcus histolyticus* in the meninges, cistern, encephalocele, and brain, but few inflammatory reactions are detected in the brain parenchyma.

The onset of disease is unknown, and its progression is slow. In its early stage, irregular low-grade fever or intermittent headache may occur, followed by continuous and progressive aggravation. The patients with weakened immune function may exhibit an acute onset. In the late stage, severe pain in the head may occur, which may even be associated with convulsions, decerebrate rigidity, and hernia cerebri. Most patients have symptoms and signs of intracranial hypertension. A small number of patients have mental symptoms such as dysphoria, personality changes, and memory decline. A large granuloma in the brain, cerebellum, or brain stem can cause focal signs such as paralysis of the limbs and ataxia. Such patients often have symptoms of double or multiple infections [17].

16.7.2 Imaging Characteristics

Brain CT lacks diagnostic specificity, in which 40–50% of cases show normal findings. The rate of positivity is related to the different stages of the disease course, with a longer disease duration providing a higher rate of positivity. The CT scans show ventricular enlargement, hydrocephalus, meningeal enhancement, and brain parenchyma with irregular sheets or miliary hypodense shadows. A few CT scans reveal a small infarction or hemorrhage. Intracranial MRI can show hypointensity in parenchymal T1-weighted images, hyperintensity in T2-weighted images, and a lump similar to a rotundity with an expanded perivascular space. In some cases, miliary nodular changes are observed (Fig. 16.8).

Classification of imaging findings based on location and imaging characteristics of the disease [18]:

1. Diffusion-limited subcortical lesions are seen in the brain area supplied by the perforator-type artery.

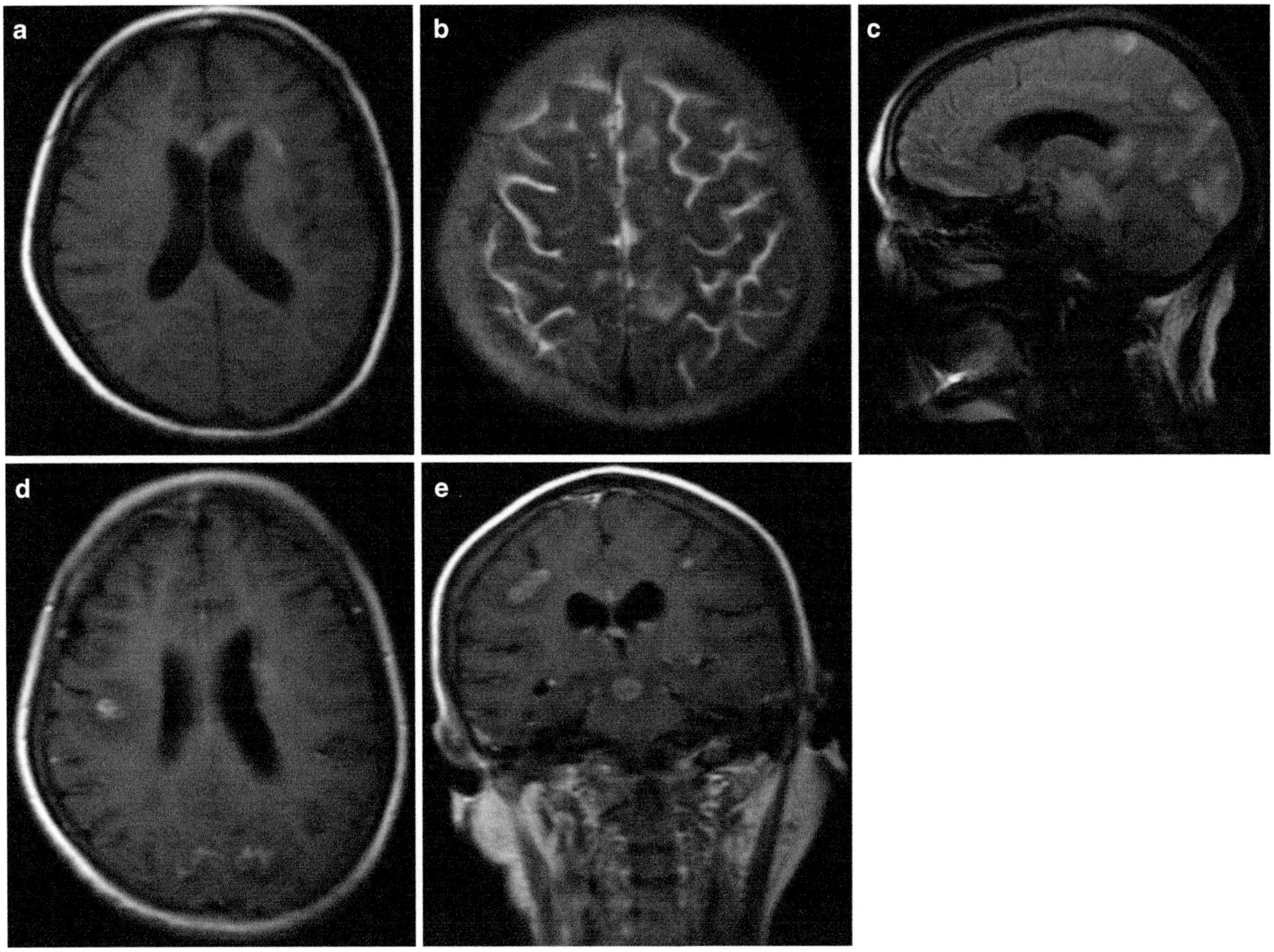

Fig. 16.8 Cerebral cryptococcosis; multiple patchy abnormal signals are observed in the bilateral brain, brain stem, corpus callosum, and cerebellum. T1-weighted image shows hypointensity (**a**) while T2-weighted image hyperintensity with a fuzzy border (**b**). On post-contrast the nodules are circular with significant enhancement and mild mass effect (**c, d**)

2. Pseudocysts: There is elevated T2 signal and reduced T1 signal in the expanded perivascular space, but diffusion is not limited.
3. Focal meningitis and meningoencephalitis: manifest as leptomeningeal thickening and pathological regional enhancement; the latter has parenchymal involvement signs.
4. "Hazy brain base" sign: The perforating arteries in the anterior, middle, and posterior arteries showing uniform and diffuse T2 signal elevation enter the basal brain parenchyma of the brain.

16.7.3 Diagnosis and Differential Diagnosis

The clinical diagnosis must be confirmed by the presence of *Cryptococcus histolyticus* in the CSF. Repeated staining of the CSF, culture, or animal inoculation should be conducted to search for the pathogen. The clinical manifestations and CSF and imaging features of the disease are very similar to those of tuberculous meningitis, and thus identification of the two diseases relies on evidence of the pathogen. In addition, the disease must be differentiated from viral encephalitis, intracerebral abscess, intracerebral tumor, and cerebral cysticercosis (cysticercosis). Other fungal diseases of the brain, such as aspergillosis and mucormycosis, should also be considered during diagnosis.

16.8 *Aspergillus* Meningitis

Aspergillus meningitis is a CNS disease caused by *Aspergillus* fungus, which is a conditional pathogenic fungus in humans and includes *Aspergillus fumigatus* and *Aspergillus flavus*. *Aspergillus* is present on the surface of a healthy body, and it does not cause human *Aspergillus* meningitis. Only when the immune function of the body is compromised can it infect the meninges and brain parenchyma of the CNS to initiate the onset of disease.

16.8.1 Clinical Presentation and Pathology

Fungal abscesses, inflammatory granulomas, and purulent and necrotic lesions are the main pathological manifestations of *Aspergillus* meningitis. The meninges and brain parenchyma of the anterior cranial fossa or middle cranial fossa may show acute exudative inflammation and a microscopic neutrophil and lymphocyte infiltrate. Fungal aneurysm, thrombosis, and embolism caused by *Aspergillus* hyphae can be observed in small arteries, with bleeding in the vessel wall and radial or coralline *Aspergillus* hyphae in the purulent brain tissue lesion. The clinical manifestations of *Aspergillus* meningitis are mostly symptoms of neurological involvement accompanied by clinical manifestations of eye and nose diseases. Examination of patients with visual impairment or blindness, accompanied by fever, headache, nausea, vomiting, neck rigidity, and other symptoms, shows the involvement of the cavernous sinus cranial nerve and signs of meningeal irritation. In addition, the disease may be accompanied by chest pain, cough, expectoration, corneal ulcer, conjunctival congestion, or ciliary body congestion [19].

16.8.2 Imaging Characteristics

The imaging performance varies according to the immune status of the patients. CT shows a focal swollen soft tissue shadow in anterior cranial fossa and intracranial low-density shadow for the inflammatory exudate lesion. MRI examination shows long T1-weighted and long T2-weighted signals in the anterior cranial fossa and intracerebral parenchymal lesions. The T2-weighted center contains an area with a weak signal (indicative of hemorrhage or paramagnetic material deposition). Necrosis, peripheral bleeding, and slight enhancement of the edge may appear similar in appearance to the coloring of "peach slices."

Intracranial aspergillus fungal infections are rare and lack specific imaging features, but some imaging features such as hemorrhage and infarcted areas in heterogeneous parenchymal lesions, hypointensity on the T2W images, bone destruction, fungal sinusitis, and blood vessels stenosis or obstruction can help the clinic make the correct diagnosis. New imaging techniques such as DWI and perfusion imaging help identify with other lesions [19].

16.8.3 Diagnosis and Differential Diagnosis

Patients can be diagnosed with *Aspergillus* meningitis if they have a medical history of chronic wasting disease, malignant tumor, or another triggering factor that can cause weakened immunity; symptoms of nervous system involvement found based on clinical manifestations in the eyes, nose, or systematic aspergillosis; a physical examination showing signs of meningeal irritation and cranial nerve dysfunction; and yellowish green *Aspergillus* that can be cultured in CSF. *Aspergillus* meningitis should be mainly differentiated from mucormycosis and bacterial meningitis. Pathogen examination can effectively identify *Aspergillus* meningitis and other diseases [20].

16.9 Candidiasis of the CNS (CNSC)

CNSC is a type of systemic candidiasis that is clinically rare. In recent years, with the extensive spread of HIV/AIDS, organ transplantation, and the extensive development of intracranial surgery as well as the increased incidence of diabetes, CNSC has also displayed an increasing trend.

16.9.1 Clinical Presentation and Pathology

Common clinical manifestations of CNCS are fever, headache, and different degrees of disturbance of consciousness (such as delirium, coma, among others) as well as signs of meningeal irritation, but edema of the optic disc and increased intracranial pressure are not obvious. Pathological changes associated with CNSC are mainly of the following types: meningoencephalitis, encephalopyosis, primary granuloma, and vascular complications.

16.9.2 Imaging Characteristics

Pathological changes are often observed together and can be reflected in the imaging characteristics. Although direct abscess formation and meningitis occur, tiny abscesses less than 3 mm that occur at the corticomedullary junction, the cerebellum, and basal ganglia are the most common, accompanied by enhancement and less associated with hemorrhage or infarction. The lesion showed hypointensity on T1WI, and the signal varied on T2WI. Granulomas are mainly formed by macrophages and foreign body giant cells, with no obvious positive performance or the performance of local small patchy short T2-weighted, equivalent T1-weighted signals in plain scanning. The enhanced MRI often shows a lumpy, irregular, small nodule shadow, with irregular enhancement, as one of the characteristic changes related to fungal infection. CNSC is often associated with intracranial vascular complications. MRI also shows corresponding changes and imaging changes mainly related to venous sinus thrombosis, cerebral infarction, and moyamoya-like alterations. Diagnosis is generally not a problem because patients often develop microabscesses in the known candidal fungemia [21].

16.9.3 Diagnosis and Differential Diagnosis

During the process of clinical diagnosis and treatment, changes in enhanced cranial MRI provide evidence for a timely diagnosis and assessment of a therapeutic strategy. Diagnosis still depends on the identification of the fungi in the sample of cerebral tissue or CSF, but it is not easy to find fungi during early examinations of the CSF, and repeated fungal smears and cultures of the CSF are needed. Meningoencephalitis and encephalopyosis types must be distinguished from bacterial meningitis and brain abscess. CNSC granulomatous lesions sometimes exhibit tuberculoid nodules or caseous necrosis, and thus can easily be misdiagnosed as tuberculous meningoencephalitis.

16.10 Cerebral Parasitosis

Cerebral parasitosis is an encephalopathy with allergic inflammation, granuloma formation, or cerebral vascular occlusion caused by the invasion of parasitic polypides, eggs, or larvae in the brain. Patients with this parasitic disease show encephalopathic symptoms during disease progression.

16.10.1 Cerebral Cysticercosis

Cerebral cysticercosis, also known as cysticercus disease, is the most common cerebral parasitosis and is caused by *Taenia solium* larvae parasitization of the brain. The incidence of this condition accounts for approximately 80% of cysticercosis.

Clinical Presentation and Pathology
Cysticercus enters the brain and forms a vesicle that contains liquid and white scolex. The dead worm is encapsulated by inflammatory cells, and the stratum externum is full of vascular collagen fibers that form a granuloma. In the latter stage, the lesion changes from collagen fibrous connective tissue to a scar, and the dead worm undergoes calcification. The lesion can be divided into cerebral parenchyma and encephalocelic, meningeal, and mixed-type lesions according to the location [22].

The main symptoms are a disturbance of consciousness and mental disorders, various types of epileptic seizure, transient paralysis of the limbs, and high intracranial pressure after the seizure. Physical examination reveals subcutaneous nodules that are located more in the head and trunk. The results of the cysticercosis complement fixation test can be positive.

Imaging Characteristics

X-Ray Plain film shows an increase in intracranial pressure. In a few cases, intracranial calcification can be observed, exhibiting a round shape with a diameter of 3–5 mm, often as multiple structures, but it can also be a single structure. The postmortem cysticercus shows shrinkage, and the calcium plaque can be irregular. Sometimes calcific cysticercus can be found in soft tissue, exhibiting a long spindle shape.

CT

Cerebral Parenchymal Type (1) Multiple sacculus types: multiple sporadic small round low-density shadows are observed in the hemisphere, with a diameter of 5-10 mm. A small nodular dense shadow can be observed in the lesion, suggesting the presence of cysticercosis scolex. Many lesions are found at the junction of gray and white matter. An enhanced CT scan is generally not enhanced or ring-enhanced. Surrounding mild edema is observed. (2) Single large capsule type: A single giant cysticercus or fused growth of multiple cysticercuses is observed. CT shows the brain as a round, oval, or lobulated low-density area, with an internal CSF density, a clear boundary, and no solid nodules. The large capsule itself is not enhanced, but the periphery can be slightly ring-enhanced due to fibrous tissue proliferation. (3) Multiple calcification types: Multiple types of calcification occur in the brain parenchyma, which can be round or oval and range in diameter from 2 to 5 mm. Sometimes only a slice of calcification can be observed, with no surrounding edema and no enhancement.

Encephalocelic Type This type is frequently observed in the fourth ventricle. It is difficult to directly observe a vesicle with the same density as CSF, which is shown as an indirect sign, such as an abnormal cerebral ventricular pattern or limited asymmetric expansion of the ventricle, the obstructive hydrocephalus. The density of the vesicle can sometimes exceed that of the CSF, and ring enhancement or calcification can be observed in the wall of the vesicle.

Meningeal Type The cistern of the fissure of Sylvius, the suprasellar cistern, is characterized by cystic enlargement with signs of slight occupation. The cavum subarachnoidale expands and deforms, and the lateral ventricle undergoes enlargement. After contrast enhancement, the wall of the vesicle displays nodular enhancement, with meningeal enhancement in some cases.

MRI

Cerebral Parenchyma Type MRI shows cystic lesions that are mostly round, range in diameter from 2 to 8 mm, and have eccentric small shadow dots attached to the walls of the vesicle that represent the cysticercosis scolex, namely, the T1- and short T2-weighted signals. Edema is slight during the survival time of cerebral cysticercus. The enhancement with Gd-DTPA shows that the walls of the vesicle can or cannot be enhanced. When the cysticercus has died, the scolex becomes unclear. Peripheral edema is aggravated, and the occupying effect is clear. Enhanced ring thickening is observed. In this case, the symptom of "white target" may be detected, that is, in the T2-weighted image, the cystic hydatid fluid and peripheral edema show hyperintensity, and the capsule wall and blurred head section of the capsule provide a weak signal.

Encephalocelic Type This type is small and round, with a diameter ranging from 2 to 8 mm. The long T1- and long T2-weighted signal often show no scolex. The adjacent brain parenchyma may have a smooth impression. Some cases show a large capsule type that is lobulated, has distinct intervals, and occasionally displays the scolex at its edge.

Meningeal Type Most patients present with cerebral sulcus cysticercus and meningeal adhesion formation.

MR spectroscopy helps to characterize the noninvasive diagnosis of the hydatid cyst. The peak at 2.4 ppm has been described as a very specific marker for intracranial cestodal infection and has been found to be a noninvasive marker of cestodal cysts [23]. Acetate and alanine peaks have also been reported, but unlike cysticercal cysts, creatine does not usually exist.

Diagnosis and Differential Diagnosis

Clinical manifestations are varied, mainly during epileptic seizure, intracranial hypertension, movement disorders, mental disorders, and meningeal irritation. A history of cestodiasis and subcutaneous nodules is observed.

The results of cysticercosis complement fixation tests or the indirect cysticercosis hemagglutination test can provide positive results.

The performance of various types of CT and MRI has been mentioned above. The encephalitis type must be identified with multiple sclerosis, multiple cerebral infarction, or subcortical arteriosclerotic encephalopathy. A single large capsular type must be identified with cutaneous cysts, epidermoid cysts, or arachnoid cysts. A multiple sacculus type must be identified with metastatic encephaloma.

16.10.2 Schistosomiasis of the CNS

Schistosomiasis is a chronic parasitic disease caused by blood flukes of the genus *Schistosoma* that invades the vascular system. It is mainly spread in 73 countries in Asia, Africa, and Latin America. It is estimated that 500–600 million people are threatened, and the number of patients reaches 200 million. CNS involvement is uncommon, and such involvement has varied consequences depending on the location of the ectopic egg laying in cerebral parenchyma and the spinal cord.

Spinal Medullary Schistosomiasis

The most common manifestation of neuroschistosomiasis is myeloradiculopathy, which is considered very rare, but the myeloradiculopathy is undoubtedly underestimated because of the prevailing social and economic conditions in the endemic area, affecting the precise diagnosis.

Clinical Presentation and Pathology

The mechanism of egg laying is not yet clear. The main pathological changes are as follows: (1) egg secretions and the release of antigenic substances cause an acute inflammatory reaction, edema, hemorrhage, and necrosis of the nerve tissue, leading to acute myelitis; (2) the epithelioid cells around the necrotic collapse of the eggs, the foreign body giant cells, and the leukomonocytes aggregate to form scattered or fused intramedullary granulomas; (3) granuloma lesions with granulomatous neurodocitis occur around the cone and the cauda equina; and (4) spinal cord infarction is caused by inflammatory spinal artery occlusion.

The basis of symptoms mainly come from the following four pathological processes, radicular, vascular, granulomatous, and myelitic processes, the latter two being the most common. Most patients have radicular and medullary involvement, with varying degrees of granulomatous inflammation, necrosis, vascular damage, thrombosis, necrotizing arteritis, and perivascular inflammation, causing severe headache, epilepsy, intracranial hypertension, etc [24].

Imaging Characteristics

MRI is more sensitive to the assessment of disease in cases of prolonged medullary atrophy, showing diffuse hyperintensity with varying degrees of the medullary cone expansion on T2-weighted images. The use of contrast agents often causes heterogeneous impregnation with the multifocal, micronodular, converging aspect. This manifestation of the individual highly suggests that the disease originated in endemic areas of schistosomiasis.

Diagnosis and Differential Diagnosis

Some clinical features of the patient observed in the epidemiological background can suggest the disease. This disease generally starts with lumbago and/or lower limb pain, which is usually radicular, followed by sensory disturbances of the lower limbs and muscle weakness, and is always accompanied by autonomic nerves, in particular vesical dysfunction. Blood and CSF analysis showed specific intrathecal antibodies and eosinophilia.

For primary intramedullary tumors, anatomical deformation of the spinal cord is more obvious, and a rough outline of the tumor and enhanced morphological diversity are rarely associated with signs of spinal cord surface strengthening or arachnoiditis. Metastatic tumors typically have a history of primary tumors, and through CSF implantation metastasis, layered or small nodular enhancement can be observed in the pia mater.

Medullitis is mostly associated with an acute onset and is usually located in the cervical and upper middle thoracic spinal cord area. In general, no enhancement or signs of mild patchy enhancement are observed, and arachnoiditis signs are rare.

Spinal TB mostly occurs in the thoracic region and can be associated with subarachnoid adhesions and localized effusion. T1-weighted images of intramedullary tuberculoma are typically not uniform. The central caseating tissue exhibits hypointensity, and central necrosis shows hyperintensity on the T2-weighted image, with annular enhancement after contrast enhancement.

Spinal cord sarcoidosis is frequently located in the cervical and upper thoracic segment. MRI shows involvement of the spinal cord thickness, with abnormal signals and irregular nodular enhancement. After hormone therapy, the size of the focus narrows, the spinal cord swelling is alleviated, and, together with chest examination, hilus of the lung with or without sarcoidosis may facilitate the diagnosis.

Cerebral Schistosomiasis

Cerebral schistosomiasis is caused by the deposition of schistosome ova in the brain tissue, resulting in granuloma formation and inflammatory reactions. It is generally believed that this condition is the main source of pulmonary lesions. The brain tissue in which eggs are deposited softens, and brain edema forms around the granuloma. This disease is more common in young people.

Clinical Presentation and Pathology

Eggs are deposited in the cerebral blood vessels of the brain embolism to stimulate the host immune response and pathological change. The cerebral pia mater and leptomeningeal subcutaneous tissue of the lesion show a granuloma of the ovum, pseudotubercle and scar nodule, glial cell response to non-specific lesions, cerebromalacia, and encephaledema. Clinically, this disease can be divided into an acute type and a chronic type. The onset of the acute type occurs after infection for approximately 6 months, and it manifests as meningoencephalitis with fever, disturbance of consciousness, paralysis, convulsions, tendon hyperreflexia, signs of meningeal irritation, and pyramidal signs. The chronic type mostly occurs in early schistosomiasis patients, and the main symptom is epileptic attack and, commonly, localized epilepsy. There are also patients with increased intracranial pressure and location signs as main manifestations.

Imaging Characteristics

The plain scan of the acute type shows mainly encephaledema with a varied size and degree of low-density lesions in the parenchyma as well as non-enhanced performance. The performance of the chronic type shows localized granuloma, iso-density, or a slight increase in density, with space-occupying signs, an unclear boundary, and peripheral edema. The contrast CT scan shows enhancement of the lesions. Cerebral schistosomiasis is mainly observed as a weak signal on the T1-weighted image and as a strong signal on the T2-weighted imaged, with bleeding. The MRI signals show different degrees of edema around the focus and some potentially heterogeneous lesions. After contrast enhancement, the lesions show obvious enhancement, such as a mottled, sand-like, or nodular appearance, which are known characteristics [25].

Diagnosis and Differential Diagnosis

Diagnosis

First, it should be determined whether the patient is suffering from schistosomiasis. Cerebral symptoms appear after infection by *Schistosoma*. Brain symptoms caused by other diseases should be excluded.

Antimonials or praziquantel treatment are effective. Sometimes a definite diagnosis requires the detection of eggs during surgery.

Differential Diagnosis

Other types of cerebral Schistosomiasis include, for example, echinococcosis of the brain, cerebral cysticercosis, cerebral amoebiasis, and cerebral toxoplasmosis. Identification is mainly dependent on epidemiological features, specific immune diagnosis, and typical imaging assessments.

Cerebral nonparasitic infectious diseases, such as encephalitis, cerebral abscess, and cerebral TB, among others, are observed.

Cerebral noninfectious diseases, such as cerebral infarction, cerebrovascular malformation, tuberous sclerosis, and multiple sclerosis, among others, are observed.

16.10.3 Cerebral Paragonimiasis

Cerebral paragonimiasis is a disease caused by mechanical damage resulting from continuous movement of imago in the brain and a pathological immune response induced by metabolin. The temporal lobes are the most common sites of damage.

Clinical Presentation and Pathology

Pathology

Period of histological destruction: Migration of the invasive worm into the brain tissue causes tunnel-like damage and hemorrhage, followed by destruction of the brain tissue to form a cave-like lesion. The surrounding brain tissue reaction then becomes obvious.

Period of granuloma or cystitis: An inflammatory reaction that occurs around the lesion, with tissue necrosis and liquefaction, and contains Charcot Leyden crystals and a large number of eggs and imagoes in the granulation tissue and the crystal wall. The worm often migrates from the cyst to the surrounding brain tissue to form new cysts. These cysts communicate with the tunnel to form a compound cyst.

Period of fibrous scar: After worm death or migration to other places, the cystic contents are gradually absorbed, with dead egg calcification, cystic wall thickening, and fibrosis.

Infection caused by *Paragonimus westermani* initially causes abdominal symptoms, such as abdominal pain and diarrhea, followed by pulmonary symptoms, such as cough, chest pain, and hemoptysis, among others. In addition, headache, convulsions, and limb movement disorder are most common neurologic symptoms, which appear during the late phases of the disease [26].

Imaging Characteristics

X-Ray Calcification of the cystic wall can be observed in the plain skull X-ray. Together with the thoracic and pulmonary type, the X-ray examination shows significant changes in the lungs.

CT A large, low-density lesion with edema and an infarction focus can be observed, with an irregular shape, size inequality, and an unclear boundary. A change in digitate impressions can be detected in the cerebral white matter. The gyri show obvious thickened edema, while the sulci are narrow, shallow, and partially disappear. The cerebral midline structures show no significant shift. Ring-shaped lesion: The CT examination shows ring-shaped lesions with an isodensity and a slightly higher density, with a range of sizes and relatively clear edges, and numerous ring-shaped lesions that accumulate like soap bubbles that are surrounded by a zone of edema with different degrees of low density. Mild space-occupying signs are observed. Enhanced examination: Annular and small patch-like enhancements are observed, and sometimes a number of ring-shaped, enhanced lesions that accumulate like soap bubbles are observed, in which the lesion is more evident [27].

MRI Large, low-density lesion of edema and an infarction focus is observed. Obvious cerebral white matter is observed, showing a long T1-weighted and a long T2-weighted change, and most of the signals are homogeneous. Ring-shaped lesion: The lesions are more clearly observed. The ring-shaped cystic wall exhibits a slightly weakened signal in the T2-weighted image, with a focus of necrosis with a strong central signal surrounded by peripheral edema. Nodular, single ring-shaped or multi ring-shaped enhancement is observed [27].

Diagnosis and Differential Diagnosis

An epidemiological history exists for this disease. The occurrence of symptoms first in the brain and then in the lungs together with laboratory tests supports the diagnosis of cerebral paragonimiasis. The eggs of *Paragonimus westermani* are found in sputum, hydrothorax, gastric juices, feces, and CSF. Larvae, imagoes, and eggs are found in subcutaneous nodules or enclosed masses, and they exhibit a positive response to intradermal tests for *Paragonimus westermani*.

Differential Diagnosis

By comparison with other meningitis, encephalitis, and space-occupying lesions, the eggs of *Paragonimus* can be found by examining the CSF, sputum, or feces, together with immunological detection methods. Combined with thoracic and pulmonary types, this condition can easily be misdiagnosed as TB or pneumonia, but the eggs can be found in the CSF, sputum, or feces, allowing identification together with immunological detection methods.

16.10.4 Amoebiasis of the CNS

The cerebral amoeba may cause human central nervous system infections with high mortality. Currently, there are two types of human meningoencephalitis caused by pathogenic free-living amoebae, that is, the primary amoebic meningoencephalitis (PAM) caused by *Naegleria* amoeba and granulomatous amebic encephalitis (GAE) caused by *Acanthamoeba* [28].

PAM

PAM is a rare acute fatal disease that is more common in children and adolescents who recently swim in contaminated ponds or swimming pools. After invading the nasal mucosa, the parasite enters the brain along the olfactory nerve, causing inflammation and destruction of the olfactory bulb and brain tissue. This is an urgent, rapid-developing disease with easy misdiagnosis.

Clinical Presentation and Pathology The incubation period of PAM varies from 2 to 7 days. It can be characterized by sore throat, nasal congestion, runny nose, headache, and mild fever at the onset of the disease, followed by a sudden increase in body temperature, aggravated headache, and the symptoms of meningeal irritation such as nausea and jet vomiting are accompanied. When the disease enters late stage, the patient suffers from disturbance of consciousness, coma, and death. The main pathological changes were purulent meningitis and hemorrhagic necrotizing encephalitis [29].

Imaging Characteristics The imaging diagnosis of PAM is difficult. Some patients have normal brain CT findings. The other part of patients show non-specific cerebral edema in the CT images. In some cases, the enhancement of leptomeninges can be seen on enhanced CT. MRI shows higher sensitivity than CT and can show initial changes.

Diagnosis and Differential Diagnosis Analysis of cerebrospinal fluid in PAM usually shows an increase in the red blood cell count, an increase in the percentage of polymorphonuclear leukocytes, an increase in protein, and a decrease in sugar content, and the amniotic trophozoites could be seen on smears as the basis for diagnosis. PAM should be differentiated from purulent meningitis, herpes simplex encephalitis, and Japanese encephalitis.

GAE

GAE is a subacute or chronic fatal disease caused by *Acanthamoeba*. This disease occurs most frequently in immunosuppressed and frail populations. And some patients may have skin lesions or keratitis. GAE occurs throughout the year without significant seasonality. It is mainly related to exposure to water or air contaminated with pathogens.

Clinical Presentation and Pathology The pathogenesis of GAE is a chronic clinical course. In addition to the symptoms of meningitis in the clinic, the symptoms of damaged brain parenchyma are very prominent. And often there are symptoms and signs of focal occupation, such as hemiplegia and aphasia. Pathological changes were necrotizing granulomatous encephalitis. Multinucleated giant cells can be seen in the granulation wall or granulation. The trophozoites and cysts that are phagocytosed can be seen in giant cells. GAE tends to erode the blood vessel wall and can develop into necrotizing arteritis or even form an aneurysm.

Imaging Characteristics The imaging manifestations of granulomatous amoebic encephalitis were non-specific. CT and MRI scans showed single or multiple low-density or mixed-density lesions in the basal ganglia, cerebral cortex, subcortical white matter, cerebellum, and pons. Enhanced and non-enhanced defects can be observed in some cases.

Diagnosis and Differential Diagnosis The diagnosis of GAE should be based on the combination of comprehensive clinical manifestations, laboratory tests, and imaging data. A large number of lymphocytes and polymorphonuclear leukocytes can be observed in the cerebrospinal fluid of patients with GAE, with slightly higher pressure, lower glucose levels, and slightly higher protein levels. The final diagnosis should be based on the detection of amoeba trophozoites and cysts at brain lesions or skin lesions or smear-based visualization of amoeba trophozoites and cysts.

GAE should be differentiated from amoebic brain abscess. In general, patients with amoeba brain abscess have a history of intestinal amebiasis or hepatic amebiasis, and most of the intracranial infections are secondary lesions, and only circular trophozoites that engulf red blood cells can be seen in the diseased tissue slice, and amoeba cysts cannot be found.

16.10.5 Toxoplasmosis of the CNS

Toxoplasma gondii is a worldwide distributed obligate intracellular parasite that can infect all mammals, including humans. Toxoplasma infection is one of the more common infections of AIDS. In immunocompetent people, *Toxoplasma gondii* infection is not easy to cause symptoms of infection, only latent presence of hidden infections. However, in the immunocompromised population, activation or reinfection of *Toxoplasma gondii* can cause obvious infection symptoms, and severe cases can be fatal. The nervous system is the main target organ of *Toxoplasma gondii*.

Clinical Presentation and Pathology

Toxoplasma gondii enters the blood from the invaded site and spreads throughout the body and quickly enters mononuclear macrophage and tissue cells. It proliferates in the cell until it ruptures and invades neighboring cells. This repeatedly causes focal necrosis of local tissue and inflammatory reaction of surrounding tissues. The common clinical manifestation of toxoplasma encephalopathy is headache, usually accompanied by changes in mental state and fever. There may also be epilepsy, cranial nerve abnormalities, visual field defects, and sensory disturbances. Focal neurological symptoms are common, including dyskinesia and speech impairment.

Imaging Characteristics

On an unenhanced CT, toxoplasmosis encephalopathy usually presents as multiple low, equal density lesions, sometimes as solid lesions. Peripheral edema and mass effects are common. After the formation of abscesses, the boundaries of the lesions were clear, mostly in the basal ganglia, the junction of the cortex and medulla, the white matter, and the area around the ventricles. Calcification is rare. On MRI, there is a low signal on T1WI, but there is a high signal on the edge and high or mixed signals on T2WI and T2-FLAIR. On the DWI, there is a high signal around the lesion indicating bleeding. However, there is usually no diffusion limitation in the central area of the lesion, which can be differentiated from abscesses. On the enhanced T1WI, the lesions were mostly ring-shaped and the surrounding edema showed low signal. "Eccentric target sign" is a typical MR manifestation of toxoplasmosis, including three layers: the innermost layer of enhanced core area (more common in eccentricity), the middle area of low-signal area, and the outermost layer of high-signal enhancement ring [30]. The MRS of toxoplasmosis in the central nervous system usually presents as an increase in lactic acid and lipids, while other peaks decrease.

Diagnosis and Differential Diagnosis
Some magnetic resonance techniques facilitate the differentiation between toxoplasma encephalopathy and other focal lesions, including DWI, MRI, and MRS. Lumbar cerebrospinal fluid examination: lymphocyte-based leukocytes increased, accompanied by eosinophils and protein increased. Anti-Toxoplasma antibodies in serum and cerebrospinal fluid can be positive. Toxoplasma trophozoites found in cerebrospinal fluid can be diagnosed. Therapeutic tests can also be conducted in clinical practice, and biopsy may be considered in the absence of an effective clinical response after treatment. Sometimes it needs to be differentiated from tuberculosis, cryptococcal meningitis, and herpes meningitis.

16.10.6 Cerebral Echinococcosis

Echinococcosis (hydatidosis) is a chronic disease of the brain, liver, lungs, heart, and kidney caused by the larval stage of *Echinococcus granulosus*, and cerebral echinococcosis accounts for about 1%. Humans infect by eating food or water contaminated with parasite eggs. The incidence of children and adolescents is relatively higher than that of adults. Since infections have nature of embolism, they are often located on the supratentorial area and involve areas of the middle cerebral artery, and cerebral hydatid cysts are usually isolated.

Clinical Presentation and Pathology

Pathology Hydatid cysts are divided into two layers. The internal capsule is the hydatid cyst, and the external capsule is the fibrous capsule, which is formed by brain tissue. Mild adhesions are present between the two, and the hydatid cyst contains the blood vessels and the nutrient supply. Most larvae survive for approximately 5 years, but many will continue to grow into a giant cyst ranging in volume from hundreds to thousands of milliliters. The cystic wall consists of the stratum corneum and corpora mucosum. The cystic fluid contains toxic albumin. If the cyst ruptures, leakage of the cystic fluid often produces varying degrees of an allergic reaction.

Clinical
Headache, nausea, vomiting, hypoplasia, and papilledema, among other symptoms, result from increased intracranial pressure and stimulate cortical seizures. Focal signs may be observed, such as hemiplegia, aphasia, and hemidysesthesia.

Imaging Characteristics
Cerebral hydatid disease generally presents as an isointense single cystic lesion in the cerebrospinal fluid, and the surrounding edema is not obvious. In the case of active inflammation, the use of contrast agent may result in the discrete enhancement around the fibrous capsule.

A hypointense loop observed in T2-weighted image is a characteristic feature of the disease, and calcifications and multivesicular cysts are not common in the brain. Except for large thin-walled cysts, there is no peripheral edema or a pronounced expansive effect that contributes to the differential diagnosis of brain abscesses and other infectious cysts (such as cysts associated with neurocysticercosis) [22].

Diagnosis and Differential Diagnosis
The disease is diagnosed on the basis of serological and radiological examinations. The liver is the most common site of involvement (74.8%), and the second site of involvement is the lung (24%). The involvement of the central nervous system is not common and is estimated to be 1–2% of all cases.

The disease must be differentiated from an intracranial tumor or intracranial arachnoid cyst and other parasitic diseases of the brain such as cerebral cysticercosis and cerebral schistosomiasis.

16.10.7 Cerebral Malaria

Malaria is a disease caused by *Plasmodium*. Cerebral malaria is the most common and most serious parasitic infection in the human central nervous system. In developing countries, cerebral malaria is an important cause of death and neurological diseases. Cerebral malaria can be transmitted by means other than mosquito bites, such as blood transfusions, contaminated needles, or organ transplantation. The disease is more common in individuals who are not immune to parasites. The incubation period varies from 1 to 3 weeks. *Plasmodium vivax* and oval malaria can recur and can cause a vicious attack of cerebral malaria [31].

Clinical Presentation and Pathology

Cerebral malaria is a rapidly fatal disease characterized by headache, seizures, and coma associated with diffuse cerebral edema. The symptoms of focal lesions are rare and mainly include hemiplegia, aphasia, hemianopia, or cerebellar ataxia. Its pathology shows a large number of red blood cells containing parasites in brain capillaries and small veins, small necrotic lesions distributed in brain tissue, and glial hyperplasia around the lesion [32].

Imaging Characteristics

The imaging results of most patients with cerebral malaria do not change their immediate therapy. And CT results have nothing to do with the degree of parasitemia, so the sensitivity of this method to the study of the disease is very low. MRI is less commonly used here, but it can show multifocal cortical or white matter infarcts and diffuse brain edema.

Recent neuroimaging studies demonstrated that brain swelling is a common feature in CM and a major contributor to death in pediatric patients. Consequently, determining the precise mechanisms responsible for this swelling could open new adjunct therapeutic avenues in CM patients. Mohanty et al. identified two distinct origins of brain swelling in both adult and pediatric patients from India, occurring in distinct parts of the brain. These support the hypothesis that both endothelial dysfunction and microvascular obstruction by *Plasmodium falciparum*-infected erythrocytes make independent contributions to the pathogenesis of CM, providing opportunities for novel therapeutic interventions [33].

Diagnosis and Differential Diagnosis

Diagnosis was established through epidemiological history, symptoms and signs, including an onset mostly during the epidemic period and an acute and high fever, chills, convulsions, and coma; through laboratory examination, mainly for the detection of *Plasmodium*; and through treatment diagnosis. The performance of multifocal petechial hemorrhage that occurs in the white matter is indistinguishable from acute multifocal hemorrhagic encephalopathy in sepsis and diffuse intravascular coagulation. The differential diagnosis of these two diseases needs to be based on clinical data.

16.11 Fatal Bacterial Granuloma After Trauma (FBGT)

Fatal bacterial granuloma after trauma (FBGT) has been observed by many domestic researchers through in-depth and meticulous clinical observation together with histological examination. FBGT is a new disease named after the discovery of the bacterium as the causal pathogen of the disease. The destruction caused by this disease is more severe than that of malignant tumors, and the pathogenesis is not clear. The same pathogenic bacteria have been successfully isolated from the skin lesions of many patients and identified as *Propionibacterium acnes* [34].

Clinical Presentation and Pathology

Histological Examination Infiltration of inflammatory cells in the dermis and nodular infiltration mainly composed of histiocytes are observed. Transmission electron microscopy shows typical *Bacillus coli* in skin lesions.

Clinical

The face and forehead have a history of microtrauma. There is a progressive increase in the dark red patches on the skin, which do not burst. New patches can appear near or far from the skin lesions. Pathological findings show a histiocytic granuloma. During the late period, consciousness disorders, and severe headache, but no obvious signs of meningeal irritation, are observed. All patients die within 1.5–4 years. The skin lesions can temporarily improve after treatment with glucocorticoids, but this treatment also significantly accelerates death. All patients are from the countryside.

Imaging Characteristics

CT The plain CT scan shows that the skull is normal, with only a patchy low-density area in the white matter of the occipital and parietal lobe and an unclear boundary suggesting inflammation.

MRI Intracranial granuloma occurs in place of the gray and white matter junction, and the gray matter shows an equal or slight hypointensity on the T1-weighted image and hyperintensity on the T2-weighted image. Bleeding in the central areas of some lesions shows hyperintensity on T1-weighted image and a somewhat strong signal on the T2-weighted image. Moderate edema is observed in the cerebral white matter around the granuloma, and edema is distributed along the subcortex, with hyperintensity on T2-weighted image and fluid-attenuated inversion recovery

(FLAIR). The granuloma shows moderate homogeneous enhancement or annular, patchy, and nodular enhancement. In some cases, meningeal line-like enhancement can be observed.

Diagnosis and Differential Diagnosis

In summary, the diagnosis of FBGT firstly relies on a patient's medical history and if the patient has a history of facial trauma with a non-healing scar after trauma. The facial scar shows an iso-intensity on the T1-weighted image and an intracranial granuloma in place of the gray and white matter junction and gray matter, which shows hyperintensity on the T2-weighted image and hypointensity on the T1-weighted image. Granuloma and peripheral meninges all show enhancement and subcortical edema around the granulomas, and in the late phase, the granuloma can involve the deep gray matter. The differential diagnosis includes tuberosa sclerosis, cerebral metastasis tumor, and multiple tuberculomas.

16.12 Primary Central Lymphomatoid Granulomatosis (LyG)

LyG is a lymphoproliferative condition that is associated with vascular wall damage disease, in which the blood vessel is central, related to EB virus infection, and may involve the whole body or more than one system. This disease is rare.

Clinical Presentation and Pathology

The pathological characteristics of LyG include lymphocyte proliferative lesions with vascular centricity and vessel damage, reactive T cell infiltration, positivity for the Epstein-Barr (EB) virus, and B lymphocyte proliferation. Proliferating B lymphocytes cross through the blood vessel wall and surround the blood vessels to form a nodular structure, with central necrosis of the lesion. However, LyG generally does not display typical pathological changes associated with granuloma, and the formation of epithelioid multinucleated giant cells is sometimes observed. The clinical manifestations of CNS LyG include personality changes, ataxia, hemiplegia, facial paralysis, headache, and blindness, with a lack of specificity. Most manifestations of the disease occur suddenly and peak within a few days [35].

Imaging Characteristics

The imaging performance of LyG can be divided into two categories of diffuse infiltration and mass lesion. MRI can reveal single or multiple lesions in the parenchyma, and the T2-weighted image shows hyperintensity and the point or linear enhancement of the lesions, with irregular enhancement of the meninges and cranial nerves. The lumpy lesions mainly show heterogeneous enhancement, surrounded by an obvious zone of edema, which could further progress to a lesion with peripheral ring enhancement. During LyG imaging, the point or linear enhancement represents the relative characteristic performance, which is related to the pathological characteristics of the vascular wall and the surrounding tissue [36].

Diagnosis and Differential Diagnosis

Imaging findings may indicate a lesion, and histopathology of lymphocyte proliferative lesions obtained by biopsy can further clarify the diagnosis. LyG and lymphoma are easy to confound in pathology, in addition to the proliferative ratio of nuclear-specific cells. The molecular pathology is an important tool for identifying the two diseases.

16.13 Non-specific Granulomatous Diseases of the CNS

Non-specific granulomatous diseases of the CNS are conditions in which a pathogenic cause cannot be determined by clinical examination or biopsy of the lesion, and the histological cerebral granuloma lesions of the inflammatory infiltrate are also known as cryptogenic granulomas. The incidence of the disease is low, and it is easy to misdiagnose as a brain tumor, affecting the choice of therapeutic method and judgment of prognosis [37].

Clinical Presentation and Pathology

The disease is a chronic proliferative pathological process, resulting in the formation of a ring structure that exhibits encapsulated necrosis in the center and can also be completely filled with inflammatory granulation tissue. The range of inflammatory granuloma form according to the number and type of invasive pathogen, and they can be fused to one another and not only confined to a small range. Edema around the lesion is common, and sometimes it is more obvious, mainly because the inflammation destroys the blood-brain barrier (BBB), allowing the blood to infiltrate the cerebral extracellular space and induce vasogenic edema. The lesions can also disrupt the pia mater and subarachnoid space and adhere to the dura mater. The incidence of this disease is low, and it occurs more often in young and middle-aged men, persists for a long duration (more than a month), and has characteristic symptoms such as headache, dizziness, epilepsy, and other symptoms of decreased hearing, decreased vision, and hemianopsia, which are caused by damage to specific functional areas.

Imaging Characteristics

CT A plain CT scan shows the distribution of the lesions close to the cerebral facies convexa or dura mater, located in the cortex or subcortex. The lesions show an iso-density or mixed density. Enhanced scanning shows irregular solidity with or without ring enhancement, and local enhancement of the adjacent meninges is observed.

MRI The lesion near the dura mater shows hyperintensity or mixed intensity on the T2-weighted image, and hypointensity on the T1-weighted image, with calcification and bleeding in a few cases. The bleeding lesion shows strong T1-weighted and strong T2-weighted signals. Edema is clearly observed around the lesion, and the space mass effect is also apparent. The enhanced scanning shows irregular homogeneous enhancement, with an inconsistent enhanced range (Fig. 16.9). The adjacent meninges show enhancement. Sometimes the lesions are located in the pineal region and cerebellar vermis compressing the aqueduct of midbrain, and this compression induces supratentorial encephalocele dilatation.

Diagnosis and Differential Diagnosis

The laboratory examination shows that the hemogram is not high and that there are no special features of the CSF. It also reveals clinical signs of the disease and specific diagnostic evidence of the laboratory examination, which can easily be misdiagnosed as a brain tumor. Therefore, the performances of CT and MRI are a major focus. This disease must be differentiated from primary tumors and solitary metastatic tumors in the brain. There is no obvious cause of cerebral primary tumor development in cortical or subcortical areas, no obvious enhancement at low levels, and reinforcement of irregular or incomplete annular enhancement at high levels, with almost no meningeal enhancement. Homogeneous enhancement can be observed in cerebral lymphadenoma, consistently at the depth of the brain, with no meningeal enhancement. The cerebral solitary metastatic tumors are mostly distributed in the cortex or subcortex, and they can also show a homogeneous enhancement. In general, the shape of the enhancement is mostly regular and similar to rotundity, and the primary lesion can be found by determining the patient's medical history.

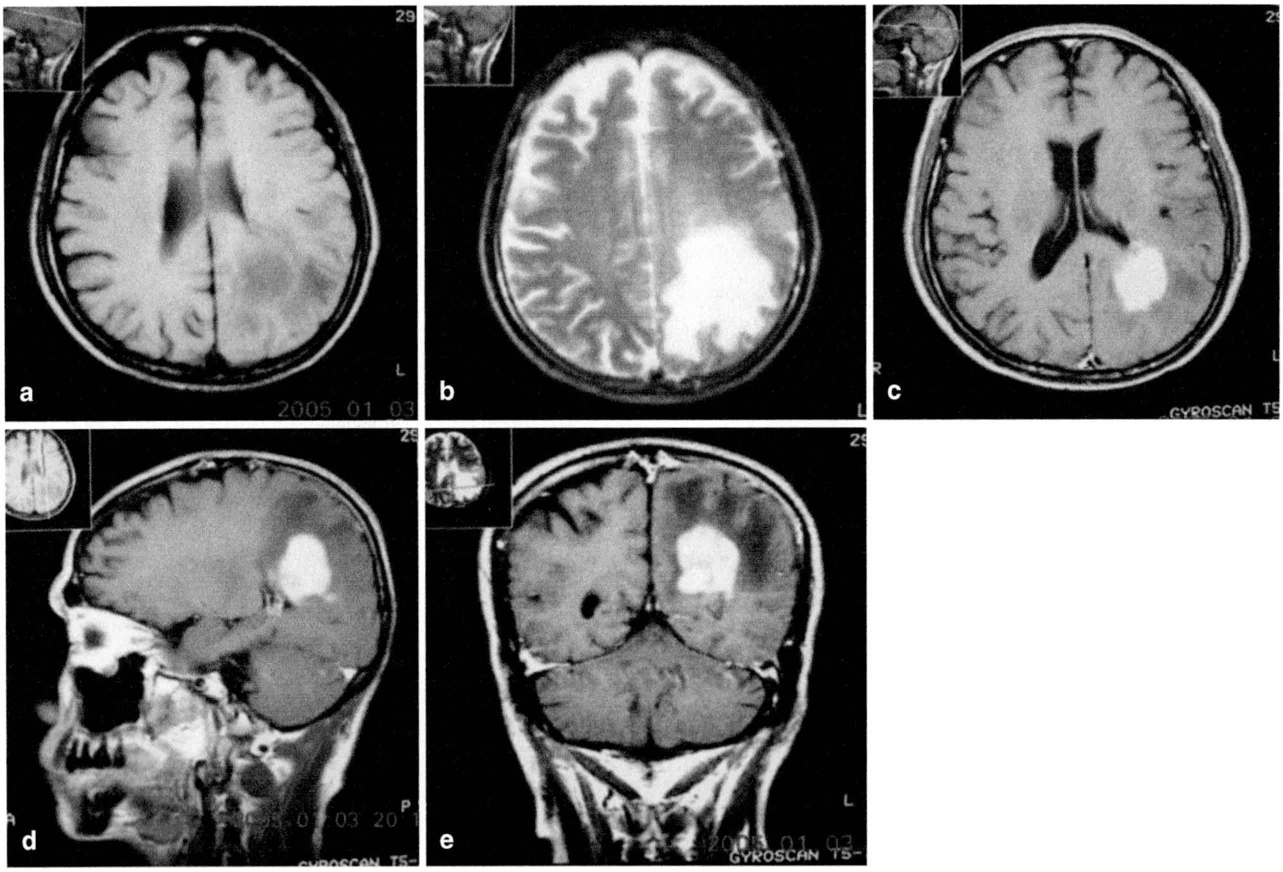

Fig. 16.9 Intracranial chronic granuloma (cryptogenic granuloma); a huge abnormal signal with an irregular signal edge is observed at the top of the occipital lobe. The T1-weighted image shows multiple weak signals (**a**), and the T2-weighted image shows a strong signal (**b**). The lesions in the enhanced scan are significantly enhanced, with surrounding edema (**c, d**). The lesions squeeze the posterior horn of the left lateral ventricle, with no abnormality in the third and fourth ventricles, and the midline structure is in the center

References

1. da Rocha AJ, Maia AC Jr, Ferreira NP, et al. Granulomatous diseases of the central nervous system. Top Magn Reson Imaging. 2005;16(2):155–87.
2. Thomas G, Murphy S, Staunton H, et al. Pathogen-free granulomatous diseases of the central nervous system. Hum Pathol. 1998;29(2):110–5.
3. Rapalino O, Mullins ME. Intracranial infectious and inflammatory diseases presenting as neurosurgical pathologies. Neurosurgery. 2017;81(1):10–28.
4. Santosh V, Mahadevan A, Chickabasaviah YT, et al. Infectious lesions mimicking central nervous system neoplasms. Semin Diagn Pathol. 2010;27(2):122–35.
5. Saini J, Gupta RK, Jain KK. Intracranial infections: key neuroimaging findings. Semin Roentgenol. 2014;49(1):86–98.
6. Thakur K, Zunt J. Neurologic parasitic infections in immigrants and travelers. Semin Neurol. 2011;31(3):231–44.
7. Han MH, Zunt JR. Neurologic aspects of infections in international travelers. Neurologist. 2005;11(1):30–44.
8. Kim HJ, Shim KW, Lee MK, et al. Tuberculous encephalopathy without meningitis: pathology and brain MRI findings. Eur Neurol. 2011;65(3):156–9.
9. Chaudhary V, Bano S, Garga UC. Central nervous system tuberculosis: an imaging perspective. Can Assoc Radiol J. 2017;68(2):161–70.
10. Raut AA, Naphade PS, Ramakantan R. Imaging spectrum of extrathoracic tuberculosis. Radiol Clin N Am. 2016;54(3):475–501.
11. Ledbetter LN, Salzman KL, Sanders RK, et al. Spinal neuroarthropathy: pathophysiology, clinical and imaging features, and differential diagnosis. Radiographics. 2016;36(3):783–99.
12. Agarwal R, Sze G. Neuro-Lyme disease: MR imaging findings. Radiology. 2009;253(1):167–73.
13. Hildenbrand P, Craven DE, Jones R, et al. Lyme neuroborreliosis: manifestations of a rapidly emerging zoonosis. AJNR Am J Neuroradiol. 2009;30(6):1079–87.
14. Beuret F, Schmitt E, Planel S, et al. Subtentorial cerebral nocardiosis in immunocompetent patients: CT and MR imaging findings. Diagn Interv Imaging. 2015;96(9):953–7.
15. Mathur M, Johnson CE, Sze G. Fungal infections of the central nervous system. Neuroimaging Clin N Am. 2012;22(4):609–32.
16. Murthy JM, Sundaram C. Fungal infections of the central nervous system. Handb Clin Neurol. 2014;121:1383–401.
17. Offiah CE, Naseer A. Spectrum of imaging appearances of intracranial cryptococcal infection in HIV/AIDS patients in the antiretroviral therapy era. Clin Radiol. 2016;71(1):9–17.
18. Katchanov J, Branding G, Jefferys L, et al. Neuroimaging of HIV-associated cryptococcal meningitis: comparison of magnetic resonance imaging findings in patients with and without immune reconstitution. Int J STD AIDS. 2016;27(2):110–7.
19. Saini J, Gupta AK, Jolapara MB, et al. Imaging findings in intracranial aspergillus infection in immunocompetent patients. World Neurosurg. 2010;74(6):661–70.
20. Starkey J, Moritani T, Kirby P. MRI of CNS fungal infections: review of aspergillosis to histoplasmosis and everything in between. Clin Neuroradiol. 2014;24(3):217–30.
21. Navarathna DH, Roberts DD, Munasinghe J, et al. Imaging candida infections in the host. Methods Mol Biol. 2016;1356:69–78.
22. Teke M, Göçmez C, Hamidi C, et al. Imaging features of cerebral and spinal cystic echinococcosis. Radiol Med. 2015;120(5):458–65.
23. Yadav VK, Sudhakar SV, Panwar J. Pathognomonic MRI and MR spectroscopy findings in cerebral hydatid cyst. Acta Neurol Belg. 2016;116(3):353–5.
24. Ross AG, McManus DP, Farrar J, et al. Neuroschistosomiasis. J Neurol. 2012;259(1):22–32.
25. Liu HQ, Feng XY, Yao ZW, et al. Characteristic magnetic resonance enhancement pattern in cerebral schistosomiasis. Chin Med Sci J. 2006;21(4):223–7.
26. Chen J, Chen Z, Lin J, et al. Cerebral paragonimiasis: a retrospective analysis of 89 cases. Clin Neurol Neurosurg. 2013;115(5):546–51.
27. Xia Y, Chen J, Ju Y, et al. Characteristic CT and MR imaging findings of cerebral paragonimiasis. J Neuroradiol. 2016;43(3):200–6.
28. Singh P, Kochhar R, Vashishta RK, et al. Amebic meningoencephalitis: spectrum of imaging findings. AJNR Am J Neuroradiol. 2006;27(6):1217–21.
29. Guarner J, Bartlett J, Shieh WJ, et al. Histopathologic spectrum and immunohistochemical diagnosis of amebic meningoencephalitis. Mod Pathol. 2007;20(12):1230–7.
30. Shih RY, Koeller KK. Bacterial, fungal, and parasitic infections of the central nervous system: radiologic-pathologic correlation and historical perspectives. Radiographics. 2015;35(4):1141–69.
31. Yusuf FH, Hafiz MY, Shoaib M, et al. Cerebral malaria: insight into pathogenesis, complications and molecular biomarkers. Infect Drug Resist. 2017;10:57–9.
32. Seydel KB, Kampondeni SD, Valim C, et al. Brain swelling and death in children with cerebral malaria. N Engl J Med. 2015;372(12):1126–37.
33. Mohanty S, Benjamin LA, Majhi M, et al. Magnetic resonance imaging of cerebral malaria patients reveals distinct pathogenetic processes in different parts of the brain. mSphere. 2017;2(3):e00193-17.
34. Qi X, Gao J, Sun D, et al. Biofilm formation of the pathogens of fatal bacterial granuloma after trauma: potential mechanism underlying the failure of traditional antibiotic treatments. Scand J Infect Dis. 2008;40(3):221–8.
35. Patil AK, Alexander M, Nair B, et al. Clinical, imaging and histopathological features of isolated CNS lymphomatoid granulomatosis. Indian J Radiol Imaging. 2015;25(1):56–9.
36. Gaha M, Souillard-Scemama R, Miquel C, et al. MR imaging of the brain and spinal cord in lymphomatoid granulomatosis: a case report and review of the literature. J Neuroradiol. 2013;40(5):364–7.
37. De Luna G, Terrier B, Kaminsky P, et al. Central nervous system involvement of granulomatosis with polyangiitis: clinical-radiological presentation distinguishes different outcomes. Rheumatology (Oxford). 2015;54(3):424–32.

17 Autoimmune Encephalitis

Jian Xu

17.1 N-Methyl-D-Aspartate (NMDA) Receptor Antibody Encephalitis

Anti-N-methyl-D-aspartate receptor (NMDAR) encephalitis was first recognized in 2007 and is the most common antibody-associated encephalitis [1]. It is associated with antibodies against GluN1 subunit of NMDAR in both CSF and serum. This disease mostly affects young women and children and mainly causes limbic encephalitis (LE). The term LE refers to an inflammatory process involving the limbic system of the brain which includes the medial temporal lobes and frontobasal and cingular regions. Patients usually present with acute psychiatric symptoms following a prodrome of flu-like symptoms, such as low-grade fever, headache, and malaise. Patients can further develop seizures, memory loss, decreased level of consciousness/catatonic symptoms, respiratory failure requiring mechanical ventilation, movement abnormality such as limb, trunk, or orofacial dyskinesias, as well as autonomic symptoms. CSF tests are often non-specific. But the anti-NMDAR antibodies can frequently be detected in both CSF and serum. Brain MRI is often unremarkable even though the frontal, parietal, and medial temporal cortex can be involved [2–4]. EEG often shows continuous delta slow waves and frontal intermittent rhythmic delta activity (FIRDA). A novel EEG feature, extreme delta brushes (EDB) was reported to be associated with a more prolonged illness in 2012 by Schmitt et al. [5]. The disease is typically associated with ovarian teratoma [2, 6] in young women, even though some recent studies indicate that it can also involve adult men as well as patients without tumor. Treatment includes tumor resection and immunotherapy. First-line immunotherapy includes corticosteroids, plasma exchange, and intravenous immunoglobulin. For patients who do not respond to first-line treatment, early engagement of second-line immunotherapy, including rituximab or cyclophosphamide or combined therapy, should be started. More than 80% of the patients acquired substantial improvement with complete recovery or mild sequelae when treated in an early stage [6].

17.2 Anti-VGKC-Complex Antibody Encephalitis

Voltage-gated potassium channel (VGKC) complexes are a group of proteins containing six transmembrane domains that are present on the neuronal membranes in both central and peripheral nervous systems. They play important roles in neuronal membrane repolarization, axonal conduction, and synaptic transmission. Anti-VGKC-complex antibodies were originally found to be associated with neuromyotonia, Morvan's syndrome, and limbic encephalitis [7–9]. However recent studies have shown that the antibodies were not directly targeting the channels but were acting against VGKC-associated proteins including leucine-rich glioma-inactivated 1 (LGI1) and contactin-associated protein-like 2 (Caspr2).

17.2.1 Anti-LGI1 Limbic Encephalitis

LGI1 antibody-associated encephalitis is the most common type of anti-VGKC-complex encephalitis. LGI1 is a secreted protein mostly found in the hippocampus and the temporal cortex. It functions as a connecting protein between presynaptic ADAM23 and postsynaptic ADAM22, an essential protein involved in the inhibitory signal transmission. The antibody to LGI1 would interfere with LGI1-ADAM interaction which results in hyperexcitability in the postsynaptic condition routes [10]. Mutations of LGI1 in human are associated with pre- and postsynaptic epilepsy-related proteins [11]. LGI1 knockout mice develop lethal epilepsy 3 weeks after birth [12]. Anti-LGI1 encephalitis typically occurs in older men, with a median onset age of 60 years. The patients

J. Xu (✉)
Department of Neurology, Detroit Medical Center, Medical School of Wayne State University,
Detroit, MI, USA

B. Gao et al. (eds.), *Imaging of CNS Infections and Neuroimmunology*, https://doi.org/10.1007/978-981-13-6904-9_17

can present with confusion, memory loss, behavioral abnormality, intractable partial or generalized epilepsy, and rapid eye movement sleep disorders. Half of the patients develop characteristic faciobrachial dystonic seizures (FBDS) where brief unilateral jerky movements of the arm and ipsilateral face or leg occur at high frequency, up to 50–100 times a day [13, 14]. Hyponatremia is another characteristic feature of the disease and can be found in about 60% of the patients. Occasionally the rapid memory deterioration as well as myoclonic movements can mimic rapid dementia such as Creutzfeldt-Jakob disease. Anti-LGI1 encephalitis is usually not associated with cancer even though thymoma and lung cancer can sometimes be found in less than 10% of the patients. CSF is usually unremarkable. Anti-LGI1 antibody can be detected in both CSF and serum. It is not clear yet which test is more sensitive than the other. Therefore it is recommended that both CSF and serum antibodies be tested. MRI at FBDS stage which precedes cognitive abnormalities is often unremarkable. However T2/FLAIR hyperintensity of medial temporal lobes including the hippocampus can be seen during the limbic encephalitis stage [3, 4, 12, 13, 15, 16]. FDG-PET also shows glucose metabolism changes in basal ganglia and temporal lobe [17, 18]. Immunotherapy has been found effective in small clinical trials. About 80% of patients showed dramatic response to the therapy. Seizures including FBDS usually disappear first, but mild cognition deficits can remain. Relapse rate is less than 20%.

17.2.2 Anti-CASPR2-Associated Encephalitis

CASPR2 is a transmembrane protein found on the cell surface of central and peripheral nervous system. Its cytoplasmic domain plays critical roles in potassium channel function at the JXP (juxtaparanodal region) in myelinated axons. Patients with CASPR2 antibodies usually develop Morvan's syndrome characterized by symptoms involving both peripheral (peripheral nerve hyperexcitability which causes muscle cramps and fasciculations, neuropathy, neuromyotonia) and central nervous system (encephalopathy, seizure, hallucination) as well as dysautonomia and insomnia. The disease almost exclusively affects male patients (80–90%) with onset age around 60 years. It is rarely associated with tumors, but lung cancer and endometrial carcinoma have been reported in patients with CASPR2 antibody encephalitis [17, 19]. Patients with the disease may also suffer from other autoimmune diseases such as myasthenia gravis. MRI of the brain usually is normal or mildly abnormal in patients with Morvan's syndrome. However, FDG-PET has shown hyper- or hypometabolism in basal ganglia, orbitofrontal cortex, anterolateral temporal region, as well as the left medial temporal lobe [17, 20, 21]. Even though large clinical trials are not available, early start of immunotherapy is recommended based on better outcome in NMDA-receptor encephalitis. Improvement of cognitive function and cerebral glucose metabolism has been reported in a CASPR2 antibody encephalitis patient who underwent 15-month of immunotherapy [20].

17.3 GAD Antibody Encephalitis

Glutamate decarboxylase (GAD) is an intracellular neuronal antigen that is essential in the formation of gamma-aminobutyric acid (GABA), an inhibitory neurotransmitter in the brain. Antibodies to GAD65 are found in patients with limbic encephalitis, stiff man syndrome, cerebellar ataxia, stiff leg syndrome, and progressive encephalomyelitis with rigidity and myoclonus (PERM). The disease is usually not considered paraneoplastic. It is rare that all the symptoms present in the same patients with GAD65 antibodies even though type 1 diabetes, stiffen syndrome, and limbic encephalitis have been reported in a young female patient with anti-GAD antibody [22]. Patients with limbic encephalitis can present with seizures, psychiatric disturbance, cognitive decline, and amnesia. Anti-GAD can be found in both CSF and serum. MRI of the brain in patients with limbic encephalitis shows characteristic T2/FLAIR hyperintensities in the medial temporal lobes, which is more prominent than the findings in anti-VGKC antibody encephalitis. Patients sometimes develop hippocampal sclerosis later even after immunotherapy [23]. Isolated cerebellum atrophy on MRI has been shown in patients with cerebellar ataxia [24]. Lesions in other locations including frontal lobe have been observed in one of our patients with anti-GAD antibody (Fig. 17.1). Patients with anti-GAD65 antibody often respond well to immunotherapy.

17.4 AMPA Receptor Antibody Encephalitis

Alpha-amino-3-hydroxy-5-methyl-4-isoxazolepropionic acid receptor (AMPAR) is an ionotropic receptor that belongs to the glutamate receptors family. It is critical in the fast excitatory synaptic transmission in the brain. Antibodies targeting GluA1 or GluA2 subunits of the receptor cause AMPAR antibody encephalitis which mostly affects female patients with median onset age of 60. Like in NMDR and LGI1 antibody encephalitis, patients frequently present with LE including memory loss, confusion, psychiatric symptoms, and seizure. Some patients can also present with hyponatremia which could be due to small cell lung cancer (SCLC)-related syndrome of inappropriate antidiuretic hormone (SIADH) or secondary to immune response alone, unlike in LGI1 antibody LE where all cases of hyponatremia are not related to SCLC. More than 70% of the patients with AMPAR antibody encephalitis are found to have underlying

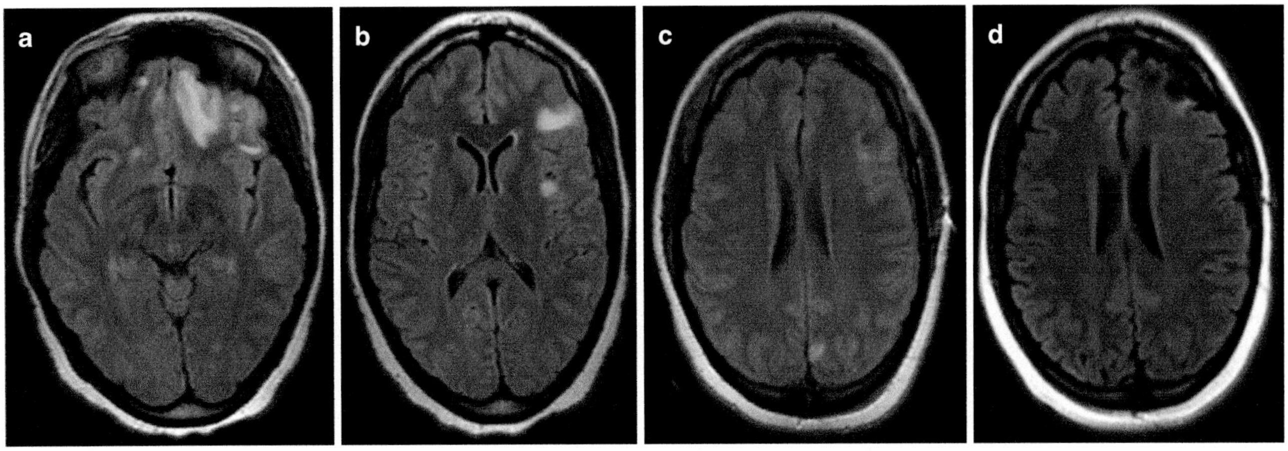

Fig. 17.1 A 20-year-old female presented with new-onset seizure and status epilepticus. Brain MRI of the brain showed multiple diffuse T2/FLAIR hyperintense lesions involving bilateral frontal lobes extending from deep and subcortical region into cortical gray-white matter (**a** and **b**). A two-stage epilepsy surgery with left subfrontal craniotomy was performed due to the location of the lesion and the severity of the seizures. However a new lesion involving the left posterior cingulate region was seen after the surgery (**c**). Anti-GAD antibody was found in both the CSF and serum. Immunotherapy with steroids was given intravenously. The new lesion disappeared after the therapy (**d**), and the seizure is well controlled with anti-epileptic medications

malignancy including SCLC, ovarian cancer, thymoma, etc. [25]. CSF often shows lymphocytic pleocytosis. Anti-AMPAR antibodies are found in both CSF and serum with higher sensitivity in CSF samples. Most of the patients have abnormal brain MRI findings where T2/FLAIR hyperintense signals are found in unilateral or bilateral mesiotemporal lobes [15, 25]. Transient changes in other areas including anterior septal nuclei and insular, occipital, or cerebellar regions have been reported [15]. More than half patients respond to immunotherapy or tumor treatment. But the improvements are not as dramatic as those observed in LGI1- or NMDR-related encephalitis. In fact, most of the patients only show partial response neurologically (48%) [25]. About half the patients who originally responded to the immunotherapy relapse possibly due to the aggressiveness of the treatment and underlying tumor types.

17.5 GABAb Receptor Antibody Encephalitis

Gamma-aminobutyric acid type B receptors (GABAbR) are a group of surface receptors that are expressed in the presynaptic and postsynaptic membranes in the hippocampus, thalamus, and cerebellum. These receptors negatively regulate synaptic plasticity which is involved in memory, cognition, and learning. Disruption of these receptors is expected to result in seizures and changes in the abovementioned functions. Indeed the theory has been proven in animal models using pharmaceutical antibodies or genetic knockout techniques [26–29]. The first cases of anti-GABAbR encephalitis in human were reported in 2010 by Lancaster et al. [30]. Patients who were considered "seronegative" based on paraneoplastic panel test results were found to express anti-GABAbR antibody in CSF, serum, or both. Since then, more cases have been reported by different groups. Patients typically present with LE with intractable seizures, memory loss, psychiatric symptoms, and autonomic dysfunction. Rare cases of ataxia, opsoclonus-myoclonus, chorea, and heart failure were reported [31]. More than half of the cases are associated with underlying tumor which is mostly SCLC even though the only reported pediatric case was not found to be associated with any malignancy [31]. CSF may show lymphocytic pleocytosis as in other types of LE. Anti-GABAbR can be found in both CSF and serum. More than 60% of the patients show typical MRI findings of LE with uni- or bilateral mesiotemporal lobe hyperintensity on T2/FLAIR. Immunotherapy can result in dramatic neurological improvements. However the prognosis is still largely dependent on the treatment of the underlying tumor.

17.6 GABAa Receptor Antibody Encephalitis

This disease was recently described by Petit-Pedrol et al. in 2014 [32]. They found high-titer CSF and serum antibodies against $\alpha1/\beta3$ subunit of gamma-aminobutyric acid A receptor (GABAa Receptor) in six patients with rapidly progressive encephalopathy and resulted refractory seizures. Five of the six patients had status epilepticus, while one had epilepsia partialis continua. All the patients experienced psychiatric symptoms or cognition deterioration before the onset of the seizure. Half of the patients were children. The ages of the patients ranged from 3 to 63 years. A 3-year-old patient developed confusion, opsoclonus, ataxia, and chorea, while another one experienced hemiparesis before the onset of the seizure. CSF showed at least one abnormality in five of the six with pleocytosis, increased protein concentration, or oligoclonal bands, whereas CSF of one patient was normal. Unlike in the other autoimmune encephalitis where brain MRI was either normal or showed abnormality in limbic system, all the six patients in this study showed extensive abnormality on FLAIR/T2 with multifocal or diffuse cortisol and subcortical involvement without contrast enhancement. No evidence of active underlying malignancy was found in any of the six patients. However, most of the patients had other autoantibodies including thyroid peroxidase antibodies (three patients), GAD65 antibodies (one patient), and GABAb receptor antibodies (two patients) indicating the tendency for autoimmune dysregulation in these patients. Half of the patients responded well to the immunotherapy despite the severity of the disease. Two patients died secondary to the epilepsy-related sepsis. One 4-year-old patient improved without immunotherapy.

In another study by Ohkawa et al. [33], antibodies are directly against the β3 subunit of the GABA. A receptor on inhibitory synapses was reported in two patients with encephalitis. Both of the patients present with cognitive impairment, while only one patient developed seizure/status epilepticus. Brain MRI showed multifocal involvement in bilateral temporal lobes as compared to unifocal involvement in limbic encephalitis. Interestingly, both of the patients had invasive thymoma. Studies of more patients are needed to provide more information regarding this novel type of autoimmune encephalitis.

17.7 Dipeptidyl-Peptidase-Like Protein-6 (DPPX) Antibody Encephalitis

DPPX is a membrane glycoprotein involved in regulating expression and conductance of Kv4.2 potassium channels. The encephalitis associated with anti-DPPX antibody was first described in four patients in 2013 by Boronat [34]. So far 28 patients with anti-DPPX encephalitis have been reported. In the original study, patients presented with severe diarrhea followed by cognition impairment and psychiatric symptoms. Patients then developed cerebellar symptoms including ataxia, nystagmus and tremor, muscle rigidity, myoclonus, and seizures. The diarrhea caused severe weight loss but no malignancy was found in these patients. The same clinical pattern was confirmed in another case report recently [35]. A subsequent study reported three patients with distinct syndrome resembling progressive encephalomyelitis with rigidity and myoclonus (PERM). Another study involving 20 patients characterized the disease with neuropsychiatric and brainstem symptoms, seizures, sleep disturbance, weight loss, dysautonomia, and central hyperexcitability (stiffness, spasms, tremulousness, and exaggerated startle). Only two patients in this study had classic findings of PERM [36]. Most of the patients had preceding prominent GI symptoms including diarrhea or constipation. The antibody can be equally detected in serum and CSF. Brain MRI showed non-specific findings such as moderate microangiopathic leukoencephalopathy but no evidence of limbic encephalitis. Most of the patients responded dramatically to the immunotherapy.

17.8 Other Disorders

Serum antibodies against dopamine-2 receptors have been recently described in children with basal ganglia encephalitis, Sydenham chorea, and Tourette syndrome [37]. MRI showed abnormality in half of the 12 patients where T2/FLAIR hyperintensity was seen in caudate, putamen, globes pallidus, and substantial nigra. Antibodies to glycine receptor were described in patients presenting with PERM or stiff person syndrome [38–41]. Brain MRI in these patients is mostly unremarkable though temporal lobe involvement, and non-specific white matter changes have been seen in a few cases. Antibodies against IgLON5, a member of cell adhesion molecule family, were found in eight patients who presented with abnormal sleep movements and obstructive sleep apnea. Video polysomnography showed undifferentiated non-REM sleep or poorly structured non-REM stage N2, as well as REM parasomnias and sleep breathing disorders [42]. The brain MRI, EEG, and CSF studies were unremarkable in all these patients. With the development of the lab and imaging techniques, more types of autoimmune encephalitis will likely be discovered in the near future, expanding the spectrum of the complicated disorder family.

17.9 Conclusion

Over the last one or two decades, a group of autoimmune encephalitis with different antibodies against intracellular or cell surface antigens have been discovered. Despite the wide range of proteins that are involved, most of the diseases, such as NMDAR, AMPAR, LGI1 receptor, and GABAbR encephalitis, present with limbic encephalitis with characteristic MRI findings of hyperintensities involving medial temporal lobes on T2/FLAIR. Tumors and other autoimmune disorders are sometimes accompanied with the distinct encephalitis. Early diagnosis and initiation of immunotherapy are important as in most of the cases, the patients respond dramatically to the therapy despite the severity of the clinical symptoms. First-line immunotherapy includes IVIG, plasmaphoresis, and IV steroids. However in cases that are resistant to first-line therapy, second-line therapy with rituximab and/or cyclophosphamide was proven to be effective in some patients. In cases with underlying tumors, resecting and treating the primary tumor is important in preventing the relapses.

References

1. Granerod J, Ambrose HE, Davies NW, et al. Causes of encephalitis and differences in their clinical presentations in England: a multicentre, population-based prospective study. Lancet Infect Dis. 2010;10(12):835–44.
2. Dalmau J, Lancaster E, Martinez-Hernandez E, et al. Clinical experience and laboratory investigations in patients with anti-NMDAR encephalitis. Lancet Neurol. 2011;10(1):63–74.
3. Irani SR, Alexander S, Waters P, et al. Antibodies to Kv1 potassium channel-complex proteins leucine-rich, glioma inactivated 1 protein and contactin-associated protein-2 in limbic encephalitis, Morvan's syndrome and acquired neuromyotonia. Brain. 2010;133(9):2734–48.
4. Irani SR, Bera K, Waters P, et al. N-methyl-D-aspartate antibody encephalitis: temporal progression of clinical and paraclinical observations in a predominantly non-paraneoplastic disorder of both sexes. Brain. 2010;133(Pt 6):1655–67.
5. Schmitt SE, Pargeon K, Frechette ES, et al. Extreme delta brush: a unique EEG pattern in adults with anti-NMDA receptor encephalitis. Neurology. 2012;79(11):1094–100.
6. Titulaer MJ, McCracken L, Gabilondo I, et al. Treatment and prognostic factors for long-term outcome in patients with anti-NMDA receptor encephalitis: an observational cohort study. Lancet Neurol. 2013;12(2):157–65.
7. Liguori R, Vincent A, Clover L, et al. Morvan's syndrome: peripheral and central nervous system and cardiac involvement with antibodies to voltage-gated potassium channels. Brain. 2001;124(Pt 12):2417–26.
8. Sinha S, Newsom-Davis J, Mills K, et al. Autoimmune aetiology for acquired neuromyotonia (Isaacs' syndrome). Lancet. 1991;338(8759):75–7.
9. Vincent A, Buckley C, Schott JM, et al. Potassium channel antibody-associated encephalopathy: a potentially immunotherapy-responsive form of limbic encephalitis. Brain. 2004;127(Pt 3):701–12.
10. Ohkawa T, Satake S, Yokoi N, et al. Identification and characterization of GABA(A) receptor autoantibodies in autoimmune encephalitis. J Neurosci. 2014;34(24):8151–63.
11. Fukata Y, Adesnik H, Iwanaga T, et al. Epilepsy-related ligand/receptor complex LGI1 and ADAM22 regulate synaptic transmission. Science. 2006;313(5794):1792–5.
12. Irani SR, Michell AW, Lang B, et al. Faciobrachial dystonic seizures precede Lgi1 antibody limbic encephalitis. Ann Neurol. 2011;69(5):892–900.
13. Irani SR, Pettingill P, Kleopa KA, et al. Morvan syndrome: clinical and serological observations in 29 cases. Ann Neurol. 2012;72(2):241–55.
14. Ismail FS, Popkirov S, Wellmer J, et al. Faciobrachio-crural dystonic seizures in LGI1 limbic encephalitis: a treatable cause of falls. Neurol Neuroimmunol Neuroinflamm. 2015;2(5):e146.
15. Lai M, Hughes EG, Peng X, et al. AMPA receptor antibodies in limbic encephalitis alter synaptic receptor location. Ann Neurol. 2009;65(4):424–34.
16. Lai M, Huijbers MG, Lancaster E, et al. Investigation of LGI1 as the antigen in limbic encephalitis previously attributed to potassium channels: a case series. Lancet Neurol. 2010;9(8):776–85.
17. Irani SR, Stagg CJ, Schott JM, et al. Faciobrachial dystonic seizures: the influence of immunotherapy on seizure control and prevention of cognitive impairment in a broadening phenotype. Brain. 2013;136(Pt 10):3151–62.
18. Shin YW, Lee ST, Shin JW, et al. VGKC-complex/LGI1-antibody encephalitis: clinical manifestations and response to immunotherapy. J Neuroimmunol. 2013;265(1-2):75–81.
19. Vynogradova I, Savitski V, Heckmann JG. Hemichorea associated with CASPR2 antibody. Tremor Other Hyperkinet Mov (NY). 2014;4:239.
20. Spinazzi M, Argentiero V, Zuliani L, et al. Immunotherapy-reversed compulsive, monoaminergic, circadian rhythm disorder in Morvan syndrome. Neurology. 2008;71(24):2008–10.
21. Toosy AT, Burbridge SE, Pitkanen M, et al. Functional imaging correlates of fronto-temporal dysfunction in Morvan's syndrome. J Neurol Neurosurg Psychiatry. 2008;79(6):734–5.
22. Sharma CM, Pandey RK, Kumawat BL, et al. A unique combination of autoimmune limbic encephalitis, type 1 diabetes, and Stiff person syndrome associated with GAD-65 antibody. Ann Indian Acad Neurol. 2016;19(1):146–9.
23. Malter MP, Helmstaedter C, Urbach H, et al. Antibodies to glutamic acid decarboxylase define a form of limbic encephalitis. Ann Neurol. 2010;67(4):470–8.
24. Honnorat J, Saiz A, Giometto B, et al. Cerebellar ataxia with anti-glutamic acid decarboxylase antibodies: study of 14 patients. Arch Neurol. 2001;58(2):225–30.
25. Hoftberger R, Titulaer MJ, Sabater L, et al. Encephalitis and GABAB receptor antibodies: novel findings in a new case series of 20 patients. Neurology. 2013;81(17):1500–6.
26. Lau CG, Zukin RS. NMDA receptor trafficking in synaptic plasticity and neuropsychiatric disorders. Nat Rev Neurosci. 2007;8(6):413–26.
27. Prosser HM, Gill CH, Hirst WD, et al. Epileptogenesis and enhanced prepulse inhibition in GABA(B1)-deficient mice. Mol Cell Neurosci. 2001;17(6):1059–70.
28. Schuler V, Luscher C, Blanchet C, et al. Epilepsy, hyperalgesia, impaired memory, and loss of pre- and postsynaptic GABA(B) responses in mice lacking GABA(B(1)). Neuron. 2001;31(1):47–58.
29. Shepherd JD, Huganir RL. The cell biology of synaptic plasticity: AMPA receptor trafficking. Annu Rev Cell Dev Biol. 2007;23:613–43.
30. Lancaster E, Lai M, Peng X, et al. Antibodies to the GABA (B) receptor in limbic encephalitis with seizures: case series and characterisation of the antigen. Lancet Neurol. 2010;9(1):67–76.
31. Kruer MC, Hoeftberger R, Lim KY, et al. Aggressive course in encephalitis with opsoclonus, ataxia, chorea, and seizures: the first pediatric case of gamma-aminobutyric acid type B receptor autoimmunity. JAMA Neurol. 2014;71(5):620–3.
32. Petit-Pedrol M, Armangue T, Peng X, et al. Encephalitis with refractory seizures, status epilepticus, and antibodies to the GABAA receptor: a case series, characterisation of the antigen, and analysis of the effects of antibodies. Lancet Neurol. 2014;13(3):276–86.
33. Ohkawa T, Fukata Y, Yamasaki M, et al. Autoantibodies to epilepsy-related LGI1 in limbic encephalitis neutralize LGI1-ADAM22 interaction and reduce synaptic AMPA receptors. J Neurosci. 2013;33(46):18161–74.
34. Boronat A, Gelfand JM, Gresa-Arribas N, et al. Encephalitis and antibodies to dipeptidyl-peptidase-like protein-6, a subunit of Kv4.2 potassium channels. Ann Neurol. 2013;73(1):120–8.
35. Piepgras J, Holtje M, Michel K, et al. Anti-DPPX encephalitis: pathogenic effects of antibodies on gut and brain neurons. Neurology. 2015;85(10):890–7.

36. Tobin WO, Lennon VA, Komorowski L, et al. DPPX potassium channel antibody: frequency, clinical accompaniments, and outcomes in 20 patients. Neurology. 2014;83(20):1797–803.
37. Dale RC, Merheb V, Pillai S, et al. Antibodies to surface dopamine-2 receptor in autoimmune movement and psychiatric disorders. Brain. 2012;135(Pt 11):3453–68.
38. Carvajal-Gonzalez A, Leite MI, Waters P, et al. Glycine receptor antibodies in PERM and related syndromes: characteristics, clinical features and outcomes. Brain. 2014;137(Pt 8):2178–92.
39. Hutchinson M, Waters P, McHugh J, et al. Progressive encephalomyelitis, rigidity, and myoclonus: a novel glycine receptor antibody. Neurology. 2008;71(16):1291–2.
40. McKeon A, Robinson MT, McEvoy KM, et al. Stiff-man syndrome and variants: clinical course, treatments, and outcomes. Arch Neurol. 2012;69(2):230–8.
41. Wuerfel E, Bien CG, Vincent A, et al. Glycine receptor antibodies in a boy with focal epilepsy and episodic behavioral disorder. J Neurol Sci. 2014;343(1-2):180–2.
42. Sabater L, Gaig C, Gelpi E, et al. A novel non-rapid-eye movement and rapid-eye-movement parasomnia with sleep breathing disorder associated with antibodies to IgLON5: a case series, characterisation of the antigen, and post-mortem study. Lancet Neurol. 2014;13(6):575–86.

18 Inflammatory Diseases of the Meninges

Fuqing Zhou

18.1 Brief Introduction of Meninges' Anatomy

The meninges which is covering and protecting the brain and spinal cord comprise the three distinct associated membranes between the skull and the brain, including dura mater, arachnoid, and pia mater (Fig.18.1).

18.1.1 Dura Mater

In the human or other mammals, the dura mater is a thick and tough double membrane, which consists of periosteal dura, meningeal dura, and dural border layer. Outer layer is the skull inside periosteum, only loose to accompany the calvarium, particularly in the occipital and temporal attached more loose, called periosteal layer. However, the craniotomy and cranial soles are more tightly attached, and they are difficult to separate. No intracranial cavity. The inner layer of the dura mater is thicker than the outer layer and is tough, and the dura mater is conjoined with the endorhachisdura lining at the foramen magnumlarge hole in the occiput, known as the meningealpleura layer.

18.1.2 Arachnoid Matter

The arachnoid mater is located in the deep part of the dura mater, where there is a latent space between the dura mater. In which that subarachnoid cavity is expand and deepened to become the subarachnoid space, filled by cerebrospinal fluid. The largest of subarachnoid space is the cerebellar medullary pool, which is connected with the fourth ventricle through the median hole and the front hole. Subarachnoid cavities that pierce the dura mater in the intravenous hard film sinus are known as arachnoid particles, and they are related to the reabsorption of the cerebrospinal fluid.

18.1.3 Pia Mater

Pia mater is a layer of transparent membrane that is attached to the surface of the brain and extends into the fissure. It is the innermost layer of the meninges, surrounding the brain and spinal cord. In some parts of the wall of the ventricle, the pia mater and its vessels form together with the ependymal epithelium choroid tissue.

18.1.4 The Role of Meninges in Inflammatory Diseases Pathogenesis

Most inflammation of meninges prominently was *Haemophilus influenzae* type B, *Neisseria meningitidis*, and *Streptococcus pneumoniae* (pneumococcus). About 80 percent of inflammation of meninges is bacterial meningitis in the United States. It is common for a small portion of healthy person to carry these germs within nasal or body surface that do not infringe on the human body, which is spread by coughing or sneezing. Some studies suggested that people are most susceptible to infections when they have a cold, because inflammation in the nose makes it extremely easy to get bacteria into the brain. Other infrequent causes may involve the meninges, including a number of systemic diseases, such as sarcoidosis or vasculitis. Meningitis infection originate from four aspects [1, 2]: (1) hematogenous spread infection; (2) Direct invasion of adjacent lesions; (3) Direct spread of intracranial lesions; (4) Iatrogenic infection.

After the bacteria enter the subarachnoid space, the antigens of the bacterial wall and some cytokines that mediate the inflammatory reaction stimulate the adhesion of endothelial cells and induce neutrophils to enter the central nervous system, triggering the inflammatory process. The inflammatory

F. Zhou (✉)
Department of Radiology, The First Affiliated Hospital, Nanchang University, Nanchang, China

B. Gao et al. (eds.), *Imaging of CNS Infections and Neuroimmunology*, https://doi.org/10.1007/978-981-13-6904-9_18

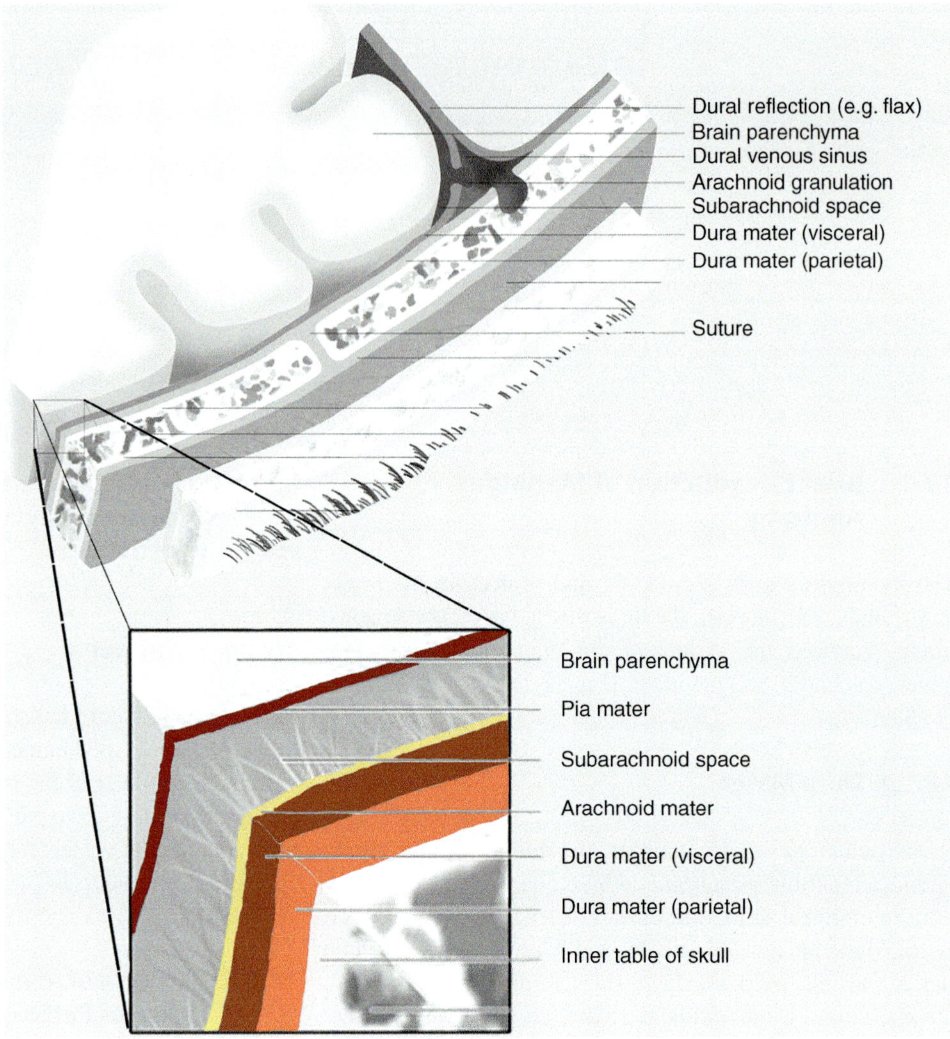

Fig. 18.1 Three layers of the meninges. The dura matter is a thick and tough layer of double membrane. The outer layer is the periosteum of the inner of the skull. It is only loosely attached to the skull cap, especially in the occipital and temporal attachment, which is called periosteum. Arachnoid membrane, a translucent membrane, is located in the deep part of the dura mater. The pia matter is a layer of transparent film that is attached to the surface of the brain and extends into the fissure

process produces a lot of purulence. The exudate in the brain can cause inflammatory adhesion of the central brain water pipe, the lateral hole of the fourth ventricle, or the arachnoid, which affects the circulation and absorption of cerebrospinal fluid and causes hydrocephalus.

The basic pathological changes of acute suppurative meningitis caused by various pathogenic bacteria are soft meningitis, cerebral vascular congestion, and inflammatory cell infiltration. In the early stages of the disease, the epidural and the superficial blood vessels of the brain are hypercharged and dilated, and the neutrophils are in the subarachnoid space. The subarachnoid cavity is full of purulent secretions containing a large number of bacteria, which makes the cerebrospinal fluid mixed. Purpureus exudate covers the surface of the brain, which is often deposited in the brain drain and brain pool and can also be found in the brain. The color of the pus can vary with the spread of the pathogenic bacteria, and the superficial soft meningeal and ependymal membrane are granulated by fibrinolytic exudate.

18.2 Purulent Bacterial Meningitis

18.2.1 Epidemiology and Clinical Manifestations

Purulent bacterial meningitis, or purulent meningitis, is still one of the most common diseases in the world. The epidemiological situation in different countries and regions is different. Higher rates in developing countries may be associated with a lack of vaccination [3]. Suppurative bacterial infection is a common suppurative infection in the central nervous system [4]. Acute onset usually occurs in infants and children and the elderly over 60.

The incubation period of this disease is 1–7 days, generally 2–3 days, clinically according to the disease and performance into three types. Infection may arise from hematogenous spread during systemic infection, from a chronic suppurative focus. Another path of infection is direct spread from brain injury with open or covered disruption of the dura mater.

The most common pathogens of suppurative meningitis are as follows [5]: *group-B Streptococcus* and *Escherichia coli* (in adults), *Streptococcus pneumoniae* and *Neisseria meningitidis* (in adolescents), *Haemophilus influenzae*, *Streptococcus pneumoniae*, and *Neisseria meningitides* (in infants) (Fig.18.2).

Most meningitis is acute onset or explosive, with similar clinical manifestations, mainly as follows:

1. Symptoms of infection: fever, chills, or upper respiratory tract infection.
2. Meningeal stimulation: It was characterized by stiff neck, Kernig, and Brudzinski. However, it is often not obvious that neonatal, elderly, or comatose patients have meningeal stimulation.
3. Increased intracranial pressure: Symptoms include severe headache, vomiting, disturbance of consciousness, etc.
4. Focal symptoms: Some of the patients may have symptoms of focal neurological impairment, such as hemiplegia, aphasia, etc.

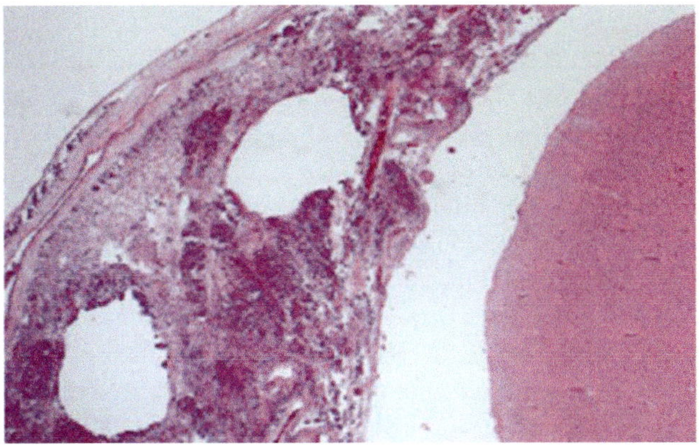

Fig. 18.2 Histopathology of bacterial meningitis: inflammatory infiltrates of the pia mater consisting of neutrophil granulocytes

5. Other symptoms: Some patients have a more specific clinical features, such as *Neisseria meningitidis meningitis*; there was a rash of bacteremia, which began to diffuse red maculopapule quickly into the skin petechiae, mainly in the trunk and lower limbs, mucosa, and conjunctiva, and accidentally found in the palm of your hand and foot. Headache is the most common symptom in meningitis, and it is found in more than 80% of the patients [5].

18.2.2 Imaging Findings

18.2.2.1 CT Imaging

Imaging findings of plain CT scan [6]: In the initial phase of purulent meningitis: might normal finding of meninges. In the advanced phase of purulent meningitis (sign of beginning in the CSF circulation): (1) mild enlargement of the ventricles including basal cistern and lateral deformation crack pool, (2) mild enlargement of the subarachnoid space, and (3) higher density in the ventricles. Imaging findings of CT enhancement: (1) partial or total occlusion of basal pool and lateral fissure pool and (2) significant enhancement or linear leptomeningeal enhancement.

18.2.2.2 MRI

Imaging findings of conventional plain MRI scan: (1) hyperintensity of the subarachnoid space on T2-weighted images or FLAIR images indicating leakage of the blood-brain barrier with hypercellularity or increased proportions of proteins in the CSF and (2) vascular or septic complications. Imaging finding of enhancement MRI: (1) more effective then contrast-enhanced CT, (2) extends into the basal cisterns and asymmetrical enhancement (Fig.18.3). Imaging finding of diffusion-weighted imaging: highly

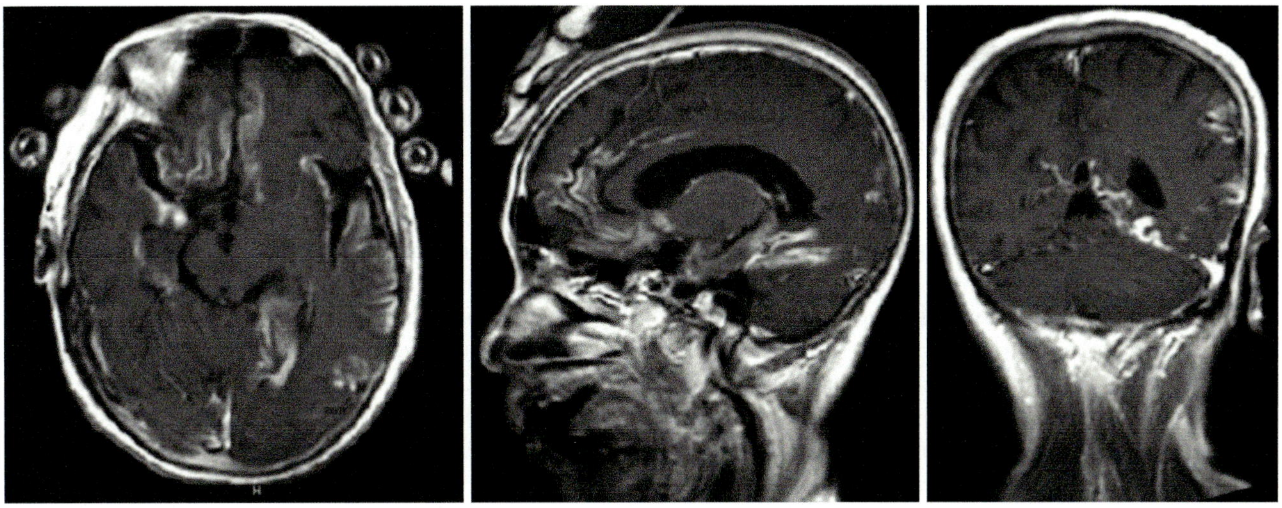

Fig. 18.3 Pneumococcal meningitis of MRI enhancement imaging in adult female. Enhanced scanning of brain trench and cerebral pool showed a line-like enhancement. Enhanced scan lesions were flaky enhancement. Inflammation of the intima of the cerebral artery caused by pneumococcus, causing stenosis of the lumen, thrombosis, focal cerebral softening, and so on

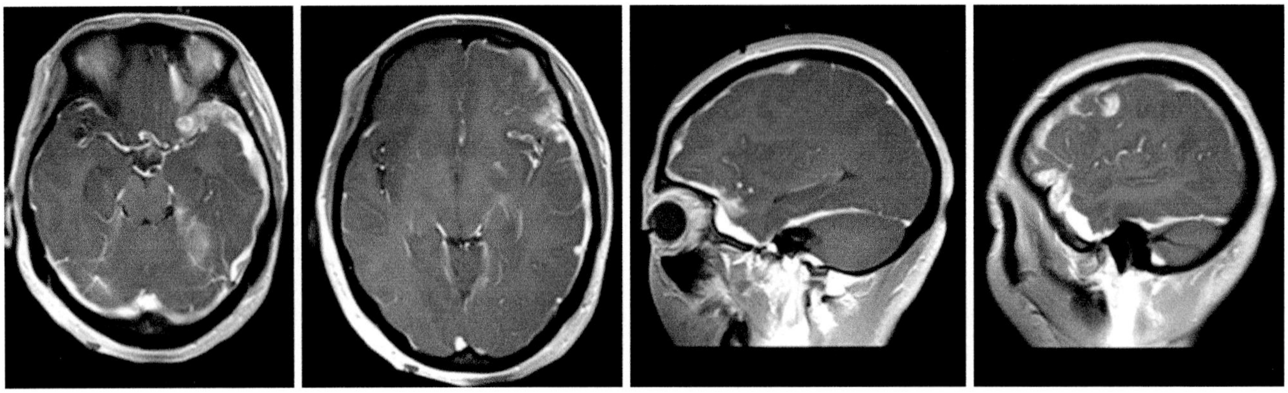

Fig. 18.4 Axial and sagittal T1-weighted image after contrast administration demonstrated thickened pachymeningeal enhancement and epidural empyema in patients with pneumococcal meningitis

sensitive to find the small infarctions of cortical or deep white matter. Imaging finding of perfusion weighted imaging: (1) functional information about hemodynamic effects, (2) influenced by septic vasculitis. MRA imaging visualized vascular changes.

Subdural or epidural empyemas are often associated with mass effect and edema (Fig.18.4), which hypointense to white matter and slightly hyperintense relative to CSF on T1-weighted images and hyperintense relative to white matter and CSF on T2-weighted images. Subdural empyema usually shows hyperintense, but epidural empyemas tend to be of hypointense or mixed signal intensity on diffusion-weighted imaging [7].

18.2.3 Diagnose and Differential Diagnosis

The diagnosis of suppurative meningitis was according to the clinical manifestations, CT or MRI findings. For imaging finding, it is more used to found the sequelae of suppurative meningitis. In suppurative meningitis, isolated enhancement is not specific imaging finding, similar findings could present in viral or fungal meningitis. But for fungal meningitis, it is more common in the subarachnoid space, such as thicker, lumpy, or nodular enhancement.

18.3 Tuberculous Meningitis

18.3.1 Epidemiology and Clinical Manifestations

Tuberculous meningitis (TBM) is a nonsuppurative inflammation of the meninges and meningiomas caused by *Mycobacterium tuberculosis* (more than 90%). About 5–15% of patients with extrapulmonary tuberculosis are involved in the nervous system, which is the most common form of TBM, about 70% of the total. In recent years, the incidence and mortality of tuberculosis in China and abroad have been increasing due to the genetic mutation of mycobacterium tuberculosis, the development of anti-tuberculosis drugs and the increase of AIDS patients.

According to the British Medical Research Council, TBM can be classified into the following three periods based on its nonspecific signs and symptoms: Stage 1, unconscious fuzziness with no neurological function impairment; Stage 2, brain stimulation, mild nervous system dysfunction (such as cerebral palsy), and abnormal motor function; and Stage 3, convulsion, lethargy or coma, and severe neurological impairment (such as paralysis or systemic paralysis).

In the early stage of TBM, due to the inflammation of the cerebral membrane, choroid plexus, and ventricular tube membrane, the generation of CSF is increased, but the absorption of arachnoid granule drops and then forms traffic hydrocephalus. In advanced stage of TBM, arachnoid, choroid plexus adhesion, form a complete or incomplete obstructive hydrocephalus. The result is increased intracranial pressure.

Clinical manifestations: most patients with onset conceals, chronic course of the disease, can also be acute or subacute onset, or lack the history of tuberculosis exposure. The natural course of the patient are as follows:

1. Symptoms of tuberculosis poisoning: low fever, night sweats, fatigue and weakness, and hypoesthesia
2. Meningeal irritation and intracranial hypertension: fever, headache, vomiting and meningeal irritation, and increased intracranial pressure (early stage); eventually leading to tonic seizure, and obstructive hydrocephalus (progressive stage)
3. Damage of brain parenchyma: lethargy, apathy, delirium or delusion, partial sex, generalized epileptic seizure or persistent state of epilepsy, lethargy, or confusion of consciousness; related symptoms of tuberculous arteritis, arachnoid of the brain and spinal cord

4. Dysfunction of cranial nerve: vision loss, diplopia, and facial paralysis (cranial nerves III, VI, and VII)

18.3.2 Imaging Findings

18.3.2.1 Thickening of Basal Cisterns, Lateral Fissure Cisterns, and Soft Meninges

It is caused by the infiltration and proliferation of the meningitis. It's showed that the inflamed meninges as distinct basal periparenchymal hyperintensity in the basal cisterns, cerebral fissure and cerebral sulcus (between CSF and parenchymal signal) on non-enhanced T1-weighted imaging. On contrast-enhanced T1-weighted images, basal meningeal enhancement is found in approximately 60% of TBM cases, obvious enhancement, homogenous or heterogeneous enhancement, or line-like reinforcement [8]. The adjacent brain parenchyma with thickening of the meninges can have inflammatory edema, which is shown as a long T1- and T2-weighted signal without contrast enhancement. Thickening of the meninges in the lateral fissure is usually wrapping with the horizontal segment of middle cerebral artery, causing secondary ischemia and infarctions. Secondary ischemic or hemorrhagic infarcts are diagnosed best with diffusion-weighted and susceptibility-weighted imaging. Further imaging findings, TBM comprise infarcts due to secondary vasculitis in 30–40% [1, 9].

CT scans showed that the thickening of the cerebral fissure and cerebral sulcus was higher than the density of cerebrospinal fluid (partial or full). The basal cistern is thickened, and it can be calcified. On contrast-enhanced CT, thickening of the meninges of basal cisterns was significantly enhanced, and the delayed 5-min scanning enhancement effect was the best. Delayed 5 min scan, the density of the thickening of the meninges increased, but in the blood vessel density in the cerebral sulcus decreased, thereby better confirming the thickening of the meninges.

18.3.2.2 Tuberculomas of Meningitis

It can be single, but usually multiple and clustered distribution in the basal cisterns, cerebral fissure and cerebral sulcus (Fig.18.5). Tuberculoma is composed of granulomatous ring and caseous necrotic center, which is circular or irregular and rarely exists independently, and is fused with thickened meninges. T2-weighted images showed slightly high signal; most of the center of the lesion is difficult to discern the caseous necrosis; thus, on the non-enhanced T1-weighted imaging, it is difficult to distinguish between the irregular thickening of the meningioma and the tuberculoma. Whether either unliquefied or liquefied cheese necrosis, on diffusion-weighted imaging, low signal is not caused by the limited diffusion of water. On CT imaging, when tuberculoma diameter is smaller, lesions are shown to have higher density than that of CSF, but similar to the density of brain parenchyma, especially in the delayed 5-min scanning, it is obviously enhanced granuloma ring and unreinforced caseous necrosis center (Fig.18.6).

18.3.2.3 Epidural or Epidural Tuberculous Abscess

The subdural abscess shows a meniscus lesion in the cranial plate, and the epidural abscess is the lesion of the double convex lens in the skull. The abscess cavity is shown as low signal in T1-weighted image, and the T2-weighted image is high signal. The wall of the abscess in T1-weighted images

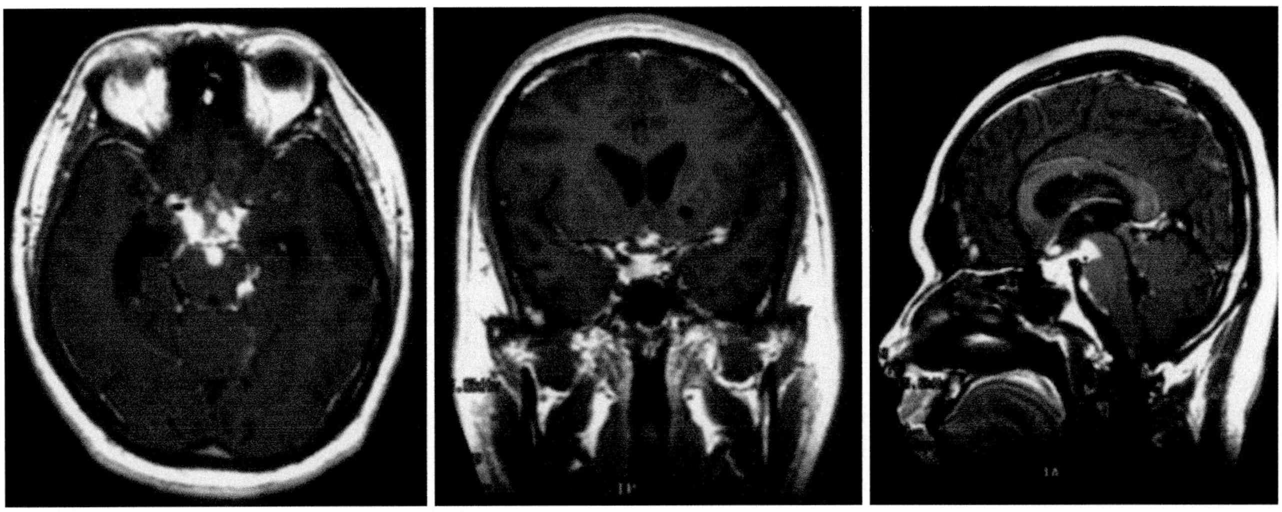

Fig. 18.5 T1-weighted image after contrast administration of tuberculous meningitis

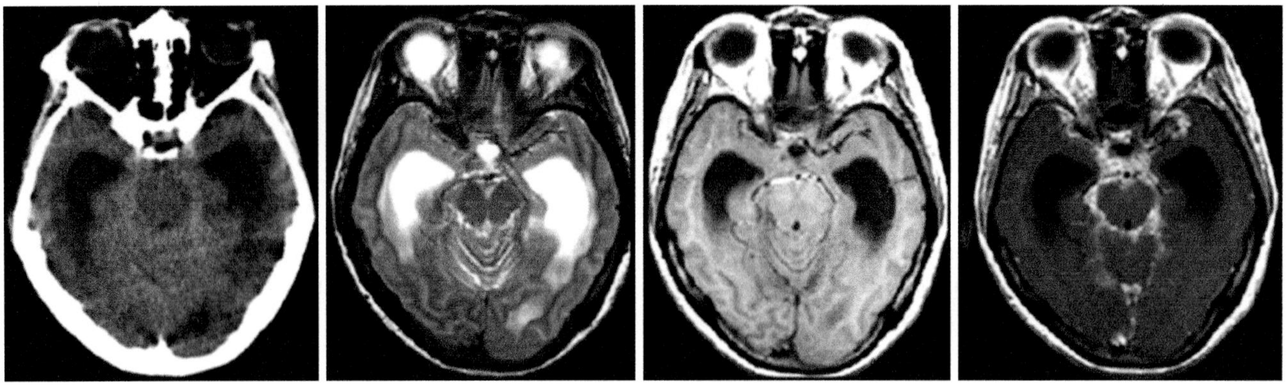

Fig. 18.6 Imaging (CT, T2WI, T1WI, and T1-CE) of tuberculous meningitis with hydrocephaly

and T2-weighted images was either equal or slightly higher signal. The abscess wall was obviously strengthened during the enhanced scan, and the abscess cavity was not strengthened. Due to the limited water diffusion, the pus can show the high signal in diffusion-weighted imaging.

18.3.3 Diagnose and Differential Diagnosis

Diagnosis of TBM is made by CSF analyses collected by lumbar puncture. Other causes of infectious meningitis have to be considered for differential diagnosis [8]. On the contrast-enhanced imaging, TBM result predominantly in basilar meningeal enhancement, while bacterial meningitis affects more often the leptomeninges of the convexities.

18.4 Viral Meningitis

18.4.1 Epidemiology and Clinical Manifestations

Viral meningitis is diffuse inflammation syndrome of the pia meninges caused by viral infection. The main clinical manifestations are fever, headache, vomiting, and meningeal irritation, which is the most common aseptic meningitis. The course of disease was benign, most of which is not more than 3 weeks, with self-limitation and good prognosis.

Most of the infections are enteroviruses, including poliovirus, coxsackievirus A and B, evironoviruses, etc., which are prevalent or sporadic. It is mainly transmitted by fecal-oral route, and few are transmitted by respiratory secretion. The second infected viruses are mumps virus, herpes virus, and adenovirus infection. Mumps virus is frequent in winter and spring season and often is self-limited. Herpes viruses include herpes simplex virus, EB virus, cytomegalovirus, and varicella zoster virus. Other viruses contain insect-borne viruses, human immunodeficiency virus (HIV), West Nile virus, etc. [10, 11].

18.4.2 Imaging Findings

In the early stages of viral meningitis, there are normality and only unspecific changes (focal or diffuse brain edema and swelling) or signal abnormalities in the subarachnoid space (increased protein content) in the brain CT or MRI. But in the later stage of HSV-1-meningoencephalitis, enhancement of the affected leptomeningeal may be visible on T2-weighted and FLAIR images in limbic structures (hyperintensity).

18.4.3 Diagnose and Differential Diagnosis

Diagnose of viral meningitis is made by testing of the CSF. The symptoms of systemic infection with acute onset of disease, meningeal stimulation, and mild and moderate increase of CSF lymphocytes could contribute to the diagnosis of the disease. The viral encephalitis of summer and autumn is diagnosed by Japanese b encephalitis, and the latter has a basal ganglia lesion in the brain CT or MRI. In case of HSV meningitis, differential diagnosis includes paraneoplastic (limbic) encephalitis, infiltrating neoplasm, and status epilepticus [11]. In addition, viral meningitis needs to be differential diagnosis with tuberculous meningitis, fungal meningitis, and bacterial meningitis.

18.5 Fungal Meningitis

18.5.1 Epidemiology and Clinical Manifestations

Fungal meningitis is an inflammation caused by fungal infection of the meninges and is often associated with brain parenchymal infection. Pathogenic fungi and opportunistic pathogens cause fungal infections in the central nervous system. The former includes *Cryptococcus neoformans*, *Pityrosporum ovale*, *Blastomyces dermatitidis*, *Sporothrix schenckii*, and

Histoplasma capsulatum. The latter has *Candida, Aspergillosis*, *Zygomycetes*, and *Trichosporum* [12, 13].

Most patient have a subacute disease course, a few are chronic onset. Symptoms include general systemic symptom (headache, fever, nausea, vomiting), nervous system symptom (cranial nerve dysfunction, conscious, and coma), and symptoms of double or multiple infections.

18.5.2 Imaging Findings

Brain edema, hydrocephalus, and focal abnormalities of the brain can be detected by imaging studies such as brain CT or MRI. Brain parenchymal granulomas can be shown as slightly T1 hypointensity and significantly T2 hyperintensity in MRI examination. For cryptococcal meningoencephalitis, the typically manifestation is diffuse meningeal enhancement and ventriculitis beside characteristic cystic. The "soap-bubble lesions" punctuate lesions in the basal ganglia due to cryptococcal invasion of the perivascular spaces. Hydrocephalus is not found more often in immunocompromised patients but often as a manifest in immunocompetent individuals as arachnoid reactions with exudates in the basal cisterns.

18.5.3 Diagnose and Differential Diagnosis

Fungal meningitis often causes meningeal thickness than bacterial or viral meningitis and significant enhancement in CT or MRI with contrast-enhanced scanning. Other meningitis, especially TBM and bacterial meningitis have to be excluded.

References

1. Rohde S. Inflammatory diseases of the meninges. Berlin: Springer; 2012. p. 127–37.
2. Kim IO. Infection and inflammatory diseases of the central nervous system. Berlin: Springer; 2014. p. 75–103.
3. Chang WN, Lu CH, Huang CR, et al. Mixed infection in adult bacterial meningitis. Infection. 2000;28(1):8–12.
4. Huang CR, Chen SF, Lu CH, et al. Clinical characteristics and therapeutic outcomes of nosocomial super-infection in adult bacterial meningitis. BMC Infect Dis. 2011;11:133.
5. Honda H, Warren DK. Central nervous system infections: meningitis and brain abscess. Infect Dis Clin N Am. 2009;23(3):609–23.
6. Packer RJ, Bilaniuk LT, Zimmerman RA. CT parenchymal abnormalities in bacterial meningitis: clinical significance. J Comput Assist Tomogr. 1983;6(6):1064–8.
7. Wang L, Zhang YG, Ya-Zhuo HU. The comparison on diagnostic values of CT and MRI in the diagnosis of central nervous system infection. Med Innov China. 2016;20:60–2.
8. Bernaerts A, Vanhoenacker FM, Parizel PM, et al. Tuberculosis of the central nervous system: overview of neuroradiological findings. Eur Radiol. 2003;13(8):1876–90.
9. Abdelmalek R, Kanoun F, Kilani B, et al. Tuberculous meningitis in adults: MRI contribution to the diagnosis in 29 patients. Int J Infect Dis. 2006;10(5):372–7.
10. Rotbart HA. Viral meningitis. Semin Neurol. 2000;20(3):277–92.
11. Logan SA, Macmahon E. Viral meningitis. Brit Med J. 2008;336(7634):36–40.
12. Gottfredsson M, Perfect JR. Fungal meningitis. Semin Neurol. 2000;20(3):307–22.
13. Chen Y, He Y, Li W, et al. The CT and MRI manifestations of intracranial fungal infection. China Med Her. 2010;17:66–8.

Inflammatory and Autoimmune Disorders of the Spinal Cord

19

Kirt Gill, Mark S. Shiroishi, Chia-Shang Liu, Alexander Lerner, and Meng Law

19.1 Introduction

Inflammatory and autoimmune disorders of the spinal cord are a heterogeneous group of myelopathies with a diverse differential diagnosis. Due to similarities in presentation and diverse associated conditions, confusion can arise in differentiating among them. The primary characteristic tying them together is an inflammatory process of the spinal cord known as transverse myelitis. Primarily this inflammatory process is associated with viral infections and autoimmune responses [1]. Particular manifestations of transverse myelitis, such as a longitudinally extensive form, are found with presentations of neuromyelitis optica, multiple sclerosis, and sarcoidosis among many others [2]. By focusing primarily on the clinical presentation followed by differentiating pathophysiology for the disorders discussed, this chapter aims to provide a foundation for differentiation based on nuances among otherwise similar presentations in these disorders. However, in many cases, the cause of transverse myelitis is unknown, and thus the topic remains an active research area. Diagnostic algorithms and select cases will be discussed with a focus on spinal cord imaging.

19.2 Transverse Myelitis

The primary clinical manifestation of inflammatory processes of the spinal cord is described as transverse myelitis (TM). TM is an acquired neuro-immune spinal cord disorder associated with numerous neuro-inflammatory disorders. It is characterized by a rapid development of bilateral neurological symptoms including weakness, sensory deficits, and autonomic dysfunction [1, 3]. Symptoms can develop within hours to days and can reach a maximum severity within 2 weeks [4].

The development of TM is a characteristic manifestation of inflammatory process in the spinal cord and has been definitively associated with a number of inflammatory diseases including demyelinating diseases such as multiple sclerosis and neuromyelitis optica, connective tissue disorders (i.e., systemic lupus erythematosus, Sjögren syndrome, Behcet syndrome, rheumatoid arthritis, etc.), sarcoidosis, paraneoplastic syndromes, and acute disseminated encephalomyelitis. It is also associated with infectious etiologies including but not limited to neurocysticercosis, HIV, herpes viruses, HTLV-1, West Nile virus, mycoplasma, and syphilis [5]. The diverse pathogenesis of TM reflects the varied associated diseases and will be discussed in more detail in later sections. However, certain pathologic features such as lymphocytic perivascular infiltration and axonal degeneration can be found in varying degrees in all manifestations [6]. Additionally, the involvement of both gray and white matter in TM indicates that it is a mixed inflammatory disorder affecting neurons, axons, oligodendrocytes, and myelin rather than a purely demyelinating condition.

TM can be classified as acute partial, acute complete, or longitudinally extensive. Acute partial TM refers to spinal cord dysfunction with mild clinical features or grossly asymmetric lesions on MRI (Fig. 19.1). Acute complete TM refers to spinal cord dysfunction with symmetric complete or near-complete neurologic deficits below the level of the lesion. Both acute partial and acute complete types show lesion extending vertically one to two vertebral segments in length along the cord on MRI. Longitudinally extensive transverse myelitis (LETM) refers to complete or partial spinal cord dysfunction that extends over three or more contiguous vertebral segments [7]. Brain MRI may help in the differential diagnosis of LETM. The brain MRI of a NMO patient is historically thought to be normal or nonspecific, especially at the onset of the disease; however, the presence of certain

K. Gill (✉) · M. S. Shiroishi · C.-S. Liu · A. Lerner
Division of Neuroradiology, Keck School of Medicine, University of Southern California, Los Angeles, CA, USA
e-mail: kirtgill@usc.edu

M. Law
Radiology and Nuclear Medicine, Alfred Health, Melbourne, VIC, Australia

Department of Electrical and Computer Systems Engineering, Monash University, Clayton, VIC, Australia

Department of Neuroscience, Monash School of Medicine, Nursing and Health Sciences, Clayton, VIC, Australia

B. Gao et al. (eds.), *Imaging of CNS Infections and Neuroimmunology*, https://doi.org/10.1007/978-981-13-6904-9_19

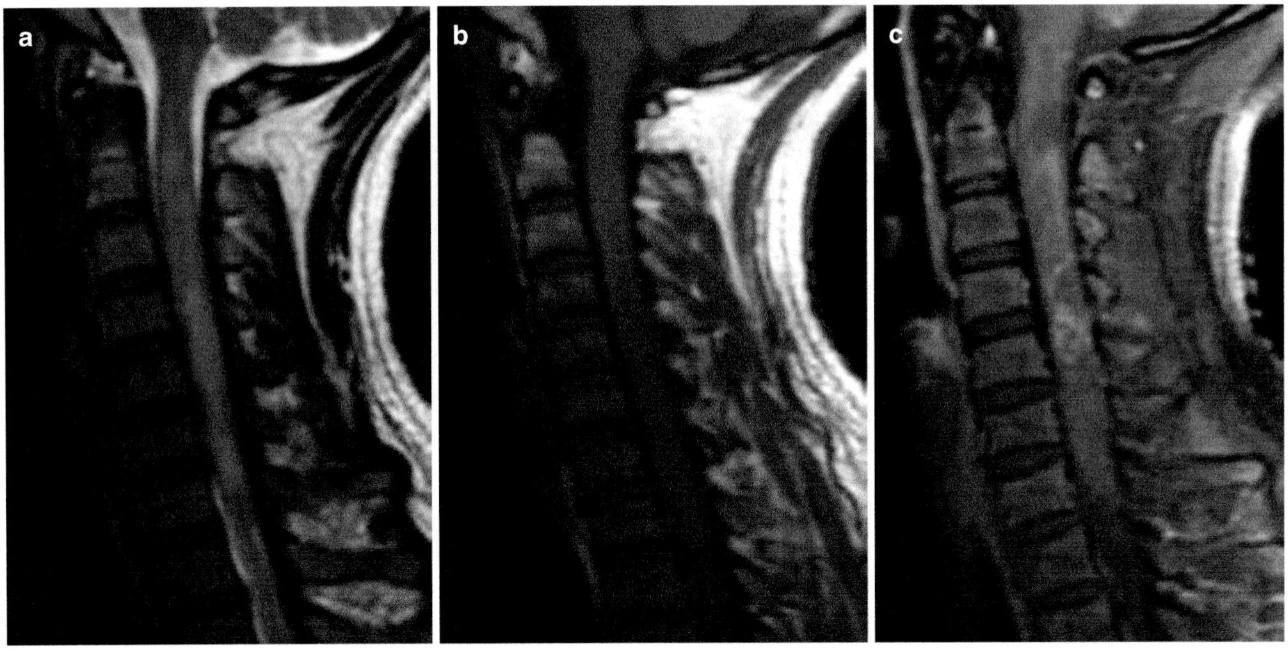

Fig. 19.1 Idiopathic transverse myelitis of the cervical cord. Sagittal T2-weighted image (**a**) demonstrates a T2 hyperintense intramedullary lesion extending from C2 through C6/C7 level in the cervical cord consistent with LETM. There is marked edema and expansion of the cord. Noncontrast- (**b**) and contrast-enhanced (**c**) sagittal T1-weighted images show heterogeneous enhancement throughout the T2 hyperintense lesion

lesions described as specific to NMO may differentiate NMO from other causes of LETM [8].

Notably, acute partial or complete TM should be differentiated from the diagnosis of intramedullary glioma, a common misread. Acute TMs range widely along the spinal cord and are associated with more mild, consistent, and sharply demarcated edema. Intramedullary tumors, however, most commonly grow slowly, demonstrate a wide area of spinal cord thickening, possess irregular tumor edges, and appear heterogenous in composition. Intramedullary gliomas can be cystic and can present with proximal or distal syringomyelia. Radiographically, perhaps the clearest differentiating factor is that gliomas show significant enhancement while TM generally does not enhance or presents with only mild patchy enhancement. If fortunate enough to have the clinical presentation as well, acute symptoms such as a viral prodrome helps differentiate TM from glioma and from other spinal edema causes such as traumatic spinal cord injury.

19.2.1 Idiopathic Transverse Myelitis

Idiopathic TM is a diagnosis of exclusion. Studies have found that about 15% of TM cases may be classified as idiopathic [9]. However, as advancements in the understanding of TM pathogenesis have been made and the specificity of assays testing for specific disease biomarkers has increased, the number of idiopathic cases has decreased. It is theorized idiopathic cases may eventually "vanish" [10].

Nonetheless, in cases currently classified as idiopathic, a preceding gastrointestinal, respiratory, or systemic illness is often present. Postinfectious TM has been postulated to be due to molecular mimicry and superantigen-mediated diseases leading to autoimmunity [11]. For instance, superantigens such as toxic shock syndrome toxin-1 and staphylococcal enterotoxins A through I prime the immune system and can activate T lymphocytes without costimulatory signals, triggering autoimmune disease via autoreactive T-cell clones [11]. The clinical features of TM develop acutely or subacutely. Symptoms vary with the associated condition and will be discussed in more detail in later sections. Idiopathic TM at baseline presents with a conglomerate of symptoms consistent with motor, sensory, and autonomic syndromes. Motor dysfunction presents initially as a flaccid condition and subsequently develops into spastic condition as time progresses. Typical sensory symptoms include pain, dysesthesia, and paresthesia. Autonomic symptoms include urinary urgency, frequency, or retention, constipation and incomplete evacuation, and sexual dysfunction [6]. Symptoms depend on the spinal level affected. Idiopathic TM is localized primarily to the cervical or thoracic spinal cord. In rare cases, spinal involvement can range from one vertebral segment to the entire spinal cord [7].

Suspicion of TM increases with acute or subacute signs of symptoms but requires exclusion of a lesion causing cord compression for diagnosis. Exclusion occurs preferably via gadolinium-enhanced MRI; however CT myelogram or high-quality spine CT can be used alternatively although CT

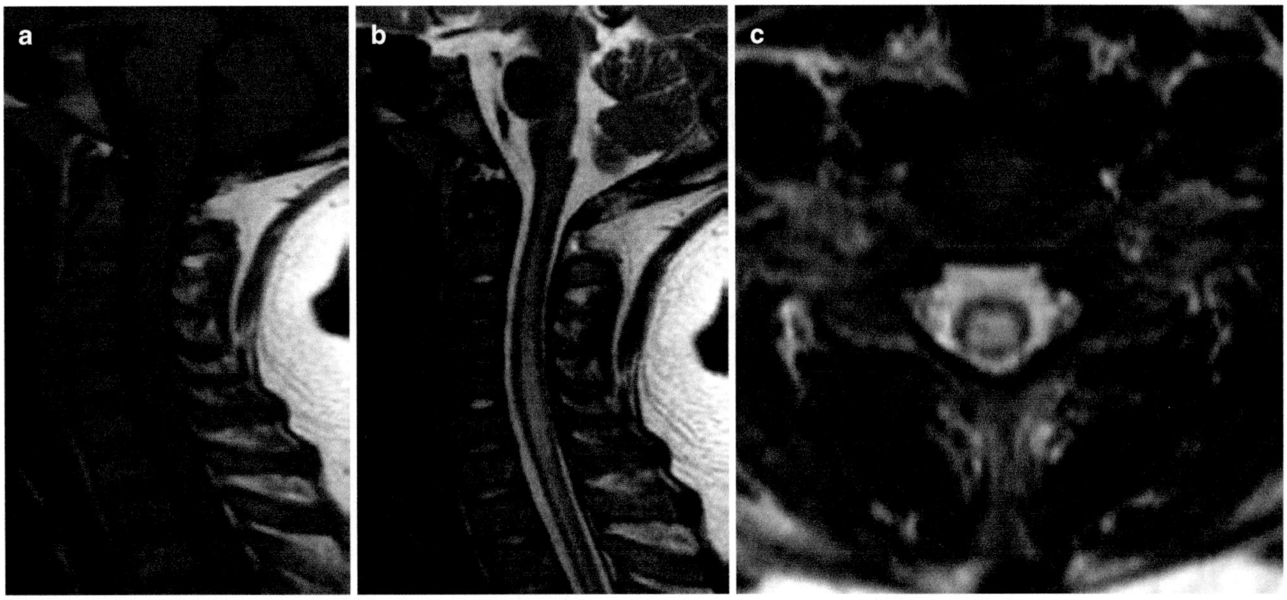

Fig. 19.2 Idiopathic transverse myelitis of the cervical cord. Sagittal T1-weighted (**a**) and T2-weighted (**b**) images demonstrate a T1 hypointense and T2 hyperintense intramedullary lesion extending throughout the cervical cord. Axial T2-weighted image (**c**) confirms central location of the lesion with moderate T2 hyperintensity. The signal intensity on these sequences allows for differentiation from syringohydromyelia which would demonstrate higher T2 signal and lower T1 signal similar to CSF

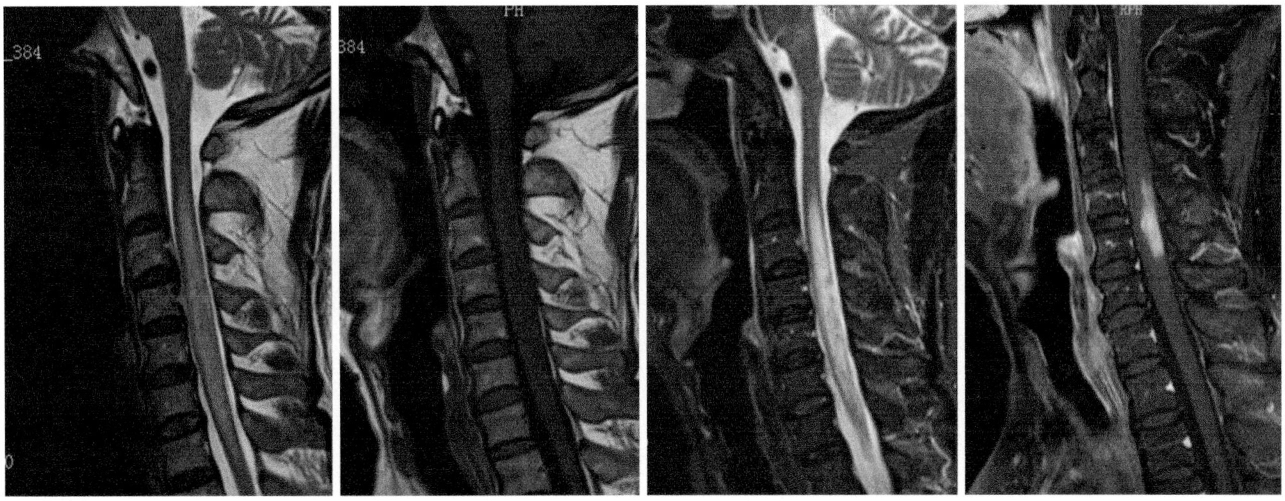

Fig. 19.3 Longitudinally extensive transverse myelitis. (**a**, **b**) On the sagittal T2WI and T1WI cervical spinal cord swollen,T2-weighted image hyperintensity and T1-weighted image hypointensity; (**c**, **d**) sagittal fat suppression image shows strip-shaped hyperintensity; post-contrast MRI shows mild patchy enhancement in cervical spinal cord (courtesy of Chenglong Ren MD., Department of Radiology, Affiliated Hospital of Shanxi University of Chinese Medicine)

is usually not definitive for this purpose. Once cord compression is ruled out, inflammatory or noninflammatory status is assessed by looking for positive gadolinium enhancement on MRI, pleocytosis, or elevated IgG index within the CSF [7].

The typical appearance of idiopathic TM on MRI is of a central T2 hyperintense lesion (Fig. 19.2) usually extending over more than two vertebral segments in length and involving more than a two-thirds cross section of the cord [12]. Enhancement patterns vary including heterogeneous, peripheral, and diffuse enhancement (Fig. 19.3). Enhancement is more frequent in the subacute stage than during initial presentation in the acute stage [3, 9].

The patients with LETM are found to have important distinctive features of NMO, of which the most useful MRI findings include the presence of bright spotty lesions (BSLs) (either punctuate or as larger cavities) and T1 dark lesions, centrally located or both centrally and peripherally located lesions, and a lesion involving ≥50% of the cord area [8]. The full investigative algorithm for idiopathic TM forms the baseline diagnostic procedure used in all situations for TM regardless of cause and assists in identifying associated disorders. These studies include MRI of the entire spine with or without contrast, brain MRI with and without contrast, CSF cell count and differential, and serum studies including but not limited to HIV antibodies, NMO-IgG antibodies, syphilis serologies, B12, methylmalonic acid levels, ANA, and TSH [7].

Brain MRI may help in the differential diagnosis of LETM. The brain MRI of a NMO patient is historically thought to be normal or nonspecific, especially at the onset of the disease; however, the presence of certain lesions described as specific to NMO may differentiate NMO from other causes of LETM [8].

19.3 Demyelinating Inflammatory Myelopathies

19.3.1 Multiple Sclerosis

Multiple sclerosis (MS) has been discussed extensively in a previous chapter; so, it will be touched on lightly here for the purposes of highlighting distinguishing features among spinal myelopathies. Acute transverse myelitis can be the first detected symptom of MS, which presents typically with a partial myelitis. Due to the partial lesions, sensory or motor symptoms will be present, but bowel and bladder dysfunction will not usually be compromised [13]. Characteristic MS symptoms include positive neurological symptoms such as Lhermitte phenomenon (sensation of paresthesia in the spine or limbs elicited by neck flexion) and paroxysmal manifestations of pruritic and tonic muscle spasms in addition to negative symptoms such as fatigue, worsening of function with heat, and blurry vision [14].

MS affecting the spinal cord is seen on MR in 70–80% of MS cases. In about 5–24% of cases, MS is confined to the spinal cord. Sixty to seventy-five percent of these lesions are cervical. Usually lesions extend less than two contiguous vertebral segments in length. T2-weighted images typically show peripheral or paracentral located lesions that are ovoid in shape. Only about 15% of cord plaques will enhance. Cord swelling is atypical and atrophy is more common. More than 50% of patients have multiple lesions, but about 50% of the lesions are clinically silent at any time. The relapsing course of MS is a key distinguishing feature from other myelopathies [15]. Notably, the imaging findings for MS can vary depending on the population. For instance, opticospinal MS with atypical longitudinal extensive spinal cord lesions three or more vertebral segments in length has been described to be more prevalent in Central and South America and in Hispanic population in the USA [16] (Fig. 19.4).

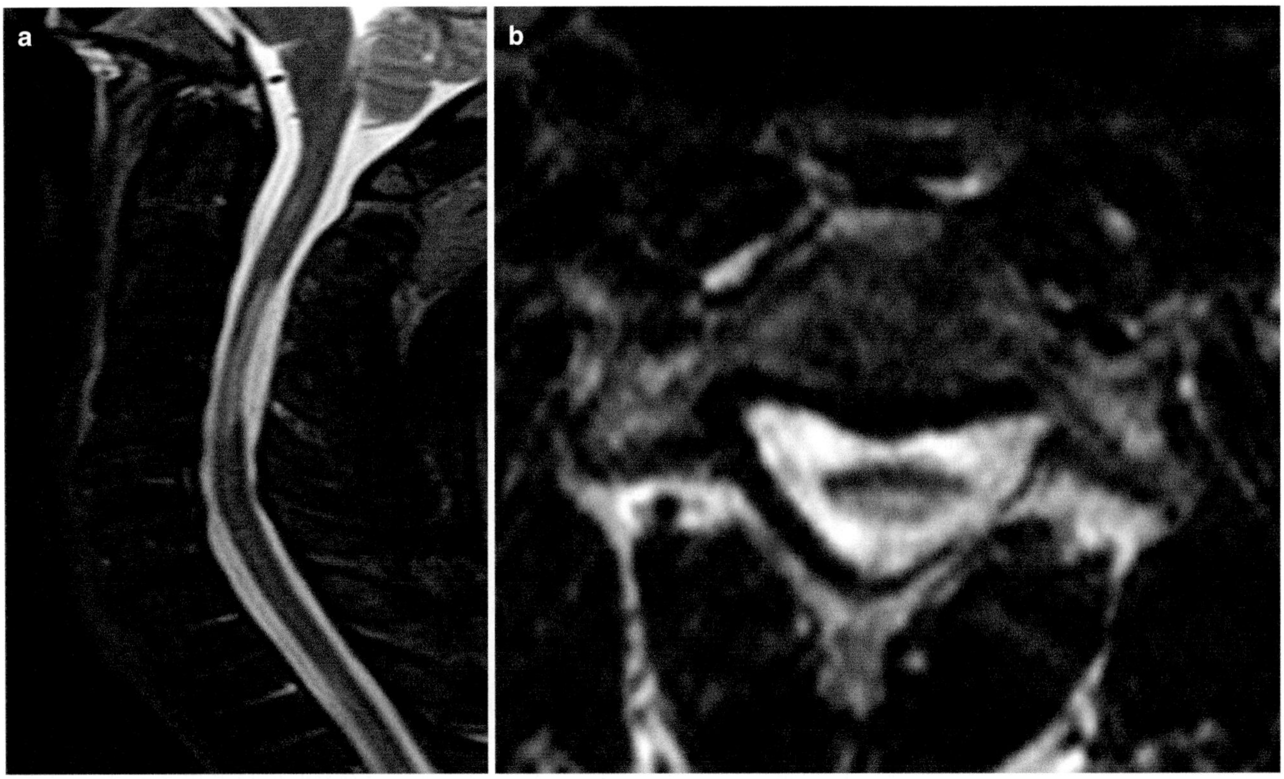

Fig. 19.4 Atypical appearance of multiple sclerosis: longitudinally extensive spinal cord lesion (LECL), alternatively referred to as longitudinally extensive transverse myelitis (LETM). Sagittal STIR image (**a**) demonstrates a dorsal hyperintense lesion extending along three vertebral body segments in length (C3 through C5 levels) representing LESCL. There is associated volume loss of the cord in this region. A more typical small focal hyperintense ventral MS lesion is seen at T2 level. Axial T2-weighted image (**b**) at C4 level confirms dorsal location of the LESCL and associated volume loss

It is important to once again note that following the diagnosis of acute TM, a brain MRI should be performed. In MS myelitis, patients whose brain MRI shows at least one lesion consistent with demyelination have an 82% chance of meeting clinical criteria for MS in the next 20 years compared to a 21% chance for patients with a normal brain MRI [17]. Additionally, to establish a diagnosis of clinically definitive MS, only one additional brain lesion and a simultaneous asymptomatic gadolinium-enhancing lesion are needed to fulfill the space and time criteria needed for diagnosis [18].

19.3.2 Neuromyelitis Optica and Neuromyelitis Optica Spectrum Disorders

Neuromyelitis optica (NMO) and the neuromyelitis optica spectrum disorders (NMOSD) comprise a group of inflammatory disorders targeting the central nervous system (CNS) via immune-mediated attacks leading to demyelination and axonal damage. These attacks are mediated by serum NMO-immunoglobulin G (IgG) antibody which selectively binds aquaporin-4 (AQP4). Previously known as Devic's syndrome or disease, the disorders, particularly NMOSD, were considered variants of MS. The discovery and description of NMO-IgG binding to AQP4 in 2004 lead to the characterization of these disorders as distinct clinically from MS [19].

Similar to MS pathogenesis, the exact autoimmune inflammatory cascade which leads to the demyelination and axonal injury occurs through many different pathways. Unlike MS which is mostly a cell-mediated disorder, NMO/NMOSD pathophysiology is mediated through a humoral autoimmune response. The NMO-IgG antibody has been shown to correlate with disease activity and with the size of lesions [20]. The target of the antibody, AQP4, is a water channel heavily concentrated in periaqueductal and periventricular regions, astrocyte foot processes at the blood-brain barrier, and within the gray matter of the spinal cord [21]. Within NMO/NMOSD, AQP4 expression decreases unrelated to any demyelination, which differentiates the process from MS, where AQP4 loss is consistent with demyelination [22]. The prevalence of NMO/NMOSD has been estimated from 0.5 to 4.5 for every 100,000 people. It is shown to be up to ten times more prevalent in females versus males, and the median presenting age is in the patients' 30s [23]. However, epidemiological studies can be difficult to interpret due to the evolving nature of the diagnostic criteria.

The international consensus on diagnostic criteria published in 2016 establishes six core clinical characteristics (optic neuritis, acute myelitis, area postrema syndrome, acute brainstem syndrome, symptomatic narcolepsy, or symptomatic cerebral syndrome with NMOSD-typical brain lesions) [24]. Of these six, the classic clinical presentation is of acute optic neuritis or transverse myelitis attacks, often following a relapsing course. Optic neuritis is the inflammation of the optic nerve. It is associated with degrees of vision loss and eye pain which worsens with ocular movement. Optic neuritis attacks in NMO/NMOSD individually are indistinguishable from other syndromes leading to optic neuritis. However, in NMO/NMOSD, vision loss is usually more severe, and sequential optic neuritis in rapid succession or bilateral cases are more suggestive of NMO/NMOSD [25]. TM is an acquired neuro-immune spinal cord disorder associated with numerous neuro-inflammatory disorders. Rapid onset of weakness, sensory alterations, and autonomic impairment below the level of the lesion are common clinical manifestations [25]. In contrast to MS, NMO/NMOSD typically has a greater extent of spinal cord demyelination, identified via recognition of three or more involved spinal cord segments on magnetic resonance imaging (MRI) [26]. In such situations, TM is characterized as longitudinally extensive transverse myelitis (LETM). Though patients with NMO/NMOSD can also present with a shorter lesion, LETM is found in a higher proportion of cases [27].

The diagnostic algorithm is contingent on whether a positive expression of NMO-IgG is detected. When not detected, MRI of the spinal cord and brain are used to confirm status. Additional requirements on MRI for diagnosis depend on the core characteristic being observed (Table 19.1).

Focusing on the spinal cord MRI findings, imaging can be indicative of acute or chronic status. In acute cases, LETM lesions show increased signal on sagittal T2-weighted sequences extending over three complete vertebral segments. These lesions have central cord predominance with over 70% of the lesion within the central gray matter. On T1-weighted sequences, gadolinium enhancement occurs with no specific pattern to the signal [24] (Fig. 19.5). Additional characteristic features that may be observed in acute cases include extension of the lesion to brainstem, cord expansion or edema, and decreased T1-signal localized over increased T2-signal areas. In chronic cases, spinal cord MRI findings show

Table 19.1 Characteristics identifiable on MRI for diagnosis

Additional MRI requirements for NMOSD without NMO-IgG or with unknown NMO-IgG status
1. Acute optic neuritis: requires brain MRI showing (a) normal findings or only nonspecific white matter lesions, or (b) optic nerve MRI with T2-hyperintense lesion or T1-weighted gadolinium enhancing lesion extending over more than one-half the optic nerve length or involving optic chiasm
2. Acute myelitis: requires associated intramedullary MRI lesion extending over ≥3 contiguous segments (LETM) or ≥3 contiguous segments of focal spinal cord atrophy in patients with history compatible with acute myelitis
3. Area postrema syndrome: requires associated dorsal medulla/area postrema lesions
4. Acute brainstem syndrome: requires associated periependymal brainstem lesions

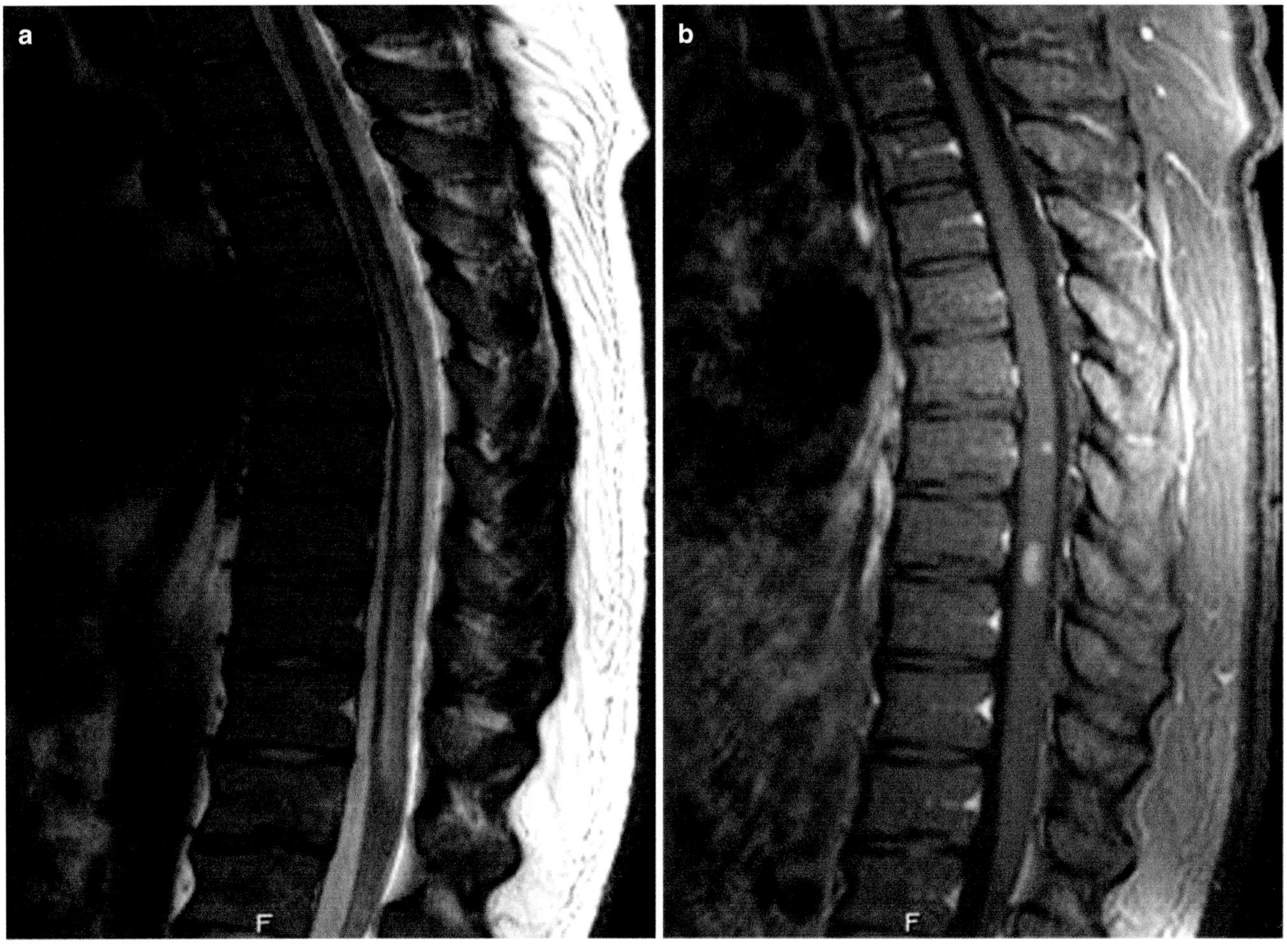

Fig. 19.5 Neuromyelitis optica (NMO) of the thoracic cord. Sagittal T2-weighted image (**a**) demonstrates a T2 hyperintense lesion extending from T5 through T11 level in the thoracic cord consistent with LETM. There is associated cord edema and expansion. Post-contrast T1-weighted sagittal image (**b**) demonstrates two nodular foci of enhancement within the large hyperintense lesion

extensive longitudinal cord atrophy with or without any change in T2 signal. Extensive longitudinal cord atrophy is characterized by sharply demarcated atrophy over three or more complete, contagious vertebral segments [24].

19.4 Myelopathies Associated with Systemic Autoimmune Disorders

A number of systemic autoimmune disorders lead to inflammatory processes which involve with the spinal cord. The primary clinical manifestation is transverse myelitis, which, as discussed above, is an acute inflammatory disease of the spinal cord. Transverse myelitis as a result of a systemic autoimmune condition has been most frequently associated with SLE and antiphospholipid syndrome. To a lesser extent, it has also been associated with Sjögren syndrome, Behcet syndrome, mixed connective tissue disease, ankylosing spondylitis, and sarcoidosis, among others.

19.4.1 Systemic Lupus Erythematous

Transverse myelitis is a rare complication of systemic lupus erythematous (SLE). Review studies have estimated this complication occurs in 1–2% of SLE patients [28]. SLE is a chronic inflammatory disease of unknown causes that affects multiple organ systems. It is characterized by immunologic findings and is associated with several antinuclear antibodies. Of the various antibodies associated with SLE, antinuclear antibodies (ANA) and antiphospholipid (aPL) antibodies are most associated with SLE myelitis. Antiphospholipid antibody is positive in 43–73% of SLE myelitis patients [29]. There is no clear designated pathologic role of this antibody in SLE myelitis. It is theorized that aPL antibodies may cause venous infarcts resulting in thrombotic events and thus SLE myelitis. Other possible mechanisms leading to immunopathogenesis in SLE include direct interaction of autoantibodies with autoantigens on neuronal cell bodies, local production of cytokines, and interference of neurotransmission. A confounding factor in SLE myelitis is that there is a well-established association between NMO-IgG antibodies and SLE-associated antibodies. Past studies have estimated that 52.6% of NMO/NMOSD patients were also ANA positive [30].

On imaging, SLE myelitis may be distinguished by an enlarged spinal cord with high T2 signal intensity involving four to five vertebral segments. Fifty percent of cases will demonstrate contrast enhancement with variable patterns. However, MRI of the spinal cord may appear normal in up to 30% of patients with clinical myelitis [28, 31].

19.4.2 Antiphospholipid Syndrome

Antiphospholipid syndrome (APS) is known for its clinical features of thrombosis leading to organ dysfunction. The most characteristic clinical manifestation is recurrent fetal loss. APS, as discussed above, is associated with an underlying autoimmune disorder, namely, SLE [32]. The autoantibody most associated with the condition is antiphospholipid antibody (aPL). CNS involvement of APS includes TM, cerebrovascular thrombosis, migraines, chorea, seizures, and cognitive dysfunction. TM specifically is a rare manifestation of APS and is reported in only 0.4–1% of patients. Pathogenesis is postulated to be due to antibody interaction with anionic phospholipid protein complexes and antigen targets on platelets, endothelial cells, or components of the coagulation cascade. aPL increases vascular tone thus increasing the risk of atherosclerosis, fetal loss, and neurological damage. Inciting events for the development of the antibody have been postulated to occur after incidental exposure to infectious agents or in the setting of active rheumatic disease. APS develops after a second inciting event. The "second hit" usually involves increase in the thromboembolic potential of a patient due to smoking, pregnancy, oral contraceptive use, hormone replacement therapy, malignancy, and nephrotic syndrome [33].

There is difficulty in differentiating between MS, SLE, and APS when it comes to TM. Patients with MS may also have higher levels of antiphospholipid antibody. Studies estimate antiphospholipid antibody is elevated in 4–44% of MS cases [34]. Additionally, MRI findings of multiple T2 hyperintense lesions in APS can be difficult to distinguish from MS. Meanwhile patients with SLE or APS may have subcortical white matter lesions on MRI reminiscent of MS. The differentiating factor may be revealed only on further imaging studies weeks to months apart. APS lesions are usually more static compared with those found in MS.

19.4.3 Sjögren Syndrome

Sjögren syndrome (SS) is a chronic inflammatory exocrinopathy with the characteristic findings of keratoconjunctivitis sicca, salivary gland inflammation, and xerostomia. Despite the localization of the characteristic findings, it is a disease that can affect any organ system. SS often goes unrecognized though it is one of the most common systemic inflammatory diseases. Most patients have positive antibodies for either ANA, anti-Ro, anti-La, or rheumatoid factor (RF), but the absence of antibodies does not exclude SS. Extraglandular manifestations of SS arise from a number of different mechanisms, including autoimmune-induced inflammation of ductal epithelial structures, immune complex deposition, and lymphoproliferation. Neurological manifestations include but are not limited to focal lesions, acute TM or LETM, chorea, subacute aseptic meningitis, and optic neuritis [35].

The history of SS and its neurological manifestations historically has had a shifting understanding leading to much controversy. Neurological manifestations often precede the diagnosis of SS, as immunological abnormalities may be lacking despite findings of xerostomia and xerophthalmia. In part due to poor initial diagnosis, many studies established that SS could mimic MS clinically and radiologically, specifically mimicking primary progressive MS (PPMS) with a steady accumulation of disease. The most common clinical presentation of PPMS involves the spinal cord with spastic paraparesis at any level of the cord [36]. Additionally, anti-Ro antibody has been detected in 2–15% of MS patients leading some to suggest that this represents cross-reactivity of antibodies against myelin or viral antigen. However, subsequent large MS studies showed no conclusive SS among the cases, indicating the mimicry may have been misrepresented. Reflecting this history and disagreements over diagnostic criteria, studies have estimated a very wide range for prevalence of neurological manifestations in SS between 0 and 70% [35].

Imaging findings on MRI characteristically include central T2 hyperintense cord lesions with expansion and variable enhancement. Multifocal lesions are a common finding [37].

19.4.4 Behcet Syndrome

Behcet syndrome (BS), also known as Behcet disease, is a systemic inflammatory disease characterized by a triad of uveitis, oral ulcerations, and genital ulcerations with any number of additional systemic manifestations including ocular disease, arthritis, skin lesions, gastrointestinal involvement, vascular disease, and neurologic manifestations. It is more prevalent in Eastern Mediterranean and Asian populations [38].

The underlying cause behind BS is still unknown. It is theorized that in genetically susceptible patients, aberrant immune activity may be triggered by infectious agents or another inciting exposure. The genetic susceptibility has been tied to certain human leukocyte antigens, particularly HLA-B51. In addition, genetic contribution has also been shown to be tied to disease severity. Possible immunological pathways contributing to pathogenesis include molecular mimicry, alterations in innate immune function, and changes in the numbers of T cell populations. Studies postulate that bacterial antigens mimic human antigens with cross-reactivity for heat shock peptides inciting T cells to propagate disease. Innate immunity through the complement cascade is affected in BS by a decrease in serum levels of mannose-binding lectin (MBL). This same finding has been found in certain cases of SLE as well. In large vessel disease, vasculitis of the vasa vasorum is a characteristic pathologic finding, but vasculitis etiology and its relation to coagulation abnormalities are unknown. More attention via further research is being paid to T-cell costimulatory molecules anti-CTLA-4 (binds CD-28), which have been shown to be associated with eye and CNS disease [39].

Neurologic symptoms develop in 5–50% of patients. Manifestations include aseptic meningitis, vascular changes such as thrombosis and arteritis, or inflammatory lesions such as encephalitis and myelitis [38]. Cases with neurological manifestations are associated with poorer prognosis. Similar to SS, BS may also clinically and radiologically mimic MS. Differentiating the two is difficult if neurological manifestations for BS develop before the systemic appearance; however, there are a few differences in course between the two diseases, namely, that MS is more polyphasic than BS and that a progressive pseudobulbar palsy is rare in MS [38, 39].

Typically MRI of the spinal cord reveals T2 hyperintense lesions extending over more than two segments in length, with preference for the posterolateral cord [40]. Some cases of myelitis occur in conjunction with meningoencephalitis, which is visualized on MRI as unilateral T2 hyperintensity, edema, and enhancement in the basal ganglia, brainstem, or thalamus [41].

19.4.5 Mixed Connective Tissue Disorder

Mixed connective tissue disorder (MCTD) is an inflammatory connective tissue disorder associated with anti-U1 ribonucleoprotein (RNP). The premise of referring to the disorder as "mixed" is based on an expected overlap between findings associated with anti-U1 RNP antibodies with clinical features of SLE, systemic sclerosis, and polymyositis, among others. Confusion in diagnosis occurs because the overlapping features tend to occur sequentially. One autoimmune rheumatic disease can evolve into another given enough time. In 25% of patients with some overlapping disease, evolution eventually occurs over several years. The diagnosis of MCTD requires the identification of key clinical findings. These characteristic signs and symptoms include Raynaud phenomenon, positive serum anti-UI RNP titer, swollen hands, synovitis, myositis, and acrosclerosis. These clinical features can take years to develop. As with other systemic inflammatory diseases discussed, this condition can affect a wide range of organ systems. Initially MCTD was not considered to have any CNS involvement in part due to the largely mild findings in many patients. The most frequent neurological manifestation is trigeminal neuropathy followed by headaches, aseptic meningitis, sensorineural hearing loss, cerebral hemorrhage, cauda equine syndrome, and TM, among others.

MCTD-associated TM is an extremely rare manifestation with only a handful of reported cases within the literature. TM appears to be an early but not presenting clinical finding in these rare cases. There is also an apparent preference for the thoracic cord. Imaging findings themselves are not unique from other systemic inflammatory diseases already discussed. Possible mechanisms of injury leading to TM include vasculitis and thrombosis of small arachnoid arteries in the cord leading to necrotizing vasculitis or an overlap with APS and SLE where aPL and another antibody lead to disease [42].

19.4.6 Ankylosing Spondylitis

Ankylosing spondylitis (AS) is a spondyloarthritis due to a chronic inflammatory disease of the axial skeleton. The classic clinical picture is of a young man in his 20s or 30s presenting with back pain and progressive stiffness. There is a strong association between AS and HLA-B27. The major sites of pathology are at the articulations of the axial skeleton and involve the fibrous or fibrocartilaginous connections of ligaments and tendons to the bone. Pathologic changes are due to inflammation leading to structural damage followed by excessive new bone formation. Eventually, part of the spine or, in severe cases, the entire spine may become fused. The inflammation is incited by microtrauma from mechanical stress. New investigations of the pathogenesis of AS are targeting the association of AS with the innate lymphoid cells from the gut. Once activated these lymphoid cells migrate and produce excess IL-23 and other cytokines to stimulate both bone erosion and new bone formation [43]. This bone formation is one of the primary differentiating factors of this disorder from RA.

Though it is a disease primarily of the musculoskeletal system, neurologic symptoms can occur as a complication. These include cord or spinal nerve compression, atlantoaxial

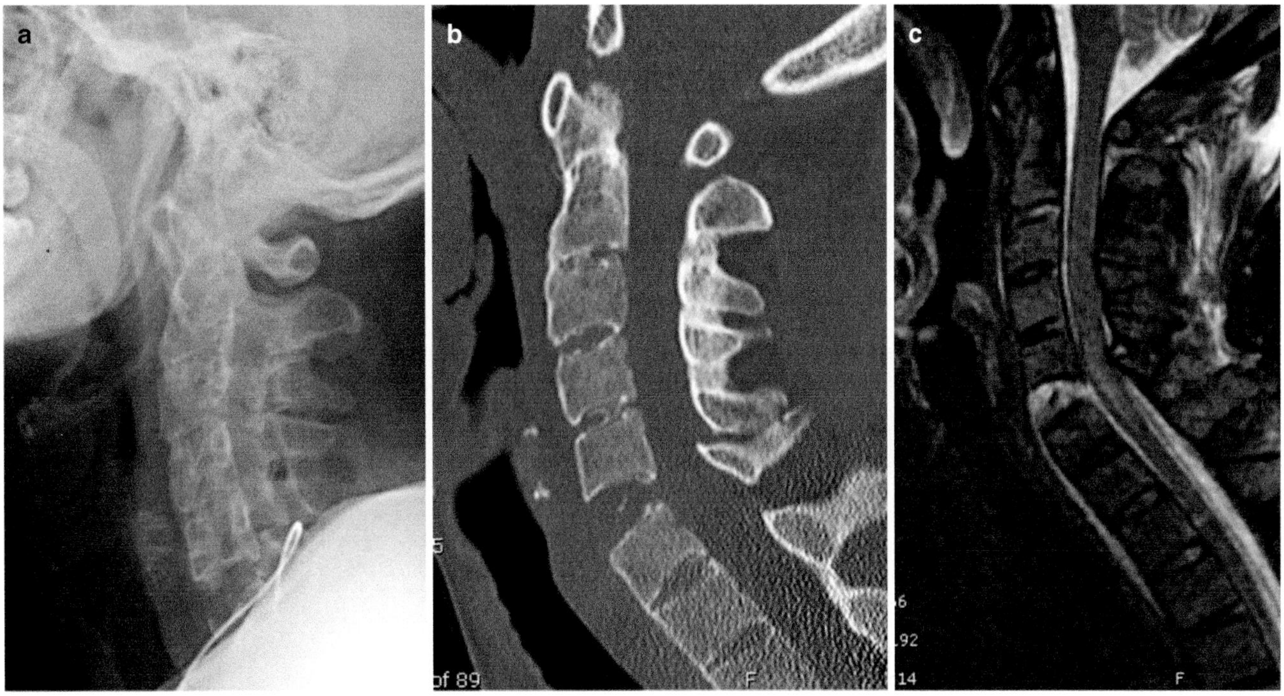

Fig. 19.6 Ankylosing spondylitis with cord contusion on MRI. Lateral cervical radiograph (**a**) and sagittal plane reconstruction CT (**b**) show extensive ankylosis of the cervical spine and thin syndesmophytes with an unstable, distracted fracture through C5/C6 fused disk space and posterior elements. Sagittal STIR image (**c**) demonstrates associated focal cervical cord expansion and hyperintensity consistent with contusion. Additionally, an extensive dorsal subdural hematoma with associated mass effect on the cord is seen extending from C6 level to the upper thoracic canal

subluxation, myelopathy, and cauda equina syndrome. These neurological injuries are usually associated with fracture, which are 11 times more common in AS [44] (Fig. 19.6), but in the cases of myelopathy or cauda equina syndrome, cord damage is secondary to long-standing arachnoiditis. For AS patients, recommended imaging begins with plain radiography followed by an MRI of the sacroiliac joints for patients that show evidence of sacroiliitis on plain films. MRI of the spine is only done in a small number of patients where neurological findings are strongly suspected [45].

19.4.7 Sarcoidosis

Sarcoidosis is a noncaseating granulomatous disease with an unknown etiology. There is a greater predominance in females, with a higher incidence in African American patients. It is a systemic disease with a strong preference for pulmonary manifestations. The diagnosis of sarcoidosis is usually made by histopathologic identification of noncaseating granulomas, compatible clinical or radiographic manifestations (i.e., bilateral hilar lymphadenopathy on chest X-ray), and exclusion of other diseases such as tuberculosis, fungal infections, and pneumoconiosis. Pathogenesis remains a mystery, as the precise antigenic stimulus that initiates the disease process has yet to be identified. The initial lesion, usually a pulmonary one, begins as a CD4 T cell alveolitis that develops into a noncaseating granuloma. The granuloma has a packed central area primarily inhabited by macrophages, multinucleated cells, and epithelioid cells. The periphery of the granuloma is composed of lymphocytes, monocytes, mast cells, and fibroblasts. Not all granulomas will lead to disease sequelae as some can resolve harmlessly or undergo change leading to interstitial fibrosis. Neurosarcoidosis occurs in up to 10% of patients with half of those presenting with a neurologic symptom. Neurosarcoidosis manifestations include facial nerve palsy, hypothalamic inflammation, seizures from granulomatous inflammation, aseptic meningitis, communicating or noncommunicating hydrocephalus, and myelopathy. Spinal involvement once thought to be rare has been shown in recent investigations to be an incidental finding for up to 40% of neurosarcoidosis cases [46].

On MRI, the most common abnormalities described are long segment T2 hyperintense lesions with patchy enhancement, associated leptomeningeal enhancement, and extradural mass lesions. However, nonenhancing lesions, multiple cauda equina lesions, and multifocal short lesions are within the range of presentation [47]. Furthermore, studies have estimated that only about 63% of myelopathy cases have a definitive abnormal MRI with the typical T2

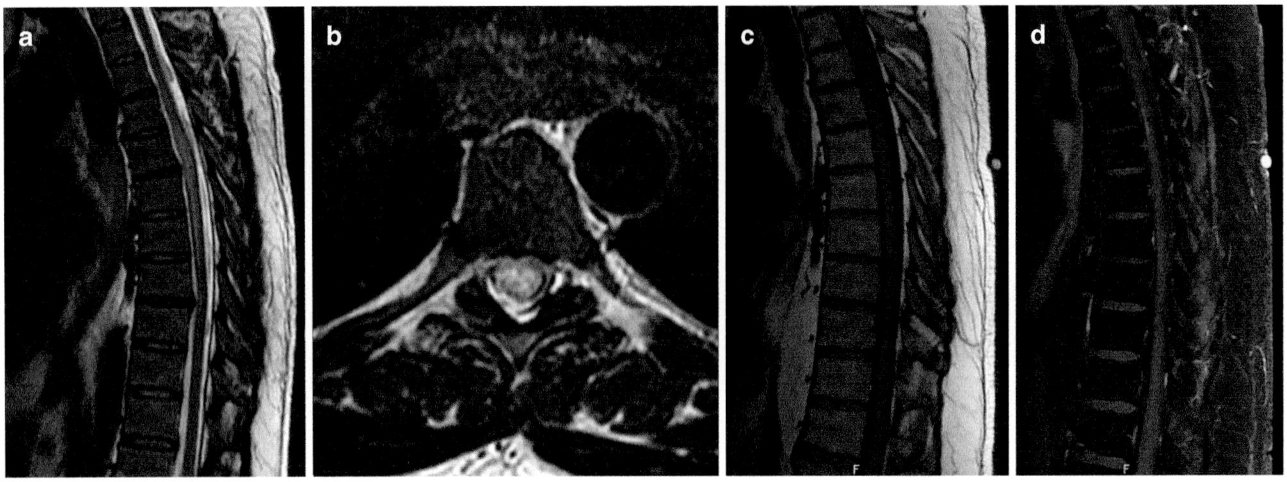

Fig. 19.7 Sarcoidosis of the thoracic cord. Sagittal (**a**) and axial (**b**) T2-weighted images demonstrate a T2 hyperintense central expansile lesion extending from T5 through T7 level in the thoracic cord consistent with LETM. Noncontrast- (**c**) and contrast-enhanced (**d**) sagittal T1-weighted images show a ventral linear region of enhancement within the larger hyperintense lesion

abnormality with patchy enhancement [46]. Additional radiologic findings include cord enlargement in up to 35% of cases and thickening of the spinal nerve roots. There is an equal predominance for cervical or thoracic spinal involvement [48] (Fig. 19.7).

After imaging, if the diagnosis remains in doubt, a meningeal, brain, or spinal cord biopsy may be indicated. A peripheral biopsy is preferred to reduce risk. A biopsy should be considered in cases where a defined systemic disease cannot be identified. It is important to note that if neurosarcoidosis is suspected, a plan chest film is recommended first. Pulmonary manifestations are very likely with any finding of sarcoidosis. Though a chest CT can better visualize pulmonary pathology, a plain film is the screening study of choice. Additional imaging modalities used for sarcoidosis include 18-F-fluoro-2-deoxy-d-glucose positron-emission tomography/computed tomography (18F-FDG PET/CT) scans and 67-Ga scintigraphy (gallium) scans [49].

19.5 Paraneoplastic Neurologic Syndromes

Paraneoplastic neurologic syndromes are a diverse group of disorders that affect the nervous system. These disorders by definition function via mechanisms other than those found in traditional cases of cancer and its treatment. These mechanisms exclude metastasis, side effects of treatment, infections, coagulopathy, and metabolic deficits. There are a number of paraneoplastic neurologic syndromes, but here only ones affecting the spinal cord will be described. Those include necrotizing myelopathy, stiff-person syndrome, subacute motor neuronopathy, and subacute sensory neuronopathy.

Pathogenesis for these syndromes is thought to be immunologic. An abnormal immune response is directed against antigens expressed by the nervous system and ectopically expressed by the tumor. There are two types of antibodies that occur in paraneoplastic disorders: antibodies against intracellular neuronal proteins or those against neuronal cell surface or synaptic proteins. The former represents the better characterized group and is a sign of underlying tumor. These antibodies include type 1 anti-neuronal nuclear antibody (ANNA-1) or Hu and type 2 anti-neuronal nuclear antibody (ANNA-2 or Ri, amphiphysin, and recoverin, among others) [50]. The latter group represents antibodies that may occur with or without an underlying cancer association. Examples include antibodies against the alpha-amino-3-hydroxy-5-methyl-4-isoxazolepropionic acid (AMPA) receptor and the anti-N-methyl-D-aspartate (NMDA) receptor [50]. In cases where an underlying tumor is not present, it is theorized that the paraneoplastic neurologic syndrome may result from immune-mediated destruction of tumor cells.

19.5.1 Necrotizing Myelopathy

Necrotizing myelopathy is a rare paraneoplastic spinal cord syndrome associated with a number of lymphomas and carcinomas. It has also been associated with a postinfectious state after viral infections, secondary to chemotherapy and radiation therapy and due to septic infarctions. Unfortunately, there are no biological markers, and the definitive diagnosis is made on autopsy when necrosis of the spine is visualized [51].

A typical clinical presentation may include ascending sensory deficits, flaccid or spastic paralysis, and autonomic dysfunction. It is usually localized to the thoracic spine. Symptoms progress quickly over days and weeks eventually culminating in respiratory failure without any intervention. Imaging on MRI may show contrast enhancement within the cord and T2 hyperintensity; however there are no truly distinctive imaging findings [52].

19.5.2 Stiff-Person Syndrome

Stiff-person syndrome (SPS), formerly called stiff-man syndrome, is a paraneoplastic spinal cord syndrome characterized by progressive muscle stiffness, rigidity, and axial muscle spasms. The spasms can lead to fractures and deformities of the extremities [53]. It is associated with antibodies against amphiphysin secondary to breast cancer, Hodgkin lymphoma, or small cell lung cancer (SCLC). Amphiphysin is a protein involved with the cytoplasmic surface of synaptic vesicles. Interestingly, in rare cases of stiff-person syndrome without an associated cancer, the antibody of note is instead against glutamic acid decarboxylase (GAD), which too is associated with the cytoplasmic surface of synaptic vesicles. It is theorized that these cytoplasmic proteins are transiently exposed during vesicle uptake allowing antibody interaction. Interference with synaptic vesicles leads to a decline in the levels of gamma-aminobutyric acid (GABA) leading to a loss of neural inhibition. There are no specific neuroimaging findings that are specific to SPS, with electromyographic studies providing better differentiating information. EMG studies show continuous motor unit activity which decreases with sleep, general anesthesia, and benzodiazepines [53].

19.5.3 Subacute Motor Neuronopathy

Subacute motor neuronopathy is a paraneoplastic neurologic syndrome that is characterized by subacute, progressive lower motor neuron weakness. Typically, the disease is pain free, produces asymmetric symptoms, and is associated with Hodgkin's and non-Hodgkin lymphoma [54]. There are few sensory deficits described. From a pathologic standpoint, the disease is known for severe neuronal degeneration of the anterior horn cells and mild axonal loss of the posterior columns of the spinal cord. The clinical course appears to be independent of the lymphoma. Imaging findings are nonspecific. Other paraneoplastic motor syndromes that are less well defined are grouped into paraneoplastic myelitis or into a diverse group of syndromes that resemble amyotrophic lateral sclerosis and primary lateral sclerosis. Only paraneoplastic myelitis has association with antibodies, namely, anti-Hu antibodies or anti-CRMP5/CV2 antibodies [55].

19.5.4 Subacute Sensory Neuronopathy

Subacute sensory neuronopathy is a paraneoplastic subacute syndrome that typically manifests first as vibratory sensation and proprioception loss followed by temperature and pain loss. Characteristically patients have ataxia exacerbated by eye closure and progressive complaints of "pins and needles." Symptoms typically predate the discovery of a malignancy. Patients with anti-Hu antibodies and SCLC are more likely to progress to paraneoplastic encephalomyelitis. In these patients, neurophysiologic studies show signs of denervation. Pathology reveals demyelination of the dorsal columns and variable involvement of the dorsal roots [56]. This sort of sensory neuronopathy can also be associated with autoimmune disorders. Imaging remains unremarkable but is useful in the identification of possible tumors in the chest, abdomen, and pelvis.

19.6 Acute Disseminated Encephalomyelitis

Acute disseminated encephalomyelitis (ADEM), also known as postinfectious encephalomyelitis, is an autoimmune demyelinating disease triggered by an environmental stimulus [57]. ADEM is a rare condition, and a precise incidence is unknown. However, there is some evidence pointing to a greater frequency of presentation in children than adults. The proposed mechanism for pathogenesis is myelin autoantigens possessing cross-reactivity with infecting pathogens. An alternative theory posits that ADEM occurs due to circulating immune complexes in response to a pathogen leading to increased vascular permeability and CNS congestion. Research of pathogenesis is still ongoing, and it is possible that these two mechanisms work in tandem [58]. ADEM is often preceded by a viral or bacterial infection; however a source is not always found. Infectious pathogens associated with ADEM include mycoplasma pneumoniae, measles, mumps, varicella, rubeola, rubella, Epstein-Barr virus, herpes simplex, human herpes virus 6, influenza, and human immunodeficiency virus [59]. Initially some postulated that ADEM could occur following immunization, but later extensive studies have shown no increased risk of developing ADEM during the primary exposure window (5–28 days after vaccination). Nonetheless coincidental findings of ADEM in exceedingly rare cases post-vaccine are still being identified.

The clinical course of ADEM begins with a pre-infectious or priming phase, anywhere from a few days to 2 months after the presence of an infectious agent, when there are no symptoms. Typically, once the lag period is over, ADEM develops quickly with the onset of acute multifocal neurologic symptoms [57]. The clinical symptoms and radiologic findings of ADEM can fluctuate in severity and evolve in the first 3 months after onset. Accordingly, a second event is defined as the development of new symptoms more than 3 months after the start of the incident illness. Data to support the biological rationale for the 3-month requirement are needed [60]. Nonspecific signs include headache, fever, and nausea. More specifically to ADEM, altered mental status is present in 30–56% of cases, indicating encephalopathy [57]. Myelitis occurs in 11–28% of cases [61]. Other neurologic manifestations include paraparesis, sensory deficits, ataxia, aphasia, optic neuritis, and seizures. The course of the disease is typically transient and self-limiting. ADEM presentations most probably vary across geographical settings or ethnicities [62].

ADEM remains a diagnosis of exclusion, always necessitating thorough consideration of alternate diagnoses. Beyond this, the new ADEM criteria require the following [60]: a first polyfocal clinical CNS event with presumed inflammatory demyelinating cause, encephalopathy (alteration in consciousness or behavior unexplained by fever, systemic illness, or postictal symptoms), brain MRI abnormalities consistent with demyelination during the acute phase (3 months), and no new clinical or MRI findings 3 months or more after the clinical onset.

Myelitis lesions associated with ADEM are of variable length and typically found in the thoracic cord. MRI T2WI reveals hyperintense multifocal lesions sometimes described as "flame-shaped" and large [63]. Enhancement patterns are variable with patchy, peripheral, or diffuse findings. Cord swelling is a common finding. However, meningeal enhancement is rare [61]. Conventional MRI cannot always capture all disease findings. Gadolinium enhancement is reported in up to 30% of patients. Serial MRIs usually play a key role on confirming the diagnosis retrospectively. However, the frequency and timing of reimaging should take into account the age of presentation and the clinical characteristics reimaging may be deferred in asymptomatic young children requiring sedation for their MRIs [60].

Recently, ADC values were found to be increased in the majority (70%) of childhood ADEM, consistent with vasogenic edema. Diffusion-weighted MRI imaging (DWI) shows hyperintensity associated with restricted diffusion confirmed by a decreased apparent diffusion coefficient (ADC) in the acute stage of the disease (within 7 days from presentation). Within a few weeks, the ADC normalizes and diffusivity increases [64]. As opposed to MS, magnetization transfer and diffusion tensor imaging findings measured in normal-appearing brain tissue were not different between ADEM and healthy controls, possibly indicating that the pathologic process of ADEM is sparing normal-appearing brain tissue [65].

References

1. Mecharles S, Herrmann C, Poullain P, et al. Acute myelitis due to Zika virus infection. Lancet. 2016;387(10026):1481.
2. Kitley JL, Leite MI, George JS, et al. The differential diagnosis of longitudinally extensive transverse myelitis. Mult Scler. 2012;18(3):271–85.
3. Misra UK, Kalita J, Kumar S. A clinical, MRI and neurophysiological study of acute transverse myelitis. J Neurol Sci. 1996;138(1–2):150–6.
4. Flanagan EP. Autoimmune myelopathies. Handb Clin Neurol. 2016;133:327–51.
5. Goh C, Desmond PM, Phal PM. MRI in transverse myelitis. J Magn Reson Imaging. 2014;40(6):1267–79.
6. Krishnan C, Kaplin AI, Pardo CA, et al. Demyelinating disorders: update on transverse myelitis. Curr Neurol Neurosci Rep. 2006;6(3):236–43.
7. Beh SC, Greenberg BM, Frohman T, et al. Transverse myelitis. Neurol Clin. 2013;31(1):79–138.
8. Pekcevik Y, Mitchell CH, Mealy MA, et al. Differentiating neuromyelitis optica from other causes of longitudinally extensive transverse myelitis on spinal magnetic resonance imaging. Mult Scler. 2016;22(3):302–11.
9. de Seze J, Lanctin C, Lebrun C, Malikova I, Papeix C, Wiertlewski S, Pelletier J, Gout O, Clerc C, Moreau C, Defer G, Edan G, Dubas F, Vermersch P. Idiopathic acute transverse myelitis: application of the recent diagnostic criteria. Neurology. 2005;65(12):1950–3.
10. Cree BA, Wingerchuk DM. Acute transverse myelitis: is the "idiopathic" form vanishing? Neurology. 2005;65(12):1857–8.
11. Kaplin AI, Krishnan C, Deshpande DM, et al. Diagnosis and management of acute myelopathies. Neurologist. 2005;11(1):2–18.
12. Choi KH, Lee KS, Chung SO, et al. Idiopathic transverse myelitis: MR characteristics. AJNR Am J Neuroradiol. 1996;17(6):1151–60.
13. Karussis D. The diagnosis of multiple sclerosis and the various related demyelinating syndromes: a critical review. J Autoimmun. 2014;48-49:134–42.
14. Sa MJ. Physiopathology of symptoms and signs in multiple sclerosis. Arq Neuropsiquiatr. 2012;70(9):733–40.
15. Desanto J, Ross JS. Spine infection/inflammation. Radiol Clin N Am. 2011;49(1):105–27.
16. Amezcua L, Lerner A, Ledezma K, et al. Spinal cord lesions and disability in Hispanics with multiple sclerosis. J Neurol. 2013;260(11):2770–6.
17. Fisniku LK, Brex PA, Altmann DR, et al. Disability and T2 MRI lesions: a 20-year follow-up of patients with relapse onset of multiple sclerosis. Brain. 2008;131(Pt 3):808.
18. Montalban X, Tintoré M, Swanton J, et al. MRI criteria for MS in patients with clinically isolated syndromes. Neurology. 2010;74(5):427–34.
19. Lennon VA, Wingerchuk DM, Kryzer TJ, et al. A serum autoantibody marker of neuromyelitis optica: distinction from multiple sclerosis. Lancet. 2004;364(9451):2106–12.
20. Jarius S, Aboul-Enein F, Waters P, et al. Antibody to aquaporin-4 in the long-term course of neuromyelitis optica. Brain. 2008;131(Pt 11):3072–80.
21. Jung JS, Bhat RV, Preston GM, et al. Molecular characterization of an aquaporin cDNA from brain: candidate osmoreceptor and regulator of water balance. Proc Natl Acad Sci U S A. 1994;91(26):13052–6.
22. Roemer SF, Parisi JE, Lennon VA, et al. Pattern-specific loss of aquaporin-4 immunoreactivity distinguishes neuromyelitis optica from multiple sclerosis. Brain. 2007;130(Pt 5):1194.
23. Pandit L, Asgari N, Apiwattanakul M, et al. Demographic and clinical features of neuromyelitis optica: a review. Mult Scler. 2015;21(7):845–53.

24. Wingerchuk DM, Banwell B, Bennett JL, et al. International consensus diagnostic criteria for neuromyelitis optica spectrum disorders. Neurology. 2015;85(2):177–89.
25. Sellner J, Boggild MM, Hintzen RQ, et al. EFNS guidelines on diagnosis and management of neuromyelitis optica. Eur J Neurol. 2010;17(8):1019–32.
26. Ghezzi A, Bergamaschi R, Martinelli V, et al. Clinical characteristics, course and prognosis of relapsing Devic's Neuromyelitis Optica. J Neurol. 2004;251(1):47–52.
27. Apiwattanakul M, Popescu BF, Matiello M, et al. Intractable vomiting as the initial presentation of neuromyelitis optica. Ann Neurol. 2010;68(5):757–61.
28. Kovacs B, Lafferty TL, Brent LH, et al. Transverse myelopathy in systemic lupus erythematosus: an analysis of 14 cases and review of the literature. Ann Rheum Dis. 2000;59(2):120–4.
29. Espinosa G, Mendizábal A, Mínguez S, et al. Transverse myelitis affecting more than 4 spinal segments associated with systemic lupus erythematosus: clinical, immunological, and radiological characteristics of 22 patients. Semin Arthritis Rheum. 2010;39(4):246–56.
30. Pittock SJ, Lennon VA, Seze JD, et al. Neuromyelitis optica and non–organ-specific autoimmunity. Arch Neurol. 2008;65(1):78–83.
31. Lu X, Gu Y, Wang Y, et al. Prognostic factors of lupus myelopathy. Lupus. 2008;17(4):323–8.
32. Mori A, Nodera H, Nakane S, et al. Transverse myelitis and polymyositis associated with antiphospholipid antibody syndrome. Clin Neurol Neurosurg. 2010;112(8):713–6.
33. Erkan D, Lockshin MD. What is antiphospholipid syndrome? Curr Rheumatol Rep. 2004;6(6):451–7.
34. Valesini G, Alessandri C, Celestino D, et al. Anti-endothelial antibodies and neuropsychiatric systemic lupus erythematosus. Ann N Y Acad Sci. 2006;1069:118–28.
35. Morgen K, Mcfarland HF, Pillemer SR. Central nervous system disease in primary Sjögren's syndrome: the role of magnetic resonance imaging. Semin Arthritis Rheum. 2004;34(3):623–30.
36. Rice CM, Cottrell D, Wilkins A, et al. Primary progressive multiple sclerosis: progress and challenges. J Neurol Neurosurg Psychiatry. 2013;84(10):1100–6.
37. Hermisson M, Klein R, Schmidt F, et al. Myelopathy in primary Sjogren's syndrome: diagnostic and therapeutic aspects. Acta Neurol Scand. 2002;105(6):450–3.
38. Yazici H, Yurdakul FS. Behçet's syndrome: disease manifestations, management, and advances in treatment. Nat Clin Pract Rheumatol. 2007;3(3):148–55.
39. Park KS, Baek JA, Do JE, et al. CTLA4 gene polymorphisms and soluble CTLA4 protein in Behcet's disease. Tissue Antigens. 2009;74(3):222–7.
40. Tali ET, Atilla S, Keskin T, et al. MRI in neuro-Behcet's disease. Neuroradiology. 1997;39(1):2–6.
41. Alaraji A, Kidd DP. Neuro-Behcet's disease: epidemiology, clinical characteristics, and management. Lancet Neurol. 2009;8(2):192–204.
42. Bhinder S, Harbour K, Majithia V. Transverse myelitis, a rare neurological manifestation of mixed connective tissue disease-a case report and a review of literature. Clin Rheumatol. 2007;26(3):445–7.
43. Ciccia F, Rizzo A, Triolo G. Subclinical gut inflammation in ankylosing spondylitis. Curr Opin Rheumatol. 2016;28(1):89–96.
44. Chaudhary SB, Hullinger H, Vives MJ. Management of acute spinal fractures in ankylosing spondylitis. ISRN Rheumatol. 2011;2011:150484.
45. Deodhar A, Mease PJ, Reveille JD, et al. Frequency of axial spondyloarthritis diagnosis among patients seen by us rheumatologists for evaluation of chronic back pain. Arthritis Rheumatol. 2016;68(7):1669–76.
46. Joseph FG, Scolding NJ. Neurosarcoidosis: a study of 30 new cases. J Neurol Neurosurg Psychiatry. 2009;80(3):297–304.
47. Spencer TS, Campellone JV, Maldonado I, et al. Clinical and magnetic resonance imaging manifestations of neurosarcoidosis. Semin Arthritis Rheum. 2005;34(4):649–61.
48. Cohen-Aubart F, Galanaud D, Grabli D, et al. Spinal cord sarcoidosis: clinical and laboratory profile and outcome of 31 patients in a case-control study. Medicine (Baltimore). 2010;89(2):133–40.
49. Braun JJ, Kessler R, Constantinesco A, et al. 18F-FDG PET/CT in sarcoidosis management: review and report of 20 cases. Eur J Nucl Med Mol Imaging. 2008;35(8):1537–43.
50. Graus F, Saiz A, Dalmau J. Antibodies and neuronal autoimmune disorders of the CNS. J Neurol. 2010;257(4):509–17.
51. Urai Y, Matsumoto K, Shimamura M, et al. Paraneoplastic necrotizing myelopathy in a patient with advanced esophageal cancer: an autopsied case report. J Neurol Sci. 2009;280(1–2):113–7.
52. Mirich DR, Kucharczyk W, Keller MA, et al. Subacute necrotizing myelopathy: MR imaging in four pathologically proved cases. AJNR Am J Neuroradiol. 1991;12(6):1077–83.
53. Helfgott SM. Stiff-man syndrome: from the bedside to the bench. Arthritis Rheum. 1999;42(7):1312–20.
54. Plante-Bordeneuve V, Baudrimont M, Gorin NC, et al. Subacute sensory neuropathy associated with Hodgkin's disease. J Neurol Sci. 1994;121(2):155–8.
55. Rosenfeld MR, Posner JB. Paraneoplastic motor neuron disease. Adv Neurol. 1991;56:445–59.
56. Camdessanché JP, Jousserand G, Ferraud K, et al. The pattern and diagnostic criteria of sensory neuronopathy: a case-control study. Brain. 2009;132(7):1723–33.
57. Gilden D, Koelman DLH, Mateen FJ. Acute disseminated encephalomyelitis in 228 patients: a retrospective, multicenter US study. Neurology. 2016;87(20):2173.2–2174.
58. Ketelslegers IA, Visser IE, Neuteboom RF, et al. Disease course and outcome of acute disseminated encephalomyelitis is more severe in adults than in children. Mult Scler. 2011;17(4):441–8.
59. Marchioni E, Ravaglia S, Piccolo G, et al. Postinfectious inflammatory disorders: subgroups based on prospective follow-up. Neurology. 2006;65(65):1057–65.
60. Pohl D, Alper G, Van HK, et al. Acute disseminated encephalomyelitis: updates on an inflammatory CNS syndrome. Neurology. 2016;87(9 Suppl 2):S38–45.
61. Tenembaum S, Chamoles N, Fejerman N. Acute disseminated encephalomyelitis a long-term follow-up study of 84 pediatric patients. Neurology. 2002;59(8):1224–31.
62. Koelman DL, Benkeser DC, Xu Y, et al. Acute disseminated encephalomyelitis in China, Singapore and Japan: a comparison with the USA. Eur J Neurol. 2017;24(2):391–6.
63. Tenembaum S, Chitnis T, Ness J, et al. Acute disseminated encephalomyelitis. Neurology. 2007;68(2):23–36.
64. Balasubramanya KS, Kovoor JME, Jayakumar PN, et al. Diffusion-weighted imaging and proton MR spectroscopy in the characterization of acute disseminated encephalomyelitis. Neuroradiology. 2007;49(2):177–83.
65. Inglese M, Salvi F, Iannucci G, et al. Magnetization transfer and diffusion tensor MR imaging of acute disseminated encephalomyelitis. AJNR Am J Neuroradiol. 2002;23(2):267–72.

Printed by Printforce, the Netherlands